Imaging of the Geriatric Patient

Guest Editor

Giuseppe Guglielmi, MD

RADIOLOGIC CLINICS OF NORTH AMERICA

www.radiologic.theclinics.com

July 2008 • Volume 46 • Number 4

SAUNDERS an imprint of ELSEVIER, Inc.

W.B. SAUNDERS COMPANY
A Division of Elsevier Inc.

1600 John F. Kennedy Boulevard • Suite 1800 • Philadelphia, Pennsylvania 19103-2899

http://www.theclinics.com

RADIOLOGIC CLINICS OF NORTH AMERICA Volume 46, Number 4
July 2008 ISSN 0033-8389, ISBN 13: 978-1-4160-6072-7, ISBN 10: 1-4160-6072-3

Editor: Barton Dudlick

Radiologic Clinics of North America (ISSN 0033-8389) is published bimonthly in January, March, May, July, September, and November by Elsevier Inc., 360 Park Avenue South, New York, NY 10010-1710. Business and Editorial Offices: 1600 John F. Kennedy Boulevard., Suite 1800, Philadelphia, PA 19103-2899. Customer Service Office: 6277 Sea Harbor Drive, Orlando, FL 32887-4800. Periodicals postage paid at New York, NY and additional mailing offices. Subscription prices are USD 290 per year for US individuals, USD 431 per year for US institutions, USD 142 per year for US students and residents, USD 339 per year for Canadian individuals, USD 530 per year for Canadian institutions, USD 394 per year for international individuals, USD 530 per year for international institutions, and USD 192 per year for Canadian and foreign students/residents. To receive student and resident rate, orders must be accompanied by name of affiliated institution, date of term and the signature of program/residency coordinatior on institution letterhead. Orders will be billed at individual rate until proof of status is received. Foreign air speed delivery is included in all *Clinics* subscription prices. All prices are subject to change without notice. **POSTMASTER:** Send address changes to *Radiologic Clinics of North America*, Elsevier Journals Customer Service, 6277 Sea Harbor Drive, Orlando, FL 32887-4800. **Customer Service:** **1-800-654-2452 (US). From outside of the United States, call (+1) 407-563-6020. Fax: 407-363-9661. E-mail: JournalsCustomerService-usa@elsevier.com.**

Reprints. For copies of 100 or more of articles in this publication, please contact the Commercial Reprints Department, Elsevier Inc., 360 Park Avenue South, New York, New York 10010-1710. Tel.: (+1) 212-633-3812; Fax: (+1) 212-462-1935; E-mail: reprints@elsevier.com.

Radiologic Clinics of North America also published in Greek Paschalidis Medical Publications, Athens, Greece.

Radiologic Clinics of North America is covered in *MEDLINE/PubMed (Index Medicus), EMBASE/Excerpta Medica, Current Contents/Life Sciences, Current Contents/Clinical Medicine, RSNA Index to Imaging Literature, BIOSIS, Science Citation Index,* and *ISI/BIOMED*.

Printed in the United States of America.

Contributors

GUEST EDITOR

GIUSEPPE GUGLIELMI, MD
Professor, Department of Radiology, University
of Foggia, Foggia; and Department of Radiology,
Scientific Institute "Casa Sollievo della
Sofferenza" Hospital, San Giovanni Rotondo, Italy

AUTHORS

ANDREA BAUR-MELNYK, MD
Associate Professor of Radiology, Department
of Clinical Radiology, University of Munich,
Grosshadern, Germany

RICCARDO BERLETTI, MD
Department of Imaging Diagnostics
and Radiological Sciences, San Martino Hospital,
Belluno, Italy

LORENZO BONOMO, MD
Professor and Chief, Department of Bioimaging
and Radiological Sciences, Catholic University of the
Sacred Heart, Policlinico Agostino Gemelli, Rome, Italy

L. BRUNESE, MD
Professor, Department of Radiology, Health
Science, University of Molise, Campobasso, Italy

FILIPPO CADEMARTIRI, MD, PhD
Departments of Radiology and Cardiology,
Erasmus Medical Center, Rotterdam, The
Netherlands; and Departments of Radiology
and Cardiology, Academic Hospital, Parma, Italy

ALESSIA CATALUCCI, MD
Staff Neuroradiologist, Department of
Neuroradiology, S. Salvatore Hospital, University
of L'Aquila, L'Aquila, Italy

MASSIMO CAULO, MD, PhD
Researcher, Itab and Department of Clinical
Science and Bioimaging, University of Chieti,
Pescara, Italy

HSUEH WEN CHEONG, MBBS, MMeD, FRCR
Registrar, Department of Diagnostic Radiology,
Changi General Hospital, Singapore, Republic
of Singapore

PIM J. DE FEYTER, MD, PhD
Departments of Radiology and Cardiology,
Erasmus Medical Center, Rotterdam,
The Netherlands

NICCOLÒ FACCIOLI, MD
Assistant Professor, Department of Radiology,
G.B. Rossi Hospital, University of Verona,
Verona, Italy

LUIGI FERRUCCI, MD, PhD
Longitudinal Studies Section, Clinical Research
Branch, National Institute on Aging, National
Institutes of Health, Bethesda, Maryland

MASSIMO GALLUCCI, MD
Professor, Department of Neuroradiology,
S. Salvatore Hospital, University of L'Aquila,
L'Aquila, Italy

FRANCESCO GIALLAURIA, MD, PhD
Longitudinal Studies Section, Clinical Research
Branch, National Institute on Aging, National
Institutes of Health, Bethesda, Maryland

R. GRASSI, MD
Professor, Section of Radiology, Department
"Magrassi-Lanzara," Second University of Naples,
Naples, Italy

GIUSEPPE GUGLIELMI, MD
Professor, Department of Radiology, University
of Foggia, Foggia; and Department of
Radiology, Scientific Institute "Casa Sollievo
della Sofferenza" Hospital, San Giovanni Rotondo,
Italy

JACK M. GURALNIK, MD, PhD
Laboratory of Epidemiology, Demography, and Biometry, National Institute on Aging, National Institutes of Health, Bethesda, Maryland

ROBERT W. HURST, MD
Interventional Neuroradiology Service, Department of Radiology, Hospital of the University of Pennsylvania, Philadelphia, Pennsylvania

SANJEEVA P. KALVA, MBBS, MD
Assistant Radiologist, Division of Cardiovascular Imaging and Intervention, Department of Radiology, Massachusetts General Hospital; and Instructor, Harvard Medical School, Boston, Massachusetts

GABRIEL P. KRESTIN, MD, PhD
Department of Radiology, Erasmus Medical Center, Rotterdam, The Netherlands

LUDOVICO LA GRUTTA, MD
Department of Radiology, University of Palermo, Piazza Marina, Palermo (PA), Italy

ANNA RITA LARICI, MD
Department of Bioimaging and Radiological Sciences, Catholic University of the Sacred Heart, Policlinico Agostino Gemelli, Rome, Italy

ANTONIO LEONE, MD
Department of Radiology, Catholic University, Rome, Italy

NICOLA LIMBUCCI, MD
Staff Neuroradiologist, Department of Neuroradiology, S. Salvatore Hospital, University of L'Aquila, L'Aquila, Italy

FABIO MAGGI, MD
Department of Bioimaging and Radiological Sciences, Catholic University of the Sacred Heart, Policlinico Agostino Gemelli, Rome, Italy

RICCARDO MANFREDI, MD
Associate Professor of Radiology, Department of Radiology, G.B. Rossi Hospital, University of Verona, Verona, Italy

PETER R. MUELLER, MD
Head, Division of Abdominal Imaging and Intervention, Department of Radiology, Massachusetts General Hospital; and Professor, Harvard Medical School, Boston, Massachusetts

SILVANA MUSCARELLA, MD
Department of Radiology, University of Foggia, Foggia; and Department of Radiology, Scientific Institute "Casa Sollievo della Sofferenza" Hospital, San Giovanni Rotondo, Italy

WILFRED C.G. PEH, MBBS, MHSM, MD, FRCPE, FRCPG, FRCR
Senior Consultant, Department of Diagnostic Radiology, Alexandra Hospital; and Clinical Professor, National University of Singapore, Republic of Singapore

M.G. PEZZULLO, MD
Section of Radiology, Department "Magrassi-Lanzara," Second University of Naples, Naples, Italy

ROBERTO POZZI-MUCELLI, MD
Professor of Radiology; and Chief, Department of Radiology, G.B. Rossi Hospital, University of Verona, Verona, Italy

A. REGINELLI, MD
Section of Radiology, Department "Magrassi-Lanzara," Second University of Naples, Naples, Italy

MAXIMILIAN REISER, MD
Professor of Radiology; and Director, Department of Clinical Radiology, University of Munich, Grosshadern, Germany

M. SCAGLIONE, MD
Department of Radiology, Clinica Pineta Grande, Castelvolturno (CE), Italy

FRANCESCO SCHIAVON, MD
Chief, Department of Imaging Diagnostics and Radiological Sciences, San Martino Hospital, Belluno, Italy

M. SCIALPI, MD
Professor, Section of Diagnostic and Interventional Radiology, Surgery and Odontostomatology Science, University of Perugia, Perugia, Italy

JOHN B. WEIGELE, MD, PhD
Interventional Neuroradiology Service, Department of Radiology, Hospital of the University of Pennsylvania, Philadelphia, Pennsylvania

Contents

interpreted erroneously as pathologies. On the other hand, the elderly tend to become ill more frequently and multipathologies are more frequent. Image diagnostics is a key element in the clarification of often blurry clinical pictures, which may make early diagnosis possible, a great advantage to timely treatment. In this sense, knowledge of heart/lung interactions makes it possible to obtain, from the onset, radiologic and clinical signs of the two physiopathologic models prevalent in the elderly, the "cardiac lung" and the "pulmonary heart."

Musculoskeletal complaints are common in the elderly population. The main concerns in geriatric orthopedics are the increased incidence of trauma, degeneration, and malignancy, commonly compounded by comorbidities and the effects of ageing. Imaging of common and important diseases of the axial and peripheral skeleton in the elderly is reviewed in this article.

Osteoporosis is a serious public health problem. The incidence of osteoporotic fractures increases with age. As life expectancy increases, social costs associated with osteoporotic fractures will multiply exponentially. The early diagnosis of osteoporosis, thanks to evermore precise devices, becomes, therefore, fundamental to prevent complications of disease and unnecessary suffering.

Gastrointestinal disorders are common in elderly patients, and the clinical presentation, complications, and management may differ from those in younger patient. Most impairment occurs in the proximal and distal tract of the gastrointestinal system. Swallowing abnormalities with a wide span of symptoms and pelvic floor pathologies involving all the pelvic compartments are common. Acute abdomen, often from small bowel obstruction or mesenteric ischemia, can pose a diagnostic challenge, because a mild clinical presentation may hide serious visceral involvement. In this setting, the radiologist often is asked to suggest the appropriate management options and to guide the management.

Aging-correlated pathologies are atherosclerosis, arterial hypertension, diabetes mellitus, bacterial infections, and malnutrition. The progressive impairment of renal function is the cause of the drug-induced renal pathologies: direct damage induced by nephrotoxic drugs or indirect damage induced by decreased renal excretion of serum molecules. In the elderly, an increase in different pathologies occurs in the genitourinary tract. Among these pathologies, an increase in neoplastic disorders is present; at the same time, several non-neoplastic pathologies are more frequent in old patients. This article considers first the neoplastic genitourinary pathologies and second the non-neoplastic genitourinary pathologies.

> Multiple myeloma is a hemato-oncologic disease in the elderly population, with a peak incidence in the eighth decade, and represents a malignant bone marrow neoplasia in which a monoclonal strain of atypical plasma cells proliferates and may result in bone destruction. Skeletal metastases represent the most common malignant bone tumor and are the third most common location for distant metastases. They occur predominantly in adults, especially in the elderly population. Chronic lymphatic leukemia is a typical malignancy of the elderly patient and aplastic anemia is a hematologic disorder characterized by pancytopenia, bone marrow hypoplasia, and lack of extramedullary hematopoiesis. Osteomyelofibrosis and sclerosis are chronic myeloproliferative diseases of the elderly, with a peak incidence in the sixth and seventh decade of life. This article addresses these oncohaematologic disorders affecting the skeleton in the elderly, examining the radiographic scanning methods, staging, and prognosis for each.

> This article outlines the changes seen using various imaging modalities in the normally aging brain and then discusses in detail the changes seen with various pathologic conditions. Entities discussed include primary degenerative dementias, extrapyramidal system diseases, and vascular dementias.

> Neurovascular diseases are major causes of disability and death in the elderly; many present as medical emergencies. With the continuing growth of the geriatric population, there has been increasing interest in the impact of aging on the cerebrovascular system. Recent advances in the clinical neurosciences have demonstrated that neurovascular emergencies in the elderly often are amenable to treatment; neuroimaging plays a critical role in diagnosis and neurointerventional techniques are becoming increasingly important therapeutic options. This article provides an overview of some of the common neurovascular disorders in the elderly that require urgent evaluation and treatment, with an emphasis on the expanding role for interventional neuroradiology in their management.

Radiologic Clinics of North America

THE CLINICS ARE NOW AVAILABLE ONLINE!

Access your subscription at:
www.theclinics.com

GOAL STATEMENT

The goal of the *Radiologic Clinics of North America* is to keep practicing radiologists and radiology residents up to date with current clinical practice in radiology by providing timely articles reviewing the state of the art in patient care.

ACCREDITATION

The *Radiologic Clinics of North America* is planned and implemented in accordance with the Essential Areas and Policies of the Accreditation Council for Continuing Medical Education (ACCME) through the joint sponsorship of the University of Virginia School of Medicine and Elsevier. The University of Virginia School of Medicine is accredited by the ACCME to provide continuing medical education for physicians.

The University of Virginia School of Medicine designates this educational activity for a maximum of 15 *AMA PRA Category 1 Credits*™. Physicians should only claim credit commensurate with the extent of their participation in the activity.

The American Medical Association has determined that physicians not licensed in the US who participate in this CME activity are eligible for 15 *AMA PRA Category 1 Credits*™.

Credit can be earned by reading the text material, taking the CME examination online at: http://www.theclinics.com/home/cme, and completing the evaluation. After taking the test, you will be required to review any and all incorrect answers. Following completion of the test and evaluation, your credit will be awarded and you may print your certificate.

FACULTY DISCLOSURE/CONFLICT OF INTEREST

The University of Virginia School of Medicine, as an ACCME accredited provider, endorses and strives to comply with the Accreditation Council for Continuing Medical Education (ACCME) Standards of Commercial Support, Commonwealth of Virginia statutes, University of Virginia policies and procedures, and associated federal and private regulations and guidelines on the need for disclosure and monitoring of proprietary and financial interests that may affect the scientific integrity and balance of content delivered in continuing medical education activities under our auspices.

The University of Virginia School of Medicine requires that all CME activities accredited through this institution be developed independently and be scientifically rigorous, balanced and objective in the presentation/discussion of its content, theories and practices.

All authors/editors participating in an accredited CME activity are expected to disclose to the readers relevant financial relationships with commercial entities occurring within the past 12 months (such as grants or research support, employee, consultant, stock holder, member of speakers bureau, etc.). The University of Virginia School of Medicine will employ appropriate mechanisms to resolve potential conflicts of interest to maintain the standards of fair and balanced education to the reader. Questions about specific strategies can be directed to the Office of Continuing Medical Education, University of Virginia School of Medicine, Charlottesville, Virginia.

The authors/editors listed below have identified no financial or professional relationships for themselves or their spouse/partner:

Andrea Baur-Melnyk, MD; Riccardo Berletti, MD; Lorenzo Bonomo, MD; Luca Brunese, MD; Filippo Cademartiri, MD, PhD; Alessia Catalucci, MD; Massimo Caulo, MD, PhD; Hsueh Wen Cheong, MBBS, MMed, FRCR; Piṅ J. de Feyter, MD, PhD; Barton Dudlick (Acquisitions Editor); Niccolo Faccioli, MD; Luigi Ferrucci, MD, PhD; Massimo Gallucci, MD; Francesco Giallauria, MD, PhD; Roberto Grassi, MD; Giuseppe Guglielmi, MD (Guest Editor); Jack M. Guralnick, MD, PhD; Theodore E. Keats, MD (Test Author); Ludovico La Grutta, MD; Anna Rita Larici, MD; Antonio Leone, MD; Nicola Limbucci, MD; Fabio Maggi, MD; Riccardo Manfredi, MD; Silvana Muscarella, MD; Wilfred C.G. Peh, MBBS, MHSM, MD, FRCPE, FRCPG, FRCR; Martina Gilda Pezzullo, MD; Roberto Pozzi-Mucelli, MD; Alfonso Reginelli, MD; Maximilian Reiser, MD; Mariano Scaglione, MD; Francesco Schiavon, MD; Michele Scialpi, MD; and John B. Weigele, MD, PhD.

The authors/editors listed below have identified the following financial or professional relationships for themselves or their spouse/partner:

Robert W. Hurst, MD is a consultant for Boston Scientific, Co.
Sanjeeva P. Kalva, MBBS, MD serves on the Speaker's Bureau for Cordin Endovascular and Johnson & Johnson, and has received a research grant from Angiodynamics.
Gabriel P. Krestin, MD, PhD is a consultant for GE-Healthcare Europe.
Peter R. Mueller, MD is a consultant for Cook.

Disclosure of Discussion of Non-FDA Approved Uses for Pharmaceutical and/or Medical Devices

The University of Virginia School of Medicine, as an ACCME provider, requires that all authors identify and disclose any "off label" uses for pharmaceutical and medical device products. The University of Virginia School of Medicine recommends that each physician fully review all the available data on new products or procedures prior to clinical use.

TO ENROLL

To enroll in the Radiologic Clinics of North America Continuing Medical Education program, call customer service at 1-800-654-2452 or sign up online at: http://www.theclinics.com/home/cme. The CME program is available to subscribers for an additional annual fee USD 205.

Preface

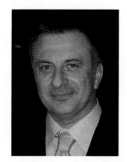

Giuseppe Guglielmi, MD
Guest Editor

Declining birth rates and increasing numbers of elderly individuals have brought about a series of social, economic, and health care problems. With increasing frequency, physicians are confronted with complex clinical scenarios arising in the same patient, which make management problematic and require special competences. In this context, diagnostic imaging plays a valuable role in the care of these patients, and in elderly and especially geriatric patients, comorbidities, a rapidly changing clinical situation, and physical and cognitive problems frequently make it difficult for radiologists to provide clinicians with the answers they expect. It is, therefore, important for the radiologist to know the most common clinical scenarios in elderly patients—which are often different from those seen in younger adults—and for the geriatrician to be aware of the potential and limitations of modern radiology and its applications in geriatric patients.

This issue of the *Radiologic Clinics of North America* includes ten review articles covering all aspects of imaging elderly patients. Each article is generously illustrated with images and explanatory diagrams and tables that, combined with the clinical information, render the discussions more effective and exhaustive.

I would like to thank the authors for their priceless contributions to this issue. With their enthusiasm and the outstanding quality of the submitted manuscripts, they have made my job as editor very easy. My special gratitude goes to Mr. Barton Dudlick from Elsevier, for inviting me to participate in this project and for his sincere determination to make it happen.

Giuseppe Guglielmi, MD
Department of Radiology
University of Foggia
Viale Luigi Pinto, 1
71100 - Foggia
Scientific Institute Hospital
San Giovanni Rotondo
Italy

E-mail address:
g.guglielmi@unifg.it (G. Guglielmi)

doi:10.1016/j.rcl.2008.07.002

radiologic.theclinics.com

Epidemiology of Aging

Luigi Ferrucci, MD, PhD[a],*, Francesco Giallauria, MD, PhD[a],
Jack M. Guralnik, MD, PhD[b]

KEYWORDS

- Aging • Epidemiology • Demographics
- Mortality • Disability • Risk factors

Over the past century, truly remarkable changes have been observed in the health of older persons throughout the world, and these changes have strongly impacted society. The growth of the older population has resulted mostly from a general increase in the overall population size but is also strongly influenced by major declines in leading causes of mortality. These demographic transformations reverberate in society, increasing medical care and social needs, which are expected to increase steeply in the years to come.[1] Based on demographic and epidemiologic perspectives, these changes were already detectable decades before and should have prompted radical changes in the structure and function of our system of health and social protection at that time. We come to this enormous challenge unprepared.

As more people live to advanced old age, these demographic changes imply much more than just an increase in chronic morbidity. The same age-related susceptibility that leads to the occurrence of multiple chronic conditions in the same individual causes decrements in functional abilities as well as social and psychologic problems that may have an impact on many facets of their well-being and quality of life. Going beyond the demographic focus of counting and projecting the number of older people in the population, epidemiology has made additional contributions to our understanding of the health status and functional trajectory of older individuals.[2–6]

Geriatric epidemiology approaches these challenges by studying the health, functional status, and quality of life of representative populations of individuals, ideally throughout the entire life span. The results of these population-based studies have often generated interventions aimed at improving the life of millions of older individuals.

DEMOGRAPHICS

Population aging is taking place throughout the world (**Fig. 1**). In 1900 only 4.1% of the 76 million persons in the United States were aged 65 years and older, and among those in this age group only 3.2% were aged 85 years and older. By 1950 more than 8% of the total population was aged 65 years and older, and by 2000 this percentage had increased to 12.6% (**Table 1**). Change in the proportion of a population that is elderly depends on changes in the survival of older persons and in the birthrate. Improved survival at older ages and a low birthrate have resulted in European countries having the oldest populations in the world. Italy and Germany are estimated to have the oldest populations in Europe and the second and third oldest in the world at approximately 19% each. Europe will continue to have the oldest populations in the world in the twenty-first century, with almost one in four Europeans projected to be aged 65 years or older by 2030.[7]

Populations have aged at different speeds in different countries, with less ability to adapt than in countries that have aged more slowly. Better survival at all ages has had a major impact on the size and age distribution of the older population, but its effect on the life of individuals is modulated

[a] Longitudinal Studies Section, Clinical Research Branch, National Institute on Aging, National Institutes of Health, MD, USA
[b] Laboratory of Epidemiology, Demography, and Biometry, National Institute on Aging, National Institutes of Health, MSC 9205, 7201 Wisconsin Avenue, Bethesda, MD 20892-9205, USA
* Corresponding author. National Institute on Aging, National Institutes of Health, Clinical Research Branch at Harbor Hospital, 3001 S. Hanover Street, Baltimore, MD 21225.
E-mail address: ferruccilu@grc.nia.nih.gov (L. Ferrucci).

Radiol Clin N Am 46 (2008) 643–652
doi:10.1016/j.rcl.2008.07.005

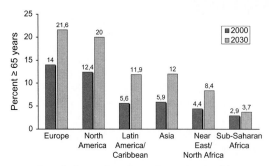

Fig. 1. Population aging throughout the world.

by parallel changes in health status (**Fig. 2**). The change observed in the shape of survival curves, which has been termed *rectangularization*, shows that more and more individuals survive to very old age, and all of them die in a very narrow time window. It has been proposed that this "compression" is due the fact that, as human life approaches its absolute biologic limits, improvements in health will contribute mostly to a reduction of morbidity but very little to further increases in life expectancy.[8]

It seems crucial to examine changes in life expectancy over the last century and life expectancy at specific ages. Life expectancy at birth was only 47.3 years in 1900 and rose to 68.2 years by 1950, affected to a large extent by improvements in infant and child mortality. Life expectancy continued to rise through the second half of the twentieth century, driven mainly by increases in survival in middle and old age.

The improvements in survival over the last century are relevant to the field of geriatric medicine. The decline in mortality rates throughout life has resulted in a population with a large proportion of individuals who survive to advanced old age. Interestingly, many of the medical interventions used in these progressively older patients were originally tested in much younger individuals; therefore, their effectiveness and safety are little understood.

Although there has always been a fascination with extreme longevity, the demographics of a very long life have been formally studied only in recent years. Studying centenarians provides a magnified view of the aging process and suggests that factors that affect a decline in health status, disability, and mortality in individuals in their nineties are quite different from those identified in younger individuals.[9–12]

Previous reports of longevity were often unsubstantiated, and pockets of the world where claims were made for general high longevity usually turned out to be no different from other parts of the world. Nevertheless, recent data from places such as Sardinia, Italy, have identified areas of increased longevity that have been meticulously validated.[13–16] There is currently no solid evidence explaining why centenarians are concentrated in these geographic areas. Although family and twin studies suggest a strong genetic predisposition to extreme longevity and candidate genes have been described, the full mechanism is not understood. The secret is probably a lucky combination of favorable genetic background and environmental factors that exert their influence in critical periods over the life span. In fact, many centenarians report that they were completely independent in self-care activities of daily living and free of disabling conditions up to their late nineties. In addition, a sizable proportion of centenarian "escapers" are totally independent and free of major medical conditions.[17–24]

MORTALITY

The increasingly greater life expectancy of the population has been driven in part by reduced mortality at older ages (**Table 2**).[8] As is true in younger individuals, heart disease is by far the most common cause of death, followed by cancer. The five leading causes of death—heart disease, cancer, stroke, chronic lower respiratory tract

Table 1
Actual and projected growth of the older US population, 1900–2050 (millions)

Year	Total Population (All Ages)	>65 Years Number	>65 Years Percent of Total	>85 Years Number	>85 Years Percent of >65 Years
1900	76.1	3.1	4.1	0.1	3.2
1950	152.3	12.3	8.2	0.6	4.9
2000	276.1	34.9	12.6	4.4	12.6
2050	403.7	82.0	20.3	19.4	23.7

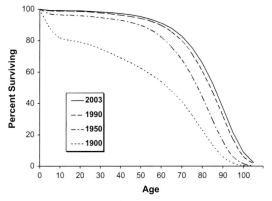

Fig. 2. Survival curves of aging population.

disease, and Alzheimer's disease—account for 69.5% of all deaths. Alzheimer's disease, only recently included on the list of leading causes of death, was the seventh leading cause of death in older persons in 2000 and in 2003 rose to the fifth leading cause of death. This ranking is still likely a gross underestimation, and the contribution of Alzheimer's disease in the future will probably grow substantially.

Age-specific mortality rates for selected leading causes of death are depicted in **Table 2**. On this logarithmic scale a straight-line increase indicates an exponential increase in mortality rate with age. An exponential increase is present for all causes of death, and parallel increases are seen for heart disease, cerebrovascular disease, pneumonia, and influenza. The exponential rise with age for Alzheimer's disease mortality is substantially steeper. The mortality rates for cancer and lower respiratory tract disease do not maintain as steep a rise with increasing age, perhaps because the people who contribute in large part to these categories are smokers who die at younger ages and are less represented in the oldest segment of the population. Diabetes mortality rates also do not show an exponential increase with advancing age, again because diabetic patients may die disproportionately at younger ages.

The first half of the twentieth century saw large declines in infant and child mortality, whereas in the second half of the century unprecedented declines in mortality occurred in the older segment of the population. Mortality change over this time period is further explored in **Table 3**, which lists 1950 and 2004 death rates and the percentage changes in these rates for heart disease, stroke, and cancer, diseases that account for 60% of deaths in older adults.[25] The total population and a subgroup of individuals aged more than 85 years showed a truly remarkable decline in heart disease and stroke, reflecting major advances in prevention and treatment as well as a secular trend that is not fully understood. Unfortunately, the mortality rate seen for cancer does not have the same trend.

Table 2
Leading causes of death among persons aged >65 years in 2004

Cause of Death	Number of Deaths	Death Rate (Per 100,000 Population)	Percent of All Deaths in Persons Aged >65 Years
Heart disease	533,302	1536.5	30.4
Malignant neoplasms	385,847	1111.6	22.0
Cerebrovascular disease	130,538	376.1	7.4
Chronic lower respiratory disease	105,197	303.1	6.0
Alzheimer's disease	65,313	188.2	3.7
Diabetes mellitus	53,956	155.5	3.1
Influenza and pneumonia	52,760	152.0	3.0
Nephritis, nephrotic syndrome, and nephrosis	35,105	101.1	2.0
All other accidents	27,939	80.5	1.6
Septicemia	25,644	73.9	1.5
Motor vehicle accidents	7081	20.4	0.4
All other causes (residual)	332,987	959.4	19.0
Total	1,755,669	5058.0	100.0

Table 3
Age-adjusted[a] and age-specific mortality in the United States, 1950 and 2004 and percent change

Cause of Death	Age (Years)	1950	2004	Change
Diseases of the heart				
Males				
	All ages	697.0	267.9	−61.6
	65–74	2292.3	723.8	−68.4
	75–84	4825.0	1893.6	−60.8
	85+	9659.8	5239.3	−45.8
Females				
	All ages	484.7	177.3	−63.4
	65–74	1419.3	388.6	−72.6
	75–84	3872.0	1245.6	−67.8
	85+	8796.1	4741.5	−46.1
Cerebrovascular disease				
Males				
	All ages	186.4	50.4	−73.0
	65–74	589.6	121.1	−79.5
	75–84	1543.6	402.9	−73.9
	85+	3048.6	1118.1	−63.3
Females				
	All ages	175.8	48.9	−72.2
	65–74	522.1	96.6	−81.5
	75–84	1462.2	374.9	−74.4
	85+	2949.4	1303.4	−55.8
Malignant neoplasms				
Males				
	All ages	208.1	227.7	9.4
	65–74	791.5	907.6	14.7
	75–84	1332.6	1662.1	24.7
	85+	1668.3	2349.5	40.8
Females				
	All ages	182.3	157.4	−13.7
	65–74	612.3	627.1	2.4
	75–84	1007.7	1023.5	1.6
	85+	1299.7	1340.1	3.1

[a] Data for "all ages" are age-adjusted using the US 2000 standard population.

DISEASE STATUS

Although there is much useful information to be gained by observing the diseases responsible for mortality, a full picture of disease status in the older population cannot be obtained by looking only at diseases that cause death. Among people aged 65 years and older in the United States, the most commonly reported condition is hypertension, followed by coronary heart disease and stroke.

Arthritis and chronic joint symptoms are reported by a large proportion of older persons, and these conditions, like many on the list, have a large impact on overall health and quality of life but do not appear on the list of the most common conditions causing death (**Table 4**).[26] Moreover, some differences occur in the prevalence rates of chronic conditions according to race and ethnicity.[26]

An important aspect of disease status that distinguishes the older population from the younger

Table 4
Most commonly reported chronic conditions per 100 persons aged >65 years in 2005

Condition	Men	Women
Hypertension	44.6	51.1
Arthritis diagnosis	40.4	51.4
Chronic joint symptoms	39.7	47.7
Coronary heart disease	24.3	16.5
Cancer (any type)	23.2	17.5
Vision impairment	14.9	18.7
Diabetes	16.9	14.7
Sinusitis	11.5	16.0
Ulcers	13.1	10.4
Hearing impairment	14.8	8.4
Stroke	8.9	8.2
Emphysema	6.3	4.1
Chronic bronchitis	4.5	6.3
Kidney disorders	4.1	3.9
Liver disease	1.4	1.4

Table 5
The ten leading causes of hospitalization in persons aged 65 years and older, first listed diagnosis in the United States, 2004

Cause of Hospitalization	Discharge Rate Per 10,000 Population
Heart disease	767.9
Acute myocardial infarction	126.6
Coronary atherosclerosis	158.6
Cardiac dysrhythmias	145.0
Congestive heart failure	225.0
Pneumonia	220.4
Cerebrovascular disease	175.6
Malignant neoplasms	172.2
Fractures, all sites	147.0
Fractures, neck of femur	79.6
Osteoarthrosis and allied disorders	117.7
Chronic bronchitis	88.9
Septicemia	78.5
Volume depletion	67.6
Psychoses	60.7

population is the high rate of co-occurrence of multiple chronic conditions, termed *comorbidity*. The concept of comorbidity is useful in considering the burden of disease in older people; however, the standardization of a definition for comorbidity depends on the number of conditions being ascertained and the intensity of the diagnostic effort to identify prevalent diseases. The longer the list of conditions and the harder one works to find prevalent diseases, the greater the prevalence of comorbidity.

According to the National Hospital Discharge Survey, heart disease is by far the most important cause of hospitalization, with congestive heart failure a slightly more common cause of hospitalization than other manifestations of heart disease (**Table 5**).[27] Other diseases that are frequent causes of death in older adults (pneumonia, stroke, and cancer) are also common reasons for hospitalization, but so are diseases not as strongly associated with mortality, including fractures, osteoarthritis, chronic bronchitis, and psychosis. Of note, the presence of septicemia and volume depletion reflects the fact that a portion of the older population is frail and at high risk for these types of illnesses.[27]

Cancer mortality rates do not always reflect the incidence rates of newly diagnosed cancers.[28–33] Data from the Surveillance, Epidemiology and End Results (SEER) survey of the National Cancer Institute and other cancer registries show that the highest incidence rates in men are seen for prostate, lung, colon and rectum, and bladder cancers and in women for breast, colon and rectum, lung, and uterine cancers. The incidence of most of these cancers rises steadily with increasing age, but several types, including prostate, breast, and lung cancers, begin to drop in incidence at the oldest ages.[34,35]

Dementia is a condition of aging for which prevalence and incidence rates cannot be validly obtained from either national survey data or registries. Because of the complexities of diagnosing dementia, data on the occurrence of the condition must rely on well-designed epidemiologic studies in local geographic areas. An even larger collection of studies on dementia incidence from around the world supports an exponential increase in dementia with age and demonstrates that rates tend to be lower in East Asia than in Europe and the United States.[4,36–44]

DISABILITY

A large body of epidemiologic studies undertaken over the past 2 decades has led to a greater understanding of the occurrence, determinants, and consequences of disability in the older population and has provided insights into strategies for the prevention of disability.[45–54] Measures of disability were originally developed for use in the clinical setting and were aimed at quantifying the impact of severe medical conditions such as stroke on physical and mental functioning, obtaining standard information on the rate and degree of recovery from these conditions and assessing work ability and the need for formal and informal care. These assessment tools were gradually applied in clinical research and population-based studies, and almost all research studies in older populations now assess disability status.

Physical limitations include basic tasks such as standing, reaching, and grasping. These tasks represent the building blocks of functioning but are not specific measures of disability. Activities of daily living (ADLs) are basic self-care tasks. Instrumental ADL (IADLs) are tasks that are physically and cognitively somewhat more complicated and difficult than self-care tasks and are necessary for independent living in the community. ADLs and IADLs are measures of disability and reflect how an individual's limitations interact with the demands of the environment.

Disability has been assessed with a wide variety of instruments, but even when instruments contain the same items, they may differ in how they assess specific aspects of performing the task or the severity of limitation in performing the task. There is no single best way to perform a disability assessment, and there is no single instrument that is ideal. Moreover, the lack of standardization that results from the use of multiple competing instruments makes it difficult to compare rates of disability across studies.[45–54]

Epidemiologic studies have clearly identified disability status to be one of the most powerful markers in predicting adverse outcomes. Disability measures are able to capture the impact of the presence and severity of multiple pathologies, including physical, cognitive, and psychologic conditions, as well as the potential synergistic effects of these conditions on overall health status.[45–61]

Longitudinal studies in older populations have revealed the presence of multiple risk factors for disability, as well as the dynamics of disability onset and progression (**Box 1**).[55–61] Interestingly, a substantial proportion of individuals who are disabled report improvement on subsequent assessments. In effect, disability is a product of the disease or diseases from which an individual suffers, a sedentary lifestyle or disuse, and physiologic declines that may be the result of aging or pathologic processes that are not specific diseases but result from factors such as inflammation or endocrine changes. As these predisposing conditions change, they have an impact on the initiation of disability and on changes in the status of already established disability.

Box 1
Risk factors for functional status decline

Behavioral risk factors and individual characteristics

    Low physical activity

    Smoking

    High and low body mass index, weight loss

    Heavy and no alcohol consumption

    Increased age

    Lower socioeconomic status (income, education)

    High medication use

    Poor self-rated health

    Reduced social contacts

Chronic conditions

    Cardiovascular disease

        Hypertension

        Coronary heart disease

        Myocardial infarction

        Angina pectoris

        Congestive heart failure

        Stroke

        Intermittent claudication

    Osteoarthritis

    Hip fracture

    Diabetes

    Chronic obstructive pulmonary disease

    Cancer

    Visual impairment

    Depression

    Cognitive impairment

    Comorbidity

In understanding the dynamics of disability progression, it is useful to consider the pace at which disability develops. The terms *progressive disability* and *catastrophic disability* have been used, indicating a slow downhill course and a rapid decline, respectively. Progressive disability results from one or more ongoing chronic conditions and causes disability over months or years, whereas catastrophic disability can occur in moments as a result of a stroke or hip fracture. The prevalence of both progressive and catastrophic severe ADL disability, defined as needing help with three or more ADLs, increases with increasing age, although progressive disability prevalence rises faster than catastrophic disability (**Fig. 3**). Among older persons with severe ADL disability, the proportion who have catastrophic ADL disability is much higher at younger ages, and the proportion who have progressive ADL disability is much higher at older ages (see **Fig. 3**). A similar age pattern has been found for the onset of severe mobility disability (inability to walk across a room); progressive disability is much more common in people who have three or more chronic conditions.

The dynamics of disability can also be approached by studying the pathologic changes that precede its onset. Most disability results from disease, and different theoretical pathways have been proposed to describe the changes that occur as a person proceeds from disease to disability. The theoretical pathway that has received substantial empirical support in aging research postulates that two intermediate steps, impairment and functional limitation, follow disease and lead to disability. Impairment describes the dysfunction and structural abnormalities in specific body systems that result from pathology. Functional limitation describes restrictions in basic physical and mental actions that result from impairments. Functional limitations are the basic building blocks of functioning, and the interaction of these components of functioning with the environmental demands faced by an individual determines whether that person is disabled.[62]

Objective measures of physical performance have received increased attention as assessments that can measure functioning in a standardized manner in research and clinical settings. These measures can be used to represent impairments or actual disability, but most are indicators of functional limitations.[63] Objective performance measures also provide a means of comparing functional status over time or across countries or cultures, whereas disability measures may lose comparability because of environmental differences or differential access to assistive devices.

Because disability status is a good way of representing overall health status in older persons with complex patterns of disease, and because disability also has direct implications for the long-term care needs of an older person, there has been much interest in evaluating disability trends over time. The National Long-Term Care Survey performed similar assessments of ADL and IADL disability from 1982 through 2005. The recent findings indicate that the decline in disability observed for the first 12 years of the study continued and actually accelerated from 1994 through 2005.[64]

There is interplay among the time of disability onset, the duration of disability, and the time of death that determines the number of years that older individuals live in the disability-free state, termed *active life expectancy*, and the number of years spent in the disabled state. As more data become available to estimate both active and disabled life expectancy, we will gain more insight into the prospects for a compression of morbidity, which is the reduction in disabled life expectancy that results from compressing chronic disease and disability into a smaller number of years between diseases or disability onset and mortality.[65]

SUMMARY

An important role for epidemiology is to elucidate risk factors for disease, injury, and disability, and many risk factors have been shown to have a large impact in older persons. Although certain risk factors that are potent predictors of major disease in middle age may have less or no impact at old age, most behavioral risk factors continue to be important throughout old age. Applying what has been learned in epidemiologic studies on older populations so that effective prevention and treatment strategies will be available to older persons is a continuing challenge for the field.

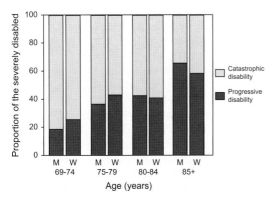

Fig. 3. Proportion of "catastrophic" and "progressive" disability stratified by age.

REFERENCES

1. Lutz W, Sanderson W, Scherbov S. The coming acceleration of global population ageing. Nature 2008;451(7179):716–9.
2. Gurven M, Kaplan H, Winking J, et al. Aging and inflammation in two epidemiological worlds. J Gerontol A Biol Sci Med Sci 2008;63(2):196–9.

3. Brach JS, Studenski SA, Perera S, et al. Gait variability and the risk of incident mobility disability in community-dwelling older adults. J Gerontol A Biol Sci Med Sci 2007;62(9):983–8.

4. Kuller LH. Dementia epidemiology research: it is time to modify the focus of research. J Gerontol A Biol Sci Med Sci 2006;61(12):1314–8.

5. Metter EJ, Schrager M, Ferrucci L, et al. Evaluation of movement speed and reaction time as predictors of all-cause mortality in men. J Gerontol A Biol Sci Med Sci 2005;60(7):840–6.

6. Metter EJ, Talbot LA, Schrager M, et al. Skeletal muscle strength as a predictor of all-cause mortality in healthy men. J Gerontol A Biol Sci Med Sci 2002; 57(10):B359–65.

7. Population Division. U.S. Census Bureau. The Census Bureau on prospects for US population growth in the Twenty-First Century. Population and Development Review 2000;26(1):197–200.

8. Miniño AM, Heron M, Smith BL, et al. Deaths: final data for 2004. National Vital Statistics Reports 2007; 55(9):1–120.

9. Willcox DC, Willcox BJ, He Q, et al. They really are that old: a validation study of centenarian prevalence in Okinawa. J Gerontol A Biol Sci Med Sci 2008;63(4):338–49.

10. Perls T, Kohler IV, Andersen S, et al. Survival of parents and siblings of supercentenarians. J Gerontol A Biol Sci Med Sci 2007;62(9):1028–34.

11. Terry DF, Wilcox MA, McCormick MA, et al. Cardiovascular disease delay in centenarian offspring. J Gerontol A Biol Sci Med Sci 2004; 59(4):385–9.

12. Terry DF, Wilcox M, McCormick MA, et al. Cardiovascular advantages among the offspring of centenarians. J Gerontol A Biol Sci Med Sci 2003;58(5): M425–31.

13. Pes GM, Lio D, Carru C, et al. Association between longevity and cytokine gene polymorphisms: a study in Sardinian centenarians. Aging Clin Exp Res 2004; 16(3):244–8.

14. Caselli G, Pozzi L, Vaupel JW, et al. Family clustering in Sardinian longevity: a genealogical approach. Exp Gerontol 2006;41(8):727–36.

15. Poulain M, Pes GM, Grasland C, et al. Identification of a geographic area characterized by extreme longevity in the Sardinia island: the AKEA study. Exp Gerontol 2004;39(9):1423–9.

16. Deiana L, Ferrucci L, Pes GM, et al. AKEntAnnos: the Sardinia Study of Extreme Longevity. Aging (Milano) 1999;11(3):142–9.

17. Peel NM, McClure RJ, Bartlett HP. Behavioral determinants of healthy aging. Am J Prev Med 2005; 28(3):298–304.

18. Karasik D, Demissie S, Cupples LA, et al. Disentangling the genetic determinants of human aging: biological age as an alternative to the use of survival measures. J Gerontol A Biol Sci Med Sci 2005; 60(5):574–87.

19. Hadley EC, Rossi WK. Exceptional survival in human populations: National Institute on aging perspectives and programs. Mech Ageing Dev 2005; 126(2):231–4.

20. Warner HR. Current status of efforts to measure and modulate the biological rate of aging. J Gerontol A Biol Sci Med Sci 2004;59(7):692–6.

21. Olshansky SJ, Hayflick L, Carnes BA. Position statement on human aging. J Gerontol A Biol Sci Med Sci 2002;57(8):B292–7.

22. Arking R, Novoseltsev V, Novoseltseva J. The human life span is not that limited: the effect of multiple longevity phenotypes. J Gerontol A Biol Sci Med Sci 2004;59(7):697–704.

23. Curb JD, Guralnik JM, LaCroix AZ, et al. Effective aging: meeting the challenge of growing older. J Am Geriatr Soc 1990;38(7):827–8.

24. Coppin AK, Ferrucci L, Lauretani F, et al. Low socioeconomic status and disability in old age: evidence from the InChianti study for the mediating role of physiological impairments. J Gerontol A Biol Sci Med Sci 2006;61(1):86–91.

25. National Center for Health Statistics. Health, United States, 2006 with chartbook on trends in the health of Americans. Hyattsville (MD): Department of Health and Human Services. Centers for Disease Control and Prevention. National Center for Health Statistics; 2006.

26. Centers for Disease Control and Prevention, National Center for Health Statistics. National Health Interview Survey, sample adult questionnaire: trends in health and aging. Available at: http://www.cdc.gov/nchs/agingact.htm. Accessed July 10, 2008.

27. Lolak LJ, DeFrances CJ, Hall MJ. National hospital discharge survey: 2004 annual summary with detailed diagnosis and procedure data. National center for health statistics. Vital Health Stat 2006; 13(162):1–218.

28. Blank TO, Bellizzi KM. A gerontologic perspective on cancer and aging. Cancer 2008;112(Suppl 11): 2569–76.

29. Extermann M, Aapro M. Assessment of the older cancer patient. Hematol Oncol Clin North Am 2000;14(1):63–77.

30. Extermann M, Hurria A. Comprehensive geriatric assessment for older patients with cancer. J Clin Oncol 2007;25(14):1824–31.

31. Balducci L. Geriatric oncology. Crit Rev Oncol Hematol 2003;46(3):211–20.

32. Wells NL, Balducci L. Geriatric oncology: medical and psychosocial perspectives. Cancer Pract 1997;5(2):87–91.

33. Balducci L, Extermann M. Cancer and aging: an evolving panorama. Hematol Oncol Clin North Am. 2000;14(1):1–16.

34. Yabroff KR, Lamont EB, Mariotto A, et al. Cost of care for elderly cancer patients in the United States. J Natl Cancer Inst 2008;100(9):630–41.

35. Hayat MJ, Howlader N, Reichman ME, et al. Cancer statistics, trends, and multiple primary cancer analyses from the surveillance, epidemiology, and end results (SEER) program. Oncologist 2007;12(1): 20–37.

36. Launer LJ, Andersen K, Dewey ME, et al. Rates and risk factors for dementia and Alzheimer's disease: results from EURODEM pooled analyses. EURO-DEM Incidence Research Group and Work Groups, European studies of dementia. Neurology 1999; 52(1):78–84.

37. Obadia Y, Rotily M, Degrand-Guillaud A, et al. The PREMAP study: prevalence and risk factors of dementia and clinically diagnosed Alzheimer's disease in Provence, France. Prevalence of Alzheimer's disease in Provence. Eur J Epidemiol 1997;13(3):247–53.

38. Lobo A, Launer LJ, Fratiglioni L, et al. Prevalence of dementia and major subtypes in Europe: a collaborative study of population-based cohorts. Neurologic diseases in the Elderly Research Group. Neurology 2000;54(11 Suppl 5):S4–9.

39. Suh GH, Shah A. A review of the epidemiological transition in dementia: cross-national comparisons of the indices related to Alzheimer's disease and vascular dementia. Acta Psychiatr Scand 2001; 104(1):4–11.

40. Rice DP, Fillit HM, Max W, et al. Prevalence, costs, and treatment of Alzheimer's disease and related dementia: a managed care perspective. Am J Manag Care 2001;7(8):809–18.

41. Chen JH, Chan DC, Kiely DK, et al. Terminal trajectories of functional decline in the long-term care setting. J Gerontol A Biol Sci Med Sci 2007;62(5): 531–6.

42. McCarten JR, Hemmy LS, Rottunda SJ, et al. Patient age influences recognition of Alzheimer's disease. J Gerontol A Biol Sci Med Sci 2008;63(6):625–8.

43. Dodge HH, Du Y, Saxton JA, et al. Cognitive domains and trajectories of functional independence in nondemented elderly persons. J Gerontol A Biol Sci Med Sci 2006;61(12):1330–7.

44. Shibata N, Ohnuma T, Higashi S, et al. Genetic association between Notch4 polymorphisms and Alzheimer's disease in the Japanese population. J Gerontol A Biol Sci Med Sci 2007;62(4):350–1.

45. Lauretani F, Semba RD, Bandinelli S, et al. Low plasma carotenoids and skeletal muscle strength decline over 6 years. J Gerontol A Biol Sci Med Sci 2008;63(4):376–83.

46. McDermott MM, Tian L, Ferrucci L, et al. Associations between lower extremity ischemia, upper and lower extremity strength, and functional impairment with peripheral arterial disease. J Am Geriatr Soc 2008;56(4):724–9.

47. Semba RD, Ferrucci L, Sun K, et al. Oxidative stress and severe walking disability among older women. Am J Med 2007;120(12):1084–9.

48. Bandeen-Roche K, Xue QL, Ferrucci L, et al. Phenotype of frailty: characterization in the women's health and aging studies. J Gerontol A Biol Sci Med Sci 2006;61(3):262–6.

49. Onder G, Penninx BW, Ferrucci L, et al. Measures of physical performance and risk for progressive and catastrophic disability: results from the Women's Health and Aging Study. J Gerontol A Biol Sci Med Sci 2005;60(1):74–9.

50. Chang M, Cohen-Mansfield J, Ferrucci L, et al. Incidence of loss of ability to walk 400 meters in a functionally limited older population. J Am Geriatr Soc 2004;52(12):2094–8.

51. Valenti G, Denti L, Maggio M, et al. Effect of DHEAS on skeletal muscle over the life span: the InCHIANTI study. J Gerontol A Biol Sci Med Sci 2004;59(5): 466–72.

52. Ferrucci L, Penninx BW, Volpato S, et al. Change in muscle strength explains accelerated decline of physical function in older women with high interleukin-6 serum levels. J Am Geriatr Soc 2002;50(12): 1947–54.

53. Guralnik JM, Ferrucci L, Balfour JL, et al. Progressive versus catastrophic loss of the ability to walk: implications for the prevention of mobility loss. J Am Geriatr Soc 2001;49(11):1463–70.

54. Simonsick EM, Newman AB, Nevitt MC, et al. Measuring higher level physical function in well-functioning older adults: expanding familiar approaches in the Health ABC study. J Gerontol A Biol Sci Med Sci 2001;56(10):M644–649.

55. Bartali B, Frongillo EA, Guralnik JM, et al. Serum micronutrient concentrations and decline in physical function among older persons. JAMA 2008;299(3): 308–15.

56. Rantanen T, Guralnik JM, Ferrucci L, et al. Compartments as predictors of severe walking disability in older women. J Am Geriatr Soc 2001;49(1): 21–7.

57. Penninx BW, Pahor M, Cesari M, et al. Anemia is associated with disability and decreased physical performance and muscle strength in the elderly. J Am Geriatr Soc 2004;52(5):719–24.

58. Cesari M, Penninx BW, Pahor M, et al. Inflammatory markers and physical performance in older persons: the InCHIANTI study. J Gerontol A Biol Sci Med Sci 2004;59(3):242–8.

59. McDermott MM, Ferrucci L, Simonsick EM, et al. The ankle brachial index and change in lower extremity functioning over time: the Women's Health and Aging Study. J Am Geriatr Soc 2002;50(2): 238–46.

60. Taaffe DR, Harris TB, Ferrucci L, et al. Cross-sectional and prospective relationships of

interleukin-6 and C-reactive protein with physical performance in elderly persons: MacArthur studies of successful aging. J Gerontol A Biol Sci Med Sci 2000;55(12):M709–715.

61. Stuck AE, Walthert JM, Nikolaus T, et al. Risk factors for functional status decline in community-living elderly people: a systematic literature review. Soc Sci Med 1999;48(4):445–9.

62. Guralnik JM, Ferrucci L. Assessing the building blocks of function: utilizing measures of functional limitation. Am J Prev Med 2003;25(3 Suppl 2):112–21.

63. Guralnik JM. Assessing the impact of comorbidity in the older population. Ann Epidemiol 1996;6(5): 376–80.

64. Manton KG, Gu X, Lamb VL. Change in chronic disability from 1982 to 2004/2005 as measured by long-term changes in function and health in the US elderly population. Proc Natl Acad Sci U S A 2006; 103(48):18374–9.

65. Fries JF. Aging, natural death, and the compression of morbidity. N Engl J Med 1980;303(3): 130–5.

Physiopathology of the Aging Heart

Filippo Cademartiri, MD, PhD[a,b,*], Ludovico La Grutta, MD[c],
Pim J. de Feyter, MD, PhD[a], Gabriel P. Krestin, MD, PhD[a]

KEYWORDS
- Heart • Coronary artery disease
- Computed tomography • Magnetic resonance imaging

Clear differences exist in the cardiovascular systems of young and older people. How much these differences can be attributed to the pathophysiologic effects of superimposed disease and how much to the physiologic effects of aging are less clear. The increased prevalence of disease with age, in particular coronary artery disease and hypertension, complicates the distinction. Changes in the heart and vasculature associated with aging, however, may interact with the effects of superimposed disease, possibly altering the effectiveness of therapy. Prevention and treatment of disease have contributed substantially to the decreasing rate of cardiovascular mortality over the past 3 decades.[1] In addition, delays in the physiologic effects of aging also may have contributed. Coronary heart disease (CHD) remains, however, the leading cause of morbidity and mortality in older adults, despite improved survival and declining mortality.[2] Many risk factors for CHD in older adults are associated with clinical and subclinical atherosclerosis, including age, hypertension, active and passive cigarette smoking, serum lipid or lipoprotein levels, diabetes mellitus, dietary antioxidant and fat intake, and hemostatic factors. Noninvasive imaging, such as carotid artery ultrasonography and calcium score quantification, are used to noninvasively evaluate atherosclerosis in several studies.[3–6] Other noninvasive techniques, such as cardiac CT (CCT) and cardiac MR imaging (CMR imaging) recently were developed. These techniques may have a clear contribution to the assessment and follow-up of CHD.

PREVALENCE AND RISK FACTORS FOR CARDIOVASCULAR DISEASE IN ELDERLY POPULATION

The importance of CHD in older adults is highlighted by the prevalence rates. In the Cardiovascular Health Study (CHS), a population-based study of 5201 men and women older than 65, the prevalence of CHD increased with age and varied by gender. Myocardial infarction (MI) was found in 11% to 18% of men and 4% to 9% of women, whereas angina pectoris was found in 15% to 17% of men and in 8% to 13% of women; congestive heart failure was present in 1% to 3% of men and women.[7] In addition, the prevalence of unreported and possibly silent MI because of ECG evidence was high (23% of men and 38% of women over 65). Overall, 28.9% of men and 19.3% of women over 65 presented with heart disease.[8]

Subclinical cardiovascular disease also is frequent in elderly people. According to CHS summary index of subclinical disease (with ECG and echocardiographic abnormalities, carotid artery wall thicknesses by ultrasonography, ankle-brachial blood pressure index, and Rose questionnaire for angina), 36.1% of women and 38.7% of men presented with subclinical disease. The prevalence of subclinical disease increased with age.

[a] Departments of Radiology and Cardiology, Erasmus Medical Center, s-Gravendijkwal 230, 3015 CE Rotterdam, The Netherlands.
[b] Departments of Radiology and Cardiology, Academic Hospital, via Gramsci 14, 43100 Parma, Italy
[c] Department of Radiology, University of Palermo, Piazza Marina, 51, 90133 Palermo (PA), Italy
* Corresponding author. Departments of Radiology and Cardiology, Erasmus Medical Center, s-Gravendijkwal 230, 3015 CE Rotterdam, The Netherlands.
E-mail address: filippocademartiri@hotmail.com (F. Cademartiri).

Radiol Clin N Am 46 (2008) 653–662
doi:10.1016/j.rcl.2008.04.011

Only 12.6% of those over 85 presented with neither clinical nor subclinical CHD.[9] Another estimate of population attributable risk showed that 9% of disability and dependency in elderly people is determined by CHD.[10] Therefore, successful prevention and treatment of CHD should include prevention of disability and loss of independence associated with aging.

Risk factors associated with the incidence of MI in people over age 65 also were assessed in the CHS. Within a 5-year follow-up period, incidence rates of MI were higher in older participants and in men (21/1000 person-years) than in women (7/1000 person-years).[11] Predictors of MI included high systolic blood pressure, cigarette smoking, and elevated serum glucose rates. Based on these results, modifiable risk factors, such as blood pressure, smoking, and serum glucose levels, are associated with an increased risk for MI, and interventions for these factors may facilitate the primary prevention of this disease in older adults. Serum lipid or lipoprotein rates were not significant predictors of MI in this group. In the CHS cohort, subclinical cardiovascular disease was associated with several risk factors: age, systolic blood pressure, fasting glucose levels, high blood pressure, smoking in women and men, and, additionally in women, diastolic blood pressure, low-density lipoprotein cholesterol levels, high-density lipoprotein cholesterol levels, and leukocyte count. Measurements of subclinical disease, including intimal medial thickness of the internal carotid artery, calcium score quantification, decreased cardiac ejection fraction, and a low ankle-arm index, are significant predictors of incident MI after adjustment for age and gender.[3,11] Factors associated with atherosclerosis included cigarette smoking, ankle-arm index, hormone replacement therapy in women, hemostatic factors, diabetes mellitus and glucose intolerance, hypertension, and left ventricular hypertrophy.[12] In the Atherosclerosis Risk in Communities study of middle-aged adults, several factors were associated with increased carotid artery wall thickness, including age, hypertension, active and passive cigarette smoking, serum lipid or lipoprotein levels, diabetes mellitus, dietary antioxidant and fat intake, and hemostatic factors.[13] These results show the importance of behavioral and clinical factors in the burden of atherosclerosis in middle-aged and older adults. The presence of subclinical cardiovascular disease identified older adults who are at high risk for progressing to clinical disease.[14] The primary prevention of subclinical cardiovascular disease is likely to have a significant impact on rates of clinical disease. Furthermore, effective secondary prevention of clinical cardiovascular disease also is critical

because of high prevalence of subclinical disease. Alternatively, follow-up of revascularization procedures is a crucial point in the prevention of new acute events. In this complicated scenario, recent noninvasive imaging, such as CCT and CMR imaging, might play an important role.

PHYSIOPATHOLOGY OF THE AGING HEART

Pathologic changes of cardiovascular system start in the third decade with an increase of epicardial adipose tissue and progressive stiffening of cardiac valves. Arterial vessel walls undergo major structural changes with age, including increased collagen deposition and hypertrophy of the smooth muscle cells (decreased vascular elasticity).[15] These structural modifications are compounded by a decrease in β-adrenergic receptor reactivity, leading to a decreased capacity for vasodilatatio, an increased systolic blood pressure, and thus afterload.[16] Potentially as detrimental, an increase in the pulse-wave velocity is reported.[16] In normal physiology, a pressure wave is referred from the aorta back to the heart during diastole, supporting coronary perfusion. The age-associated increase in pulse-wave velocity produces the referred pressure wave during systole, further increasing afterload. The increases in systolic pressure and pulse-wave velocity contribute to the age-associated structural and functional changes in the myocardium, which affect primarily the diastolic function. The increased afterload causes connective tissue deposition and increased myocyte size, which lead to left ventricular wall thickening and decreased left ventricular compliance.[17,18] The systolic function is less affected by the aging process and the resting ejection fraction does not seem to change with age.[19]

Changes in the heart and vasculature, however, associated with aging interact with the effects of superimposed disease, such as atherosclerosis of coronary arteries, hypertension, and diabetes. The first sign of atherosclerosis is the accumulation of fatty material, which is grossly visible and is called fatty-streak lesion.[20] Mature atherosclerotic plaque develops over the years from this initial lesion. It consists of a central lipid core circumscribed by a fibrous cap containing smooth muscle cells and collagen fibers. In the early stages, the sequence of disease is predictable, specific, and uniform; advanced lesions may progress in different morphogenetic stages, resulting in various lesion types and clinical syndromes. The accumulation of lipid within the arterial wall affects the diameter of the vessel only at a later stage. A previous adaptive process, known as positive remodeling, has been shown to take place, whereby the plaque grows within the vessel wall without producing significant stenoses.[21] The erosion of pathologic intimal thickening and the rupture of a thin fibrous cap atheroma may develop thrombosis and result in acute coronary syndromes, and they may heal spontaneously. Healed lesions still may rupture or become fibrocalcific and may determine lumen narrowing at the end stage.[22,23] This means that coronary stenosis is the expression of advanced disease and that the disease should be characterized at an earlier stage.[24]

NONINVASIVE IMAGING TECHNIQUES

Noninvasive techniques, such as CCT and CMR imaging, may offer a clear contribution to the assessment and follow-up of clinical and subclinical heart disease, even in elderly people.

Cardiac CT

With the introduction of the electron beam CT, noninvasive examination of a moving structure, such as coronary arteries, seemed possible but its spatial resolution allowed exploring only the proximal portion of the coronary arteries. The main application for this technique was the quantification of coronary artery calcium. The development of multislice CT (MSCT) technology brought systems with more than a single row of detectors (2-, 4-, 16-, and 64-detector rows) and equipped with faster gantry rotation speed. The resulting improvement in temporal and spatial resolution has placed CT in the field of cardiac clinical applications.[25] A high temporal resolution of the 64-slice CT scanner has been achieved by combining a fast gantry rotation speed (330 milliseconds) with a "half scan" reconstruction algorithm that provides a temporal resolution of half the rotation time (165 milliseconds). A bolus of contrast material (80 to 100 mL) with high iodine concentration (350–400 mg per mL of iodine) is injected through the brachial vein with a flow rate of 4 to 5 mL per second. A test bolus or a bolus-tracking technique may be used to synchronize the arrival of contrast in the coronary arteries with the initiation of the scan.[26] The ECG track is acquired during the scan and afterwards the image reconstruction is performed with retrospective gating. After acquisition of the CT data, an operator may set the reconstruction window at any point within the cardiac cycle by selecting the motionless dataset throughout the entire RR interval (usually the mid to end diastole or the end-systolic phase for the right coronary artery [RCA]). Reconstruction is performed with 0.6/0.75-mm–effective slice thickness, medium-smooth to medium-sharp

convolution algorithm, and the field of view as small as possible to cover the heart and vessels of interest. The reconstructed contiguous axial slices are stacked in a volume to generate a 3-D dataset from which any plane can be created. Multiplanar reformatting, curved multiplanar reformatting, maximum intensity projection, and volume rendering technique are the tools used to obtain a diagnostic 3-D view of the coronary artery tree. Calcium score and left ventricular systolic function also can be evaluated with dedicated software.

Coronary calcium can be quantified using the Agatston score.[27] Recently, the Agatston score has proved an independent predictor of risk as compared with conventional risk assessments.[28,29] Coronary calcium is an indicator of coronary atherosclerosis and it is related directly to the extent of the underlying atherosclerotic plaque burden. The amount of calcium underestimates, however, the total atherosclerotic plaque burden.[5] The higher rate of adverse cardiovascular events in patients who have increased coronary calcium is a reflection of the higher extent of underlying coronary atherosclerosis.[5] The American College of Cardiology and the American Heart Association suggest that the use of calcium score for screening asymptomatic patients is inappropriate in low- and high-risk subjects, although it is useful in intermediate-risk subjects to refine clinical risk prediction and to select patients for more aggressive target values for lipid-lowering therapies.[4] Most elderly people, however, are patients who have high pretest probabilities regardless of calcium score, and treatment of risk factors are more appropriate than screening.[30]

The literature shows a progressive improvement in the results of detection of significant coronary stenosis.[25,31] Studies with 64-slice CT confirm a high diagnostic accuracy and negative predictive value for detection of greater than 50% coronary artery stenosis in selected patient populations. The negative predictive value is between 96% and 99% in all major MSCT published series.[32–35] MSCT coronary angiography may be used to exclude the presence of significant stenosis in patients who have intermediate pretest probability because of the high negative predictive value (**Fig. 1**). In these settings, the proper use of MSCT is after an inconclusive or borderline stress test or in patients who have atypical chest pain (these situations are frequent in elderly people). MSCT has a negative predictive value of 100% in patients who have stable angina.[31] MSCT can detect chronic total occlusion adding important information as compared with conventional coronary angiography (CCA), such as the morphology of

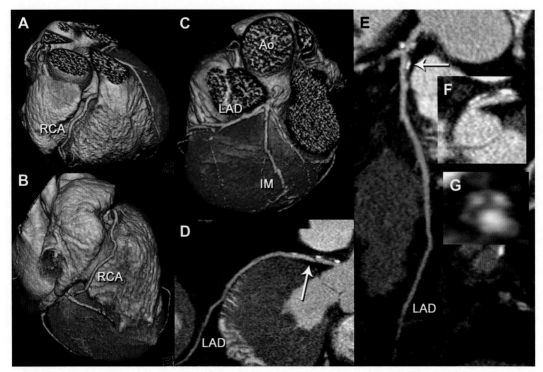

Fig. 1. A 71-year-old man who had atypical chest pain and dyspnea and no possibility for exercise stress ECG undergoing CCT. The 3-D reconstructions with volume rendering (A–C) show the presence of atherosclerosis at the level of all coronary segments. The RCA appears patent (A–B) whereas the disease appears concentrated on the left coronary artery (C). The curved multiplanar reconstructions (D–E) of the left main and left anterior descending (LAD) arteries show extensive mixed atherosclerosis with eccentric pattern. In particular, the CCT shows the presence of 50% stenosis at the level of left main (E–D) (arrow). The magnified images of the left main (F–G) show the actual extension of disease at that level. IM, intermediate branch.

the occlusion trajectory and the amount of calcium in the stump.[36] Numbers of revascularization procedures and bypass surgery interventions increase in older age.[2] MSCT also is useful for assessing stent patency and evaluating in-stent restenosis in the proximal coronary segments.[37–39] Several studies have shown that MSCT allows the assessment of coronary bypass graft occlusion and patency with high accuracy (Fig. 2). In many studies, the accuracy of detecting bypass occlusion approached 100%. A 64-slice CT scanner has the potential not only to assess the patency of the bypass graft but also the presence of coronary stenoses in the course of the bypass graft or at the anastomotic site and in the native coronary artery system.[40–42] Given the high sensitivity and negative predictive value of the technique, CT could represent an alternative to CCA in patients who have dilated cardiomiopathy of unknown origin and before cardiac valve surgery or transplant and major noncoronary cardiac surgery.[43] A preclinical application of coronary MSCT is plaque imaging, which might become a relevant diagnostic tool for risk stratification.[6,24,44,45] The introduction of MSCT could be useful in the emergency work-up of noncardiac thoracic pain, such as aortic dissection, pericarditis, or mediastinum disease. The possibility of scanning the entire thorax, visualizing the thoracic aorta, pulmonary arteries, and coronary arteries, could provide a new approach to the triage of acute chest pain.[46] If CT scanners with cardiac state-of-the-art capabilities are installed in emergency departments, early diagnosis of acute coronary syndromes with still-negative enzymes and non-diagnostic ECG alterations also would be allowed.[47]

Beyond research applications, appropriateness criteria and recommendations for CCT recently have been published.[4,48] Some assumptions must be taken into account for CCT. Patients who have significant respiratory failure, major allergy to iodine-containing contrast material, and renal failure are not eligible for the scan or may be treated accordingly. Persistent arrhythmia (ie, atrial fibrillation) precludes MSCT coronary imaging. A heart rate greater than 70 bpm results

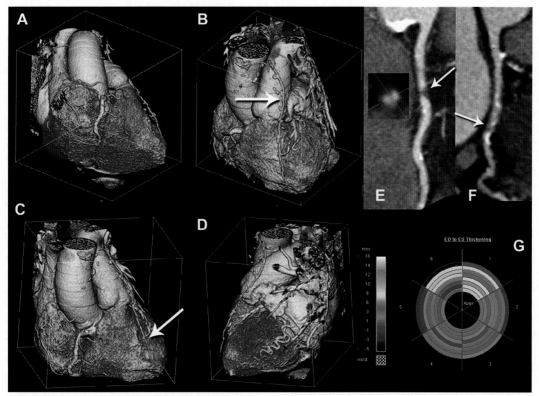

Fig. 2. A 75-year-old woman who had previous coronary artery bypass graft (12 years before) and recurrent typical angina undergoing CCT for the assessment of graft patency and eventually progression of coronary artery disease on the native coronary arteries (heart rate = 78 bpm with flutter). The 3-D reconstruction with volume rendering shows the presence of one mammary artery grafted on the LAD artery with good caliber and runoff (A–D) (arrow). The proximal LAD artery was occluded. The RCA shows on curved multiplanar reconstructions a significant stenosis in the middle tract (E) (arrow) due to a mixed eccentric atherosclerotic plaque (see vessel cross section [E]). Also, the left circumflex artery shows a significant stenosis of the middle tract (F) (arrow), close to the origin of a marginal branch, resulting from a mixed atherosclerotic plaque. The ejection fraction on CCT was 49% (height 168 cm, weight 70 kg, and body surface area 1.8 m²) and the left ventricle shows a diffused mild hypokinesia (G).

in poor image quality; therefore, lowering the heart rate is recommended with administration of β-blockers before the scan (ie, 100 mg metoprolol 1 hour before the scan). Unstable patients who have heart failure are excluded because of their incapacity to lie in a supine position. Patients who are candidates for MSCT need to be able to breath-hold for up to 12 seconds with the 64-slice scanner.[35] All these limitations should be considered carefully for MSCT coronary angiography in elderly people. Major limitations (eg, allergy to contrast material and renal failure), however, also affect invasive CCA. The high radiation exposure associated with CCT scanning still is of great concern when compared with that of CCA. The attributable lifetime risk for a single small dose of radiation varies, however, according to age at time of exposure (lower in patients older than 45) because of long latency periods of radiogenic cancers.[49] CCA is the gold standard for evaluation of the vascular lumen and provides excellent results in demonstrating stenotic lesions of coronary artery disease; however it is an invasive procedure with a small risk for fatal events. Although the incidences of significant morbidity and mortality are low, CCA may cause major complications (1.7%) and, thus, the benefits must outweigh the risks. Age generally is considered a significant factor related to cardiovascular mortality during CCA.[50] CCA is a lumen-oriented technique, which does not allow a direct evaluation of coronary artery wall. Despite the high prevalence of disease in elderly people, MSCT coronary angiography might be used to avoid the risk for invasive catheterism of CCA in subjects who do not have significant coronary artery stenoses. MSCT coronary angiography also may permit, in this group of subjects, the assessment of plaques that determine mild lume narrowing and may better address medical therapy. It is reported that a high coronary calcium score may affect diagnostic accuracy and, therefore, patients should be excluded from MSCT based on their Agatston score. The difference in the diagnostic accuracy of MSCT between low calcium score and high calcium score patients, however, is not significant for detecting any stenosis of 50% or greater, with no change in the negative predictive value.[51] Similarly, other highly attenuating materials, such as surgical clips of bypass grafts or metallic mash of coronary stents, may cause blooming artifacts and preclude a reliable assessment.[4]

MSCT coronary angiography is a technique that requires considerable training and remains operator dependent. The introduction of software able to provide a reproducible quantification of the degree of coronary stenoses may help resolve this issue. New generations of CT scanner, such as the dual-source CT, could provide better results, because of improved temporal resolution and reduction of motion artifact.[52]

Cardiac MR Imaging

CMR imaging has developed significantly in recent years and now is firmly established in clinical and research cardiovascular medicine in larger centers. This implementation and acceptance depends on several factors, including technical advances (speed, reliability, and easiness), robust image quality, and excellent reproducibility of CMR images. The last factor, excellent reproducibility, has encouraged extensive implementation by research centers and the drug industry to set up trials with reduced sample sizes and lower costs. Furthermore, MR imaging technology shares with ultrasound an advantage over x-ray techniques, as it uses nonionizing radiations. From this perspective, echocardiography is simple, fast, and less expensive, whereas CMR imaging typically provides superior image quality at a higher cost. These techniques, therefore, are effective and complementary. CMR imaging may be performed when echocardiography displays inadequate images because of a limited acoustic window.

CMR imaging equipment and operators must have the minimal technical capabilities required for the indication. Images are obtained with at least a 1.5-T magnet using standard fast sequences (spin echo, gradient echo, steady-state free precession [SSFP], and fast imaging employing steady-state acquisition [FIESTA]). Use of gadolinium contrast is needed for studies involving perfusion, angiograms, and contrast enhancement. Patients are assumed not to present with general CMR imaging contraindications, including severe claustrophobia, or specific metallic contraindications (such as pacemakers, defibrillators, and certain aneurysm clips).[48] Most metallic devices are MR imaging compatible, including prosthetic cardiac valves and vascular stents. MR imaging can be performed at any time after implantation of stents with no risk for patients.[53]

CMR imaging may assess structure and function by evaluation of ventricular and valvular function. Procedures may include evaluation of left/right ventricular mass and volumes, left ventricular function after MI or in heart failure patients, MR angiography, quantification of valvular disease, and delayed contrast enhancement.[48] CMR imaging is well validated for quantifying the volumes and mass of the ventricles, and it has become the gold standard against which other techniques are measured because of its 3-D nature, which is not dependent on geometric assumptions.[54] An important feature of CMR imaging is the excellent interstudy reproducibility of volume and mass measurements, considerably superior to that of 2-D echocardiography.[55] CMR imaging is valuable for assessment (cine-mode) of regional contractile function by quantification of wall motion and thickening.[56] Another appropriate application of CMR imaging is the evaluation of specific cardiomyopathies, including dilated, siderotic, arrhytmogenic right ventricular, infiltrative (amyloid or sarcoid), and myocarditis.[57–63] CMR imaging may assess MI areas and myocardial viability by using a protocol known as late gadolinium enhancement. Gadolinium is injected intravenously and examination is performed after a delay (10 to 15 minutes) using an inversion recovery sequence. The extracellular compartment is expanded in areas of MI due to cellular rupture. Therefore, gadolinium, an extracellular contrast agent, presents a delayed distribution in MI areas.[64] The assessment of myocardial scar and viability is relevant before revascularization because it ascertains the likelihood of recovery of function with revascularization (percutaneous coronary intervention or coronary artery bypass graft) or medical therapy (**Fig. 3**). CMR imaging seems useful especially in elderly people when viability assessment by SPECT has provided equivocal or indeterminate results.[65] Stress CMR imaging using dobutamine is clinically established for diagnosing obstructive coronary artery disease through induction of new wall motion abnormalities[66] and it is superior to dobutamine stress echocardiography.[67] Stress CMR imaging is effective in the diagnosis of coronary artery disease in patients who are unsuitable for

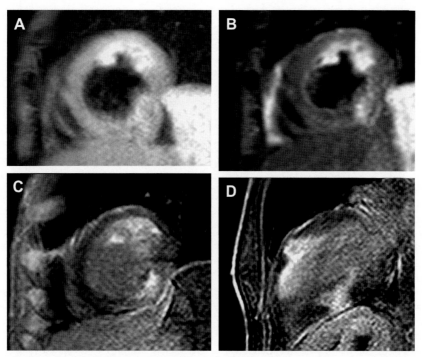

Fig. 3. A 71-year-old woman presenting at the authors' institution with acute coronary syndrome (ST segment elevation MI) and undergoing early CMR imaging for the assessment of damage extension. The proton density fat-suppressed image (A) and the T2-weighted fat-suppressed image (B) show subendocardial regions (with some segments showing transmural involvement) of hyperintensity on the lateral and inferior wall of the left ventricle indicating edema. In the same segments, the inversion recovery images 10 minutes after intravenous administration of gadolinum (C–D) show the presence of hyperenhancement in the same regions, indicating myocardial necrosis. In this case, no areas of no-reflow (ie, microvascular obstruction) are demonstrated.

dobutamine echocardiography.[68] Perfusion CMR imaging using adenosine as a pharmacologic stress agent achieved good results in the assessment of perfusion reserve measurements.[69,70] Despite successful evaluation of functional and perfusional features, coronary CMR imaging angiography (with 3-D navigator-echo sequences) is considered inappropriate for confident evaluation of coronary arteries stenoses and follow-up of coronary stents and bypass grafts.[4,48,71]

DISCUSSION

Trends in society are bringing more and more elderly people toward advanced imaging and treatment. Therefore, the capability of diagnostic modalities to investigate the advanced stages of diseases will become important in the clinical context. CCT and CMR imaging already are key modalities for the assessment of morphologic and functional disorders, but they will become even more important because the developing types of treatments in cardiovascular medicine are becoming less and less invasive. The stratification of risk and the assessment of prognostic

parameters will be of paramount importance for the decision to treat. The degree of specialization of radiologists involved in this type of imaging and integration with cardiologists' competence will determine the outcome of most patients. A turf battle for cardiac imaging will develop, in the best scenario, into an integrated approach to cardiovascular disease, which should include CCT, CMR imaging, positron emission tomography (PET)/single photon emission CT (SPECT), echocardiography, and CCA (with the addition of hybrid techniques, such as PET-SPECT/CT and others) performed by an integrated team of professionals.

SUMMARY

CCT could be used as a first-line, noninvasive approach in elderly people to avoid the risk for CCA invasive catheterism. CCA would be avoided in subjects who do not have significant coronary artery stenoses. CCT also could play an important role in the follow-up of revascularization procedures. CMR imaging is an appropriate technique in elderly people as a functional approach, when echocardiography is not sufficient, and for evaluation of MI scars before revascularization procedures. Noninvasive imaging approach is advisable for detection of clinical and subclinical CHD in the elderly population.

REFERENCES

1. Hunink MG, Goldman L, Tosteson AN, et al. The recent decline in mortality from coronary heart disease, 1980–1990. The effect of secular trends in risk factors and treatment. JAMA 1997;277(7): 535–42.
2. Rosamond W, Flegal K, Friday G, et al. Heart disease and stroke statistics—2007 update: a report from the American Heart Association Statistics Committee and Stroke Statistics Subcommittee. Circulation 2007;115(5):e69–171.
3. O'Leary DH, Polak JF, Wolfson SK Jr, et al. Use of sonography to evaluate carotid atherosclerosis in the elderly. The Cardiovascular Health Study. CHS Collaborative Research Group. Stroke 1991;22(9): 1155–63.
4. Budoff MJ, Achenbach S, Blumenthal RS, et al. Assessment of coronary artery disease by cardiac computed tomography: a scientific statement from the American Heart Association Committee on Cardiovascular Imaging and Intervention, Council on Cardiovascular Radiology and Intervention, and Committee on Cardiac Imaging, Council on Clinical Cardiology. Circulation 2006;114(16):1761–91.
5. Greenland P, Bonow RO, Brundage BH, et al. ACCF/ AHA 2007 clinical expert consensus document on coronary artery calcium scoring by computed tomography in global cardiovascular risk assessment and in evaluation of patients with chest pain: a report of the American College of Cardiology Foundation Clinical Expert Consensus Task Force. Circulation 2007;115(3):402–26.
6. Naghavi M, Falk E, Hecht HS, et al. From vulnerable plaque to vulnerable patient—part III: executive summary of the Screening for Heart Attack Prevention and Education (SHAPE) Task Force report. Am J Cardiol 2006;98(2A):2H–15H.
7. Mittelmark MB, Psaty BM, Rautaharju PM, et al. Prevalence of cardiovascular diseases among older adults. The Cardiovascular Health Study. Am J Epidemiol 1993;137(3):311–7.
8. Ettinger WH Jr, Fried LP, Harris T, et al. Self-reported causes of physical disability in older people: the Cardiovascular Health Study. CHS Collaborative Research Group. J Am Geriatr Soc 1994;42(10): 1035–44.
9. Kuller L, Borhani N, Furberg C, et al. Prevalence of subclinical atherosclerosis and cardiovascular disease and association with risk factors in the Cardiovascular Health Study. Am J Epidemiol 1994;139(12):1164–79.
10. Guccione AA, Felson DT, Anderson JJ, et al. The effects of specific medical conditions on the functional limitations of elders in the Framingham Study. Am J Public Health 1994;84(3):351–8.
11. Pearte CA, Furberg CD, O'Meara ES, et al. Characteristics and baseline clinical predictors of future fatal versus nonfatal coronary heart disease events in older adults: the Cardiovascular Health Study. Circulation 2006;113(18):2177–85.
12. Manolio TA, Furberg CD, Shemanski L, et al. Associations of postmenopausal estrogen use with cardiovascular disease and its risk factors in older women. The CHS Collaborative Research Group. Circulation 1993;88(5 Pt 1):2163–71.
13. Heiss G, Sharrett AR, Barnes R, et al. Carotid atherosclerosis measured by B-mode ultrasound in populations: associations with cardiovascular risk factors in the ARIC study. Am J Epidemiol 1991;134(3): 250–6.
14. Kuller LH, Shemanski L, Psaty BM, et al. Subclinical disease as an independent risk factor for cardiovascular disease. Circulation 1995;92(4):720–6.
15. Lakatta EG, Mitchell JH, Pomerance A, et al. Human aging: changes in structure and function. J Am Coll Cardiol 1987;10(2 Suppl A):42A–7A.
16. Renlund DG, Gerstenblith G. Exercise and the aging heart. Cardiol Clin 1987;5(2):331–6.
17. Lie JT, Hammond PI. Pathology of the senescent heart: anatomic observations on 237 autopsy studies of patients 90 to 105 years old. Mayo Clin Proc 1988;63(6):552–64.
18. Gardin JM, Siscovick D, Anton-Culver H, et al. Sex, age, and disease affect echocardiographic left ventricular mass and systolic function in the free-living elderly. The Cardiovascular Health Study. Circulation 1995;91(6):1739–48.
19. Rodeheffer RJ, Gerstenblith G, Becker LC, et al. Exercise cardiac output is maintained with advancing age in healthy human subjects: cardiac dilatation and increased stroke volume compensate for a diminished heart rate. Circulation 1984;69(2):203–13.
20. Stary HC, Chandler AB, Dinsmore RE, et al. A definition of advanced types of atherosclerotic lesions and a histological classification of atherosclerosis. A report from the Committee on Vascular Lesions of the Council on Arteriosclerosis, American Heart Association. Circulation 1995;92:1355–74.
21. Glagov S, Weisenberg E, Zarins CK, et al. Compensatory enlargement of human atherosclerotic coronary arteries. N Engl J Med 1987;316:1371–5.
22. Virmani R, Kolodgie FD, Burke AP, et al. Lessons from sudden coronary death: a comprehensive morphological classification scheme for atherosclerotic lesions. Arterioscler Thromb Vasc Biol 2000;20: 1262–75.
23. Naghavi M, Libby P, Falk E, et al. From vulnerable plaque to vulnerable patient: a call for new

definitions and risk assessment strategies: part I. Circulation 2003;108:1664–72.

24. Cademartiri F, La Grutta L, Palumbo A, et al. Imaging techniques for the vulnerable coronary plaque. Radiol Med 2007;112(5):637–59.

25. Nieman K, Cademartiri F, Lemos PA, et al. Reliable noninvasive coronary angiography with fast submillimeter multislice spiral computed tomography. Circulation 2002;106:2051–4.

26. Cademartiri F, Nieman K, van der Lugt A, et al. Intravenous contrast material administration at 16-detector row helical CT coronary angiography: test bolus versus bolus-tracking technique. Radiology 2004; 233:817–23.

27. Agatston AS, Janowitz WR, Hildner FJ, et al. Quantification of coronary artery calcium using ultrafast computed tomography. J Am Coll Cardiol 1990;15: 827–32.

28. Greenland P, LaBree L, Azen SP, et al. Coronary artery calcium score combined with Framingham score for risk prediction in asymptomatic individuals. JAMA 2004;291:210–5.

29. Shaw LJ, Raggi P, Schisterman E, et al. Prognostic value of cardiac risk factors and coronary artery calcium screening for all-cause mortality. Radiology 2003;228:826–33.

30. Clouse ME. How useful is computed tomography for screening for coronary artery disease? Noninvasive screening for coronary artery disease with computed tomography is useful. Circulation 2006; 113:125–46.

31. Mollet NR, Cademartiri F, Nieman K, et al. Multislice spiral computed tomography coronary angiography in patients with stable angina pectoris. J Am Coll Cardiol 2004;43:2265–70.

32. Leschka S, Alkadhi H, Plass A, et al. Accuracy of MSCT coronary angiography with 64-slice technology: first experience. Eur Heart J 2005;26:1482–7.

33. Raff GL, Gallagher MJ, O'Neill WW, et al. Diagnostic accuracy of noninvasive coronary angiography using 64-slice spiral computed tomography. J Am Coll Cardiol 2005;46:552–7.

34. Leber AW, Knez A, von Ziegler F, et al. Quantification of obstructive and nonobstructive coronary lesions by 64-slice computed tomography a comparative study with quantitative coronary angiography and intravascular ultrasound. J Am Coll Cardiol 2005;46:147–54.

35. Mollet NR, Cademartiri F, van Mieghem CA, et al. High-resolution spiral computed tomography coronary angiography in patients referred for diagnostic conventional coronary angiography. Circulation 2005;112:2318–23.

36. Mollet NR, Hoye A, Lemos PA, et al. Value of preprocedure multislice computed tomographic coronary angiography to predict the outcome of percutaneous recanalization of chronic total occlusions. Am J Cardiol 2005;95:240–3.

37. Gilard M, Cornily JC, Rioufol G, et al. Noninvasive assessment of left main coronary stent patency with 16-slice computed tomography. Am J Cardiol 2005;95:110–2.

38. Schuijf JD, Bax JJ, Jukema JW, et al. Feasibility of assessment of coronary stent patency using 16-slice computed tomography. Am J Cardiol 2004;94: 427–30.

39. Cademartiri F, Schuijf JD, Pugliese F, et al. Usefulness of 64-slice multislice computed tomography coronary angiography to assess in-stent restenosis. J Am Coll Cardiol 2007;49(22):2204–10.

40. Nieman K, Pattynama PM, Rensing BJ, et al. Evaluation of patients after coronary artery bypass surgery: CT angiographic assessment of grafts and coronary arteries. Radiology 2003;229:749–56.

41. Martuscelli E, Romagnoli A, D'Eliseo A, et al. Evaluation of venous and arterial conduit patency by 16-slice spiral computed tomography. Circulation 2004;110:3234–8.

42. Malagutti P, Nieman K, Meijboom WB, et al. Use of 64-slice CT in symptomatic patients after coronary bypass surgery: evaluation of grafts and coronary arteries. Eur Heart J 2007;28(15):1879–85.

43. Meijboom WB, Mollet NR, Van Mieghem CA, et al. Pre-operative computed tomography coronary angiography to detect significant coronary artery disease in patients referred for cardiac valve surgery. J Am Coll Cardiol 2006;48(8):1658–65.

44. Leber AW, Knez A, Becker A, et al. Accuracy of multidetector spiral computed tomography in identifying and differentiating the composition of coronary atherosclerotic plaques: a comparative study with intracoronary ultrasound. J Am Coll Cardiol 2004; 43:1241–7.

45. Achenbach S, Ropers D, Hoffmann U, et al. Assessment of coronary remodeling in stenotic and nonstenotic coronary atherosclerotic lesions by multidetector spiral computed tomography. J Am Coll Cardiol 2004;43:842–7.

46. White CS, Kuo D, Kelemen M, et al. Chest pain evaluation in the emergency department: can MDCT provide a comprehensive evaluation? AJR Am J Roentgenol 2005;185:533–40.

47. Runza G, La Grutta L, Alaimo V, et al. Comprehensive cardiovascular ECG-gated MDCT as a standard diagnostic tool in patients with acute chest pain. Eur J Radiol 2007;64(1):41–7.

48. Hendel RC, Patel MR, Kramer CM, et al. ACCF/ACR/SCCT/SCMR/ASNC/NASCI/SCAI/SIR 2006 appropriateness criteria for cardiac computed tomography and cardiac magnetic resonance imaging: a report of the American College of Cardiology Foundation Quality Strategic Directions Committee Appropriateness Criteria Working Group, American College of Radiology, Society of Cardiovascular Computed Tomography, Society for Cardiovascular

Magnetic Resonance, American Society of Nuclear Cardiology, North American Society for Cardiac Imaging, Society for Cardiovascular Angiography and Interventions, and Society of Interventional Radiology. J Am Coll Cardiol 2006;48(7):1475–97.

49. Picano E. Sustainability of medical imaging. BMJ 2004;328:578–80.

50. Scanlon PJ, Faxon DP, Audet AM, et al. ACC/AHA guidelines for coronary angiography: executive summary and recommendations. A report of the American College of Cardiology/American Heart Association Task Force on Practice Guidelines (Committee on Coronary Angiography) developed in collaboration with the Society for Cardiac Angiography and Interventions. Circulation 1999;99(17): 2345–57.

51. Cademartiri F, Mollet NR, Lemos PA, et al. Impact of coronary calcium score on diagnostic accuracy for the detection of significant coronary stenosis with multislice computed tomography angiography. Am J Cardiol 2005;95:1225–7.

52. Weustink AC, Meijboom WB, Mollet NR, et al. Reliable high-speed coronary computed tomography in symptomatic patients. J Am Coll Cardiol 2007; 50(8):786–94.

53. Schroeder AP, Houlind K, Pedersen EM, et al. Magnetic resonance imaging seems safe in patients with intracoronary stents. J Cardiovasc Magn Reson 2000;2(1):43–9.

54. Bellenger NG, Burgess MI, Ray SG, et al. Comparison of left ventricular ejection fraction and volumes in heart failure by echocardiography, radionuclide ventriculography and cardiovascular magnetic resonance; are they interchangeable? Eur Heart J 2000; 21(16):1387–96.

55. Grothues F, Smith GC, Moon JC, et al. Comparison of interstudy reproducibility of cardiovascular magnetic resonance with two-dimensional echocardiography in normal subjects and in patients with heart failure or left ventricular hypertrophy. Am J Cardiol 2002;90(1):29–34.

56. Young AA, Axel L. Three-dimensional motion and deformation of the heart wall: estimation with spatial modulation of magnetization–a model-based approach. Radiology 1992;185(1):241–7.

57. Anderson LJ, Holden S, Davis B, et al. Cardiovascular T2-star (T2*) magnetic resonance for the early diagnosis of myocardial iron overload. Eur Heart J 2001;22(23):2171–9.

58. McCrohon JA, Moon JC, Prasad SK, et al. Differentiation of heart failure related to dilated cardiomyopathy and coronary artery disease using gadolinium-enhanced cardiovascular magnetic resonance. Circulation 2003;108(1):54–9.

59. Moon JC, Reed E, Sheppard MN, et al. The histologic basis of late gadolinium enhancement

cardiovascular magnetic resonance in hypertrophic cardiomyopathy. J Am Coll Cardiol 2004;43(12): 2260–4.

60. Burke AP, Farb A, Tashko G, et al. Arrhythmogenic right ventricular cardiomyopathy and fatty replacement of the right ventricular myocardium: are they different diseases? Circulation 1998;97(16): 1571–80.

61. Vignaux O, Dhote R, Duboc D, et al. Clinical significance of myocardial magnetic resonance abnormalities in patients with sarcoidosis: a 1-year follow-up study. Chest 2002;122(6):1895–901.

62. Fattori R, Rocchi G, Celletti F, et al. Contribution of magnetic resonance imaging in the differential diagnosis of cardiac amyloidosis and symmetric hypertrophic cardiomyopathy. Am Heart J 1998; 136(5):824–30.

63. Wagner A, Schulz-Menger J, Dietz R, et al. Long-term follow-up of patients paragraph sign with acute myocarditis by magnetic paragraph sign resonance imaging. 1: MAGMA 2003;16(1):17–20.

64. Kim RJ, Fieno DS, Parrish TB, et al. Relationship of MRI delayed contrast enhancement to irreversible injury, infarct age, and contractile function. Circulation 1999;100(19):1992–2002.

65. Kitagawa K, Sakuma H, Hirano T, et al. Acute myocardial infarction: myocardial viability assessment in patients early thereafter comparison of contrast-enhanced MR imaging with resting (201)Tl SPECT. Radiology 2003;226(1):138–44.

66. Nagel E, Lorenz C, Baer F, et al. Stress cardiovascular magnetic resonance: consensus panel report. J Cardiovasc Magn Reson 2001;3(3):267–81.

67. Nagel E, Lehmkuhl HB, Bocksch W, et al. Noninvasive diagnosis of ischemia-induced wall motion abnormalities with the use of high-dose dobutamine stress MRI: comparison with dobutamine stress echocardiography. Circulation 1999;99(6):763–70.

68. Hundley WG, Hamilton CA, Thomas MS, et al. Utility of fast cine magnetic resonance imaging and display for the detection of myocardial ischemia in patients not well suited for second harmonic stress echocardiography. Circulation 1999;100(16): 1697–702.

69. Schwitter J, Nanz D, Kneifel S, et al. Assessment of myocardial perfusion in coronary artery disease by magnetic resonance: a comparison with positron emission tomography and coronary angiography. Circulation 2001;103(18):2230–5.

70. Saadi N, Nagel E, Gross M, et al. Noninvasive detection of myocardial ischemia from perfusion reserve based on cardiovascular magnetic resonance. Circulation 2000;101(12):1379–83.

71. Kim WY, Danias PG, Stuber M, et al. Coronary magnetic resonance angiography for the detection of coronary stenoses. N Engl J Med 2001;345(26):1863–9.

Vascular Imaging in the Elderly

Sanjeeva P. Kalva, MBBS, MD[a,b,*], Peter R. Mueller, MD[b,c]

KEYWORDS

- Geriatrics • Atherosclerosis • Peripheral arterial disease
- Renovascular disease • Carotid artery stenosis
- Venous thromboembolism • Segmental arterial mediolysis
- Giant cell arteritis • Varicose veins

The geriatric population is affected by a myriad of vascular diseases. The incidence of atherosclerosis increases with age. Though men are affected more often, the incidence of atherosclerosis in women increases sharply after menopause. A few contributing factors increase the risk of atherosclerosis in the elderly. These include hypertension, diabetes, hyperlipidemia, smoking, obesity, and a sedentary lifestyle. In addition to atherosclerosis, other vascular diseases, such as venous thromboembolism, varicose veins, and a few types of vasculitis, are also common in the elderly. The clinical presentation of vascular disease varies from acute emergency (ie, aortic rupture or pulmonary embolism) to asymptomatic disease (ie, carotid artery stenosis). Signs of disease may be observed as an incidental finding on other imaging studies. A few patients may present with symptoms specific to decreased perfusion; for example, patients who have peripheral arterial disease may present with claudication or gangrene.

Imaging of vascular diseases in the elderly is complicated by the presence of coexistent diseases. In general, image quality is degraded with obesity. Kidney disease precludes use of contrast materials during CT and MR imaging examinations. Coexistent cardiopulmonary diseases, such as congestive heart failure, arrhythmias, and chronic obstructive pulmonary diseases, limit the ability of the elderly to hold breath during image acquisition. Additionally, these cardiopulmonary diseases may preclude use of some of the imaging modalities because of inherent contraindications; for example, MR examinations are contraindicated in patients who have pacemakers, and coronary CT arteriography is of limited use in the presence of severe arrhythmias. Vascular calcifications, often encountered in the elderly, affect the diagnostic accuracy of CT arteriography. Though stochastic effects of radiation exposure are of little clinical significance in the elderly, the deterministic effects, such as skin erythema, epilation, and skin burn, can occur during catheter angiography, because interventions in tortuous arteries may demand longer procedure times.

In this article, the authors discuss the common vascular diseases affecting the elderly and the role of imaging, protocols, and findings on various imaging modalities. The authors also discuss the role of interventional procedures in the management of vascular disorders. For the purpose of this article, the authors have categorized vascular diseases in two broad categories: arterial disease and venous disease. Arterial diseases have been subcategorized to include atherosclerotic and non-atherosclerotic diseases. Atherosclerosis may result in arterial stenosis, occlusion, or aneurysm formation, but a combination of these is seen often in many patients. Atherosclerosis is

[a] Division of Cardiovascular Imaging and Intervention, Department of Radiology, Massachusetts General Hospital, 55 Fruit Street, Boston, MA 02114, USA
[b] Harvard Medical School, 25 Shattuck Street, Boston, MA 02115, USA
[c] Division of Abdominal Imaging and Intervention, Department of Radiology, Massachusetts General Hospital, 55 Fruit Street, Boston, MA 02114, USA
* Corresponding author. Division of Cardiovascular Imaging and Intervention, Department of Radiology, Massachusetts General Hospital, GRB 290, MGH, 55 Fruit Street, Boston, MA 02114.
E-mail address: skalva@partners.org (S.P. Kalva).

Radiol Clin N Am 46 (2008) 663–683
doi:10.1016/j.rcl.2008.04.009

considered separately for each vascular territory, because this facilitates detailed discussion of imaging protocols and pitfalls inherent to the region. Remeber that atherosclerosis is a systemic disease, and presence of atherosclerosis in one vascular territory almost always suggests its presence in other vascular territories and warrants examination to detect occult disease. More often, asymptomatic disease in other vascular territories may be more life threatening than symptomatic atherosclerotic disease in one vascular region. Other diseases, such as giant cell arteritis and segmental arterial mediolysis, have been included for completion. Two specific venous diseases–venous thromboembolism and varicose veins–are discussed.

ARTERIAL DISEASES
Atherosclerosis

Atherosclerosis affects medium and large sized vessels and is considered a proximal arterial disease, though distal small vessels may be affected by atheroemboli. Atherosclerotic plaques characteristically occur at vessel branching points and at sites where sudden changes in velocity and direction of blood flow occur. Progressive changes in the plaque size usually are accompanied by vessel wall changes (positive remodeling) to accommodate the blood flow, but later, various degrees of stenoses ensue. Such stenoses lead to flow turbulence and increased blood flow velocities, which in turn lead to more shear stress on the vessel wall and plaque formation. Decreased end-organ perfusion results in various clinical symptoms. Sudden changes in the configuration and size of atherosclerotic plaque may occur with rupture of the fibrous cap or intra-plaque hemorrhage. Such events result in acute clinical presentation (such as myocardial infarction and stroke).

The true incidence of atherosclerosis is not well known because of the asymptomatic nature of the disease in its early stages. In general, the incidence is higher as age advances, and it is more common in men. In women, the incidence increases and reaches that of men 5 years after menopause. Risk factors for atherosclerosis include high blood pressure, diabetes, impaired glucose tolerance, metabolic syndrome, dyslipoproteinemia, obesity, tobacco smoking, sedentary lifestyle, stress, and family history of coronary heart disease.[1] In addition, elevated serum homocysteine, C-reactive protein, serum lipoprotein A, and fibrinogen levels also are associated with increased incidence of atherosclerosis.

Imaging plays an important role in the diagnosis of symptomatic and asymptomatic atherosclerosis.

Diagnosis of steno-occlusive disease can be inferred from clinical symptoms and a few simple nonimaging tests (such as retinal examination, measuring ankle-brachial index, and so forth). However, imaging is required for proper assessment of the extent and degree of severity of the narrowing, the hemodynamic significance of such narrowing, collateral pathways in vascular occlusions, the status of the distal vascular tree, and the extent of end-organ damage. It also guides the clinician to choose proper therapy—medical therapy or endovascular surgery or open surgery for restoration of blood flow. Imaging also plays a role in surveillance of treated vascular segments and provides prognostic information. Current research focuses on identifying vulnerable plaque based on plaque composition to provide better assessment of clinically relevant asymptomatic (but potentially high risk) atherosclerotic plaques.

Peripheral Arterial Disease

The prevalence of lower extremity peripheral arterial disease increases with age. Intermittent claudication, often described as the hallmark of peripheral arterial disease, occurs in 2% of the geriatric population. However, asymptomatic or symptomatic peripheral arterial disease (defined as an ankle-brachial index [ABI]) of less than 0.9 occurs at a frequency of 7%, 12.5%, and 23.2% among people aged 60–69, 70–79, and 80 and older, respectively.[2] The symptoms of peripheral arterial disease, described as the "five P's", include pain, pulselessness, paralysis, paraesthesia, and pallor. The location of intermittent claudication depends on the level of the occlusive process in the arterial system. Patients who have aortoiliac disease often complain of pain in the buttocks and thighs, whereas patients who have femoropopliteal disease complain of calf pain. Progression of the occlusive disease results in rest pain, tissue loss, and neurologic symptoms.

A few office-based tests may provide information about the presence and location of peripheral arterial disease. The ABI is measured by dividing the highest ankle systolic blood pressure with the highest arm systolic blood pressure. The normal ABI is greater than 1, and a value of less than 0.95 is considered abnormal. An ABI of less than 0.9 suggests peripheral arterial disease, whereas less than 0.5 suggests a severe form of peripheral arterial disease. An ABI of less than 0.3 suggests poor wound healing of distal ischemic ulcers. The ABI is less reliable in heavily calcified arteries and in the presence of distal small vessel disease. Pulse-volume recoding (or plethysmography) provides segmental pulse volume recordings by applying pneumatic cuffs around the thighs, calves, ankles, feet, and toes. These tracings provide information about the location of arterial occlusion or stenosis. The ABI and plethysmography can be performed after exercise, which provides hemodynamic information about subclinical occlusive disease.[3]

Duplex ultrasound provides anatomic and physiologic information of the blood flow to the lower extremities. However, evaluation of the aorta and iliac arteries may be limited because of a poor acoustic window from body habitus or gas filled bowel loops. The femoropopliteal and tibial arteries are well visualized with high frequency ultrasound. Atherosclerotic plaques may be seen as focal wall adherent hypoechoic, mixed echogenic, or hyperechoic masses causing luminal narrowing. Calcified plaques result in shadowing, which may limit the use of Doppler examination. In addition, ultrasound studies are dependent on the experience of the operator. Doppler interrogation of normal patent peripheral arteries demonstrates a triphasic flow pattern (**Fig. 1**). Stenosis results in a change in the peak systolic velocity, a loss of flow reversal, and spectral broadening.[4] A focal stenosis of 50% or more is considered hemodynamically significant and is diagnosed when the peak systolic velocity increases by 100% or more, compared with the peak systolic velocity in the proximal segment of the artery (**Fig. 2**). Occlusion is diagnosed when there is no demonstrable flow on color Doppler at appropriate velocity settings. It is important to assess the flow in the distal vascular bed once a focal stenosis or occlusion is diagnosed. Distal to a hemodynamically significant stenosis, the vessels demonstrate a tardus parvus pattern with decreased peak systolic velocity. Sometimes, it may be difficult to detect slow flow in the distal vascular bed, and thus, ultrasound has decreased sensitivity to detect distal stenoses in the presence of a multifocal occlusive process.[5] Overall, a screening duplex study is useful in 80% of patients to effectively diagnose aortoiliac and femoropopliteal disease.[6] The reported sensitivity of duplex ultrasound for detecting stenosis and occlusion is 92% and 95% with a specificity of 95% and 97%.[7] A Color Doppler study aids in selection of patients for endovascular[8] or open surgical procedures[9] and provides prognostic information following such procedures.[10] Duplex studies also are useful to assess the patency of femoropopliteal bypass grafts. A hemodynamically significant stenosis in the bypass graft is diagnosed if the peak systolic velocity is more than 300 cm/s or if the peak systolic velocity ratio between the site of interrogation and the proximal segment is greater than 3.5.[11]

With recent advances in multi-detector row CT (MDCT), imaging of the entire aortoiliac, femoropopliteal, and tibial arteries following the administration of a single bolus of contrast material is now feasible. In addition, the data for the entire scan range can be acquired during a single breathhold. These CT scanners allow thin-section acquisition and provide high quality multi-planar reformations and three-dimensional reconstructions. Compared to ultrasound, CT angiography (CTA) is less operator dependent, can evaluate the entire extent of the stenosis or occlusion, can depict the collaterals, and can slow flow in the distal vascular bed (see **Fig. 2**). Compared to digital subtraction angiography (DSA), the CT is less invasive and less expensive and provides assessment of the luminal plaques, thrombus, inflammation, and peri-arterial disease.[12] Compared to magnetic resonance angiography (MRA), CTA is quicker, and the results are less influenced by vessel tortuousity and slow flow. In addition, CT has higher spatial resolution and provides anatomic bony landmarks, which are useful in planning therapy. Postoperative patients who have metallic clips and vascular stents are evaluated better with CT rather than MR imaging. However, elderly patients who have decreased kidney function, cardiopulmonary disease, or an allergy to iodinated contrast material may not be well suited for contrast enhanced CT. CT is less specific in detecting stenosis in the presence of calcifications. CT is associated with radiation exposure, but it has less compared with DSA. Tailoring the CT studies

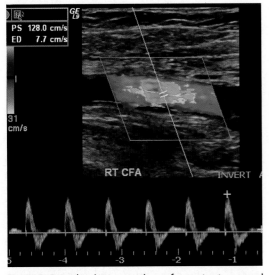

Fig. 1. A Doppler interrogation of a patent, normal right common femoral artery demonstrates triphasic flow pattern.

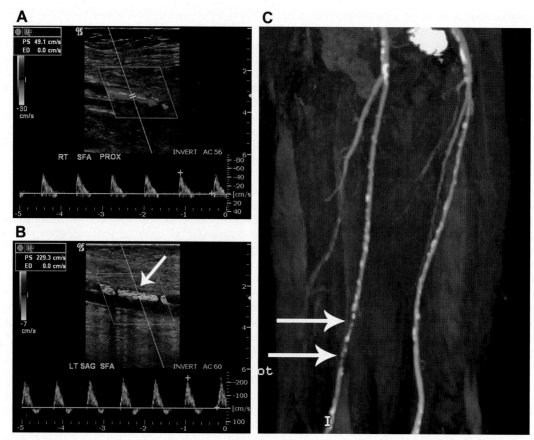

Fig. 2. A 67-year-old male who has right leg claudication. (*A*) Color Doppler of proximal right superficial femoral artery (SFA) demonstrates normal flow pattern with a peak systolic velocity of 49 cm/sec. (*B*) In the mid-distal SFA, there is flow turbulence (*arrow*) with increased peak systolic velocity (229 cm/sec). (*C*) Corresponding CTA shows focal high grade stenoses (*arrows*) in the same arterial segment.

to the patient requirements can minimize the radiation exposure. The recommended scanning range is usually from the level of the diaphragm to the feet, which can be covered in 15–20 seconds on a 16-slice or 64-slice CT scanner with the following technical parameters: detector thickness of 1–1.5 mm, pitch of 1 (table feed equivalent to the total beam width during one gantry rotation), gantry rotation time of 350–500 ms, kVp of 120 with automated tube current settings. Noncontrast CT generally is not required unless intramural hematoma or parenchymal hemorrhage is suspected. Usually, 100–120 mL of iodinated contrast material (300 mg/mL or 370 mg/mL of iodine) is administered through an 18G peripheral intravenous (IV) cannula at a rate of 4 mL/sec. Saline infusion at the end of contrast material administration is useful to flush the contrast material from the venous system and can help minimize the volume of the contrast material required for the same acquisition.[13] Similarly, total volume of contrast material may be decreased if high concentration of iodine is

used.[14] Data is acquired after a scanning delay, which is calculated with either a test bolus or through an automatic bolus triggering in the abdominal aorta. The images are reconstructed at standard algorithm at a slice thickness of 1–2.5 mm at 0%–50% overlap. Images are reconstructed in various orthogonal planes, user-defined curved planes along the long axis of the vessel, and 3D reformations, including maximum intensity projections and color-coded volume rendered images. CTA is useful in diagnosing the location, multiplicity, and extent of steno-occlusive disease, the degree of arterial calcifications, the diameter of normal adjacent arteries, collateral flow, and the patency of distal vasculature. Recent meta-analysis of 12 studies comparing multi-detector CTA with DSA revealed a pooled sensitivity and specificity of 92% and 93%, respectively, for detecting a stenosis of at least 50% per segment.[15] In the same study, the authors pointed out that the diagnostic performance of MDCT in evaluating the infra-popliteal arteries was inferior but not significantly different from that in the aortoiliac and femoropopliteal arteries. CTA aids in selecting patients for endovascular and open surgical repair.[16] CTA also is useful in the assessment of bypass grafts[17] and recurrent disease following endovascular repair.

MRA of the peripheral arteries has certain advantages in elderly patients. Unlike CT, calcifications in the arterial wall do not hamper the evaluation of the arterial lumen. In patients who have iodine allergy, MRA with gadolinium is a viable alternative technique. Contrast-enhanced MRA (CE-MRA) provides rapid, multi-phasic assessment of abdominal and peripheral vasculature. There is no radiation exposure associated with MR imagaing. The hemodynamic significance of luminal narrowing can be assessed with phase contrast imaging. However, in the presence of renal impairment, gadolinium is considered unsafe, because recent reports linked nephrogenic systemic fibrosis to gadolinium.[18] Non-contrast MRA sequences (such as time-of-flight [TOF] and phase contrast techniques) are useful in patients who have severe renal dysfunction. MR imaging is contraindicated in patients who have pacemakers and intracranial aneurysmal clips. MRA cannot be used to evaluate the patency of arterial segments treated with metallic stents. The spatial resolution of MRA is inferior to that of CTA and DSA; however, recent advances in MR (including 3T scanners, parallel imaging with multiple-element phased array coils, and dynamic imaging with time resolved imaging) have improved image quality and spatial resolution.[19] At Massachusetts General Hospital (Boston, Massachusetts), TOF images are routinely obtained for the foot and lower leg before CE-MRA is performed. TOF imaging of the leg and foot is obtained with an inferior saturation band to suppress signals from the veins, and the inflow signal from arteries is imaged. These are useful in the assessment of patency of arterial segments in these areas, because CE-MRA at these locations is often associated with venous contamination and poor delineation of arteries. Currently, the CE-MRA is the work-horse of peripheral MRA. During CE-MRA, multi-station (usually, the first station is the abdomen and the pelvis, the second station is the thighs, and the third station is the legs), 3D (or volumetric) spoiled gradient echo sequences with heavy T1 weighting are applied.[20] To minimize the acquisition time, parallel imaging and coronal plane acquisition with short time of echo (1–1.5 ms), short TR (3–4.5 ms), and small flip angle (20°) are applied. The spatial resolution is usually less than 1.5 cm. First, multi-station MRA is acquired without the administration of the contrast material (these are

called "mask" images and are akin to the DSA). These images are used to ensue that 1) the region of interest has been properly included, 2) enough overlap between the stations has been applied, 3) the patient could hold breath for the duration of the scanning, and 4) the images are artifact free. Usually, 0.1–0.2 mmol/kg of gadolinium contrast material is injected through peripheral IV cannula at a rate of 2 mL/sec followed by 30 mL of saline flush at the same rate. Images are acquired after a scanning delay, which usually is determined by a test bolus (1–2 mL of contrast material injected at 2 mL/sec followed by 10 mL of saline flush) or through an automated triggering in the abdominal aorta. All three stations are imaged sequentially from abdomen to the feet (often referred to as "bolus chasing") (**Fig. 3**). The sequence is repeated in reverse order to obtain delayed images. The leg images often may be degraded by venous opacification. A few strategies have been recommended to reduce venous contamination.[21] Tongdee and colleagues[22] advocated a hybrid MRA technique, wherein the calf vessels are imaged first, following contrast

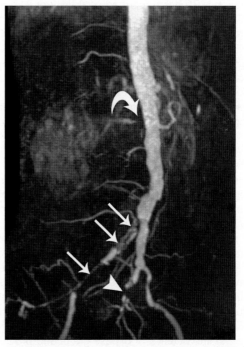

Fig. 3. A 67-year-old male who has buttock and thigh claudication. Coronal oblique maximum intensity projection contrast-enhanced MRA demonstrates steno-occlusive disease (*arrows*) affecting the right common and external iliac arteries and short segment occlusion (*arrowhead*) of the left internal iliac artery. The right internal iliac artery is occluded. Incidental high grade stenosis (*curved arrow*) of the right renal artery is also seen.

material administration. This is followed by a multi-station MRA of the abdomen and thighs after administering a second dose of contrast material. A few authors advocated application of mid-thigh blood pressure cuffs inflated to 50 mm Hg during data acquisition to decrease venous contamination.[23] Another technique to obtain high-resolution, fast, contrast enhanced, dynamic images of the calf vessels is time resolved imaging (time resolved intravascular contrast kinetics [TRICKS], GE Healthcare, Milwaukee, Wisconsin). In this technique, a small volume (5–6 mL) of gadolinium contrast material is injected, and the region of interest is imaged with TRICKS sequence. The scan duration is usually 10–12 seconds, and the sequence can be repeated as needed. This provides dynamic information about the flow pattern, filling of collateral vessels, and the dominant arterial supply to the region. Compared to traditional multi-station MRA, TRICKS MRA is superior in evaluating the calf and pedal vessels for luminal narrowing.[24] TOF MRA has been reported to be 85%–92% sensitive in peripheral arteries for detecting arterial stenoses greater than 50%, with a specificity of 81% to 88%.[25,26] Dynamic multi-station MRA has a reported sensitivity of 81% to 95% with a specificity of 91% to 98% for detecting arterial stenoses of greater than 50%. TRICKS MRA of the infrapopliteal and pedal arteries is better than conventional multi-station MRA when planning endovascular and surgical revascularization procedures.[27] MRA also is useful to assess patency of surgically placed bypass grafts, except for its limited use in the presence of metallic clips or metal stents. MRA has a sensitivity and specificity of 90% and 98% respectively for detecting graft stenoses greater than 69%.[28]

Catheter-based DSA remains the gold standard for evaluation of peripheral arterial disease. It offers an accurate depiction of the number, extent, and severity of arterial stenoses and occlusions. It provides dynamic information about the collateral pathways and the status of distal vascular tree and aids in planning endovascular and open revascularization procedures. It is part of endovascular procedures. It is also useful to accurately quantify recurrent stenosis following angioplasty or stent placement (**Fig. 4**). It can accurately assess the patency of bypass grafts and provide information about the cause of graft failure. Though iodinated contrast materials are used routinely during DSA, carbon dioxide can be used as contrast material in patients who have renal disease or an iodine allergy. This is important for elderly patients who cannot tolerate the iodinated contrast material because of renal or cardiopulmonary disease. Generally, carbon dioxide

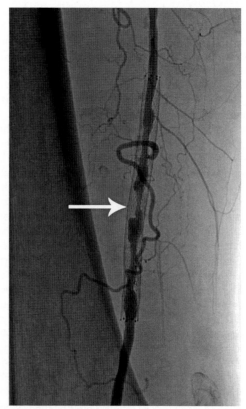

Fig. 4. A catheter angiography in a 75-year-old male who presented with recurrent claudication after 2 years of right superficial femoral artery revascularization with angioplasty and stent placement. Angiography demonstrates instent restenosis (*arrow*).

angiography is tolerated well, and it provides diagnostic quality images in the proximal vessels, though the quality of distal calf and pedal vessels may be degraded.[29] The main disadvantages of DSA include its invasive nature, its need for experienced technical and medical staff, its cost, and the complications associated with the procedure (such as hematoma, pseudoaneurysm, and arterial injury).

Renovascular Disease

Similar to peripheral arterial disease, the true incidence of renovascular disease is unknown, partly because many patients are asymptomatic, the differing definitions that are used, and the population studied varies widely.[30] Renovascular disease may manifest as asymptomatic renal artery stenosis, intractable or uncontrollable hypertension requiring multiple medications, or ischemic nephropathy with progressive loss of renal function. There are two main causes of renovascular disease: atherosclerosis and fibromuscular dysplasia; the former being more common in the elderly. Renovascular hypertension accounts for 0.5% to 5% of patients who have hypertension. Most often, ostial or proximal renal artery atheromatous plaques are responsible for renal artery stenosis.

Color Doppler ultrasound generally is regarded as the first screening modality for evaluation of renovascular disease. The main advantages of color Doppler ultrasound include ready availability, a noninvasive nature, a lack of ionizing radiation, repeatability, assessment of functional rather than morphologic data, and feasibility of bedside examination. However, it suffers from a few disadvantages, including operator dependency and difficulty in examining patients who are obese or uncooperative. Every effort should be made to visualize the proximal renal arteries. The Doppler criteria for diagnosing renal artery stenosis (**Fig. 5**) of more than 60% include peak systolic velocity of greater than 200 cm/s in the proximal renal artery and a renal-aortic ratio of peak systolic velocity greater than 3.5.[31] Absence of color flow and Doppler signal in an otherwise normal looking renal artery suggest occlusion. Indirect signs in the distal arterial bed (ie, in the intra-renal parenchymal arteries) may add confidence to the diagnosis of renal artery stenosis. Such signs include

a parvus tardus flow pattern in the segmental or arcuate arteries, an increased acceleration time (greater than 0.08 second), and a change in the resistive index of 5% or greater between the right and left kidneys.[32] The reported sensitivity and specificity of color Doppler ultrasound in the diagnosis of renal artery stenosis of more than 60% varies from 84%–98% and 90%–98%, respectively.[33,34]

Angiotensin converting enzyme (ACE) inhibitor scintigraphy with captopril is another method used to detect renovascular hypertension. It is based on the principle that glomerular filtration (or the renal function) is dependant on the circulating angiotensin II in patients who have renovascular disease, and inhibition of ACE will result in decreased renal function that is demonstrable on scintigraphy.[35] Along with color Doppler ultrasound, this study is becoming more relevant now for diagnosis of renal artery stenosis, because decreased renal function is a relative contraindication for use of CT and MR contrast materials. Technetium-99m labelled diethylenetriaminepentaacetic acid (DTPA) or mercaptoacetyltriglycine is injected through a peripheral IV, and scintigraphy of the kidneys is performed at baseline following the administration of the ACE inhibitor. Time activity curves of the renal cortex and pelvis are

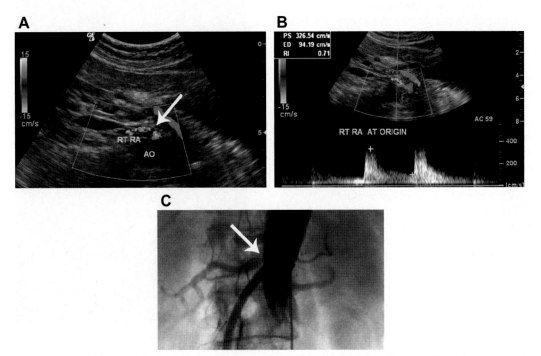

Fig. 5. A 55-year-old female who has uncontrollable hypertension. (*A*) Color flow imaging shows focal narrowing (*arrow*) of the proximal right renal artery with increased peak systolic velocity of 326 cm/sec and turbulence on Doppler (*B*). (*C*) Catheter angiography confirms the ultrasound findings—there is an osteal stenosis (*arrow*) with poststenotic dilatation.

obtained. Criteria associated with a high probability of renovascular hypertension[36] include worsening of the renogram curve, a reduction in the relative uptake, prolongation of the renal and parenchymal transit time, an increase in the 20-minute/peak-uptake ratio, and prolongation of time to maximum velocity. ACE inhibitor scintigraphy has a sensitivity of 68% with a specificity of 92% for detecting renal artery stenosis of greater than 50%.[37] The sensitivity of ACE inhibitor scintigraphy is affected by concurrent use of ACE inhibitors, urinary obstruction, and impaired renal function. Captopril infusion is associated with a precipitous fall in blood pressure in few patients who have renal artery stenosis. Some authors recommended using acetyl salicylic acid (aspirin) instead of an ACE because of reported similar sensitivity and specificity of Tc-99m DTPA aspirin scintigraphy for detecting renal artery stenosis.[38]

Multi-detector CT angiography provides operator-independent, high-resolution, thin section images of the renal arteries. CT protocol is similar to that described for peripheral arterial disease evaluation except for the extent covered—only the abdomen is included for evaluation of renovascular hypertension. A delayed phase CT of the abdomen may be performed to assess nephrographic and urographic abnormalities. Calcified plaques limit the CT evaluation of luminal narrowing. CT is used to identify the location and extent of atheromatous plaque, the true extent of luminal narrowing, post-stenotic dilatation of the renal artery, and associated parenchymal changes as a result of distal emboli (such as infarcts) or chronic hypoperfusion (eg, small size of the kidney, delayed persistent nephrogram, and periureteric and pericapsular collaterals). Overall, the sensitivity and specificity of MDCT for detecting renal artery stenosis exceeds 95%.[39] CT is useful when assessing the anatomy of the renal artery for choosing the proper emboli-protecting device during endovascular intervention. MDCT also is useful in assessing in-stent restenosis.[40]

MRA is well suited for evaluation of renal artery stenosis in the elderly. Calcified atheromatous plaques do no hamper the assessment of the arterial lumen. Phase contrast imaging can be used to assess the peak systolic velocity at the site of stenosis and the gradient across the stenosis. MRA provides information about the size of the kidney, changes in nephrogram, periureteric collaterals, and post-stenotic dilatation. It is less dependent on the operator, unlike the color Doppler ultrasound, and provides morphologic and functional information about the presence, location, and severity of renal artery stenosis. MR contrast materials are linked to nephrogenic systemic fibrosis

in the presence of reduced renal function and caution should be exercised with regards to their use in the presence of renal dysfunction. A phase contrast study is useful in patients who cannot receive gadolinium. Recently, noncontrast MRA using steady state free precision technique was found to be useful in assessing renal artery stenosis with an accuracy of 85% when compared with contrast enhanced MRA.[41] CE-MRA (**Fig. 6**) has a sensitivity of 93%–98% and a specificity of 91%–95% for the detection of a main renal artery stenosis of greater than 50%.[42] MRA is of little use in assessing the patency of stents, because metal artifacts result in loss of signal (**Fig. 7**).

DSA remains the gold standard for the diagnosis of renal artery stenosis (see **Fig. 5**). It provides accurate assessment of luminal narrowing and aides in planning endovascular intervention. It also is useful in detecting stenosis of accessory small renal arteries and branch vessel stenoses. It is possible to measure the gradient across the stenosis to evaluate hemodynamic significance of such

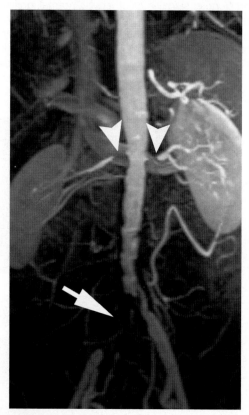

Fig. 6. A 75-year-old patient who has uncontrollable hypertension and is taking three medications. Coronal maximum intensity projection CE-MRA shows bilateral high grade stenosis (*arrowheads*) affecting the renal arteries. A long segment occlusion (*arrow*) of the right common iliac artery is also seen.

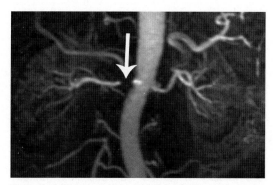

Fig. 7. Gadolinium-enhanced MRA of the renal arteries following right renal artery stent placement. Patency of the stent cannot be assessed on MRA because of signal void (*arrow*) from a metallic stent.

stenosis. DSA is part of any endovascular intervention. It also provides accurate assessment of in-stent stenosis. In patients who have renal impairment, carbon dioxide can be used as contrast material for the diagnosis and therapy of renal artery stenosis.[43]

Mesenteric Ischemia

Chronic mesenteric ischemia results from atherosclerotic narrowing of the mesenteric arteries. It is uncommon but accounts for 5% of all ischemic intestinal illnesses. It is more common in the elderly (mean age of 60 years) and affects both sexes equally. It is associated often with other foci of atherosclerosis, diabetes, and hypertension. Asymptomatic, greater than 50%, stenosis of the mesenteric artery is found in as many as 18% of patients over 65 years of age.[44] Asymptomatic stenoses generally progress and lead to symptomatic disease in more than 80% of patients. The classically described symptom is epigastric pain following a meal (known as intestinal angina). There are extensive collateral pathways between the celiac artery and the superior mesenteric and inferior mesenteric arteries. Unless two of the three vessels are severely stenotic, it is unusual to develop symptoms of mesenteric ischemia. The pancreaticoduodenal arcades, arc of Buhler, and epiploic arcades provide collateral pathways between the celiac axis and the superior mesenteric artery. The arc of Riolan and the marginal artery of Drummond form the collateral pathways between the superior mesenteric and inferior mesenteric arteries.

Doppler evaluation of mesenteric arteries is useful when assessing the celiac axis and superior mesenteric arteries. However, an adequate examination is possible in less than 60% of the general population because of a poor acoustic window from body habitus and bowel gas. In addition,

the Doppler velocity parameters are affected by the presence of diffuse atherosclerotic disease in the aorta and by tortuosity of the mesenteric arteries with consequent elevation of the peak systolic velocity in even normal patent mesenteric arteries. A stenosis of greater than 50% in celiac axis is diagnosed if the peak systolic velocity is more than 200 cm/sec. Post-stenotic dilatation of the celiac artery and reversal of flow in the gastroduodenal or common hepatic artery suggest hemodynamically significant stenosis. Superior mesenteric artery stenosis of greater than 50% is suspected if the peak systolic velocity is more than 275 cm/sec with an associated increase in end diastolic velocity (of greater than 45 cm/sec).[45] The sensitivity and specificity of ultrasound for diagnosis of mesenteric arterial stenosis of greater than 50% exceed 80%.

CTA and MRA provide precise morphologic information about the stenosis and status of the distal vascular segments. It is possible to assess the size, extent of the atheromatous plaque, severity of luminal narrowing, post-stenotic dilatation, and enlarged collateral vessels.[46] The protocols are similar to those for renal artery evaluation, except that the region of interest for scanning should include the mesenteric vascular territory. Two phases, arterial and portal venous phases, are obtained routinely. During CTA, high attenuation oral contrast medium is avoided to enable quick 3D maximum intensity projection reconstructions. Low attenuation oral contrast material, such as water or milk, can be used if bowel wall changes are suspected. Generally, a focal narrowing with greater than 50% luminal narrowing is considered hemodynamically significant (**Fig. 8**). In addition, CT enables evaluation of the bowel. Both CTA and MRA provide information about vessel tortuosity and aid in planning endovascular or open revascularization procedures. CTA also is useful when assessing in-stent restenosis following endovascular procedures. Patency of the surgical grafts is better assessed with CTA, because surgical clips often obscure the anastomotic regions on MR imaging. The overall sensitivity and specificity of both modalities approach 95%–100% in diagnosing mesenteric artery stenosis of greater than 50%.[47] DSA is the gold standard for accurate localization and grading of luminal narrowing, and it is part of any interventional procedure. It also aids in the diagnosis of recurrent stenosis following endovascular or open repair.

Carotid Artery Stenosis

Accurate diagnosis of carotid artery stenosis is clinically relevant, because recent studies have

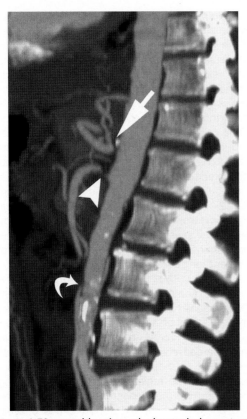

Fig. 8. A 70-year-old patient who has typical symptoms of abdominal angina. Sagittal maximum intensity of CTA data shows high grade stenosis of the celiac axis (*arrow*) and superior mesenteric artery (*arrowhead*). Mild stenosis (*curved arrow*) of the inferior mesenteric artery is also seen.

demonstrated a significant reduction in subsequent ipsilateral stroke with carotid endarterectomy in patients who have 70%–99% symptomatic carotid artery stenosis[48] and in some patients who have 50%–69% stenosis.[49] Asymptomatic patients who have carotid artery stenosis of at least 60% showed a 5.8% risk reduction of stroke following endarterectomy.[50] The incidence of carotid artery stenosis increases with age, and it is estimated that approximately 10% of people over 80 years of age have carotid artery stenosis of more than 50%. Generally, evaluation for carotid artery stenosis is requested in symptomatic patients who had stroke or transient ischemic attack and in asymptomatic elderly (greater than 60 years) patients before open heart surgery.

Color Doppler ultrasound is well suited for initial evaluation of the carotid arteries, because these vessels run superficially in the neck. High frequency linear probes provide high-resolution images of the intima and media of the carotid artery and allow characterization of the plaque morphology and surface (**Fig. 9**). Normal intima-media thickness is usually less than 0.8 mm and any value above 1.1 mm is considered abnormal, representing atherosclerotic disease. Atheromatous plaques are classified based on their echogenicity, surface, and hemodynamic effects.[51] Ulcerated and hypoechoic plaques often are associated with ischemic symptoms. Color Doppler provides information about the flow turbulence, peak systolic and end-diastolic velocities and allows grading of stenosis (see **Fig. 9**). A peak systolic velocity of greater than 230 cm/s (primary criterion), an end diastolic velocity of greater than 100 cm/s, and a peak systolic velocity ratio of greater than 4 between the internal carotid and common carotid arteries (secondary criteria) suggest a stenosis of more than 70%.[52] Near total occlusions may demonstrate a variable flow pattern but severe luminal narrowing when large atheroma is observed on gray scale imaging. Occluded arteries demonstrate no flow. Other signs of occluded internal carotid artery include increased diastolic flow in the ipsilateral external carotid artery and increased velocities in the contralateral internal carotid artery. The differentiation of near total occlusion from complete occlusion may be improved with the use of ultrasound contrast materials. The limitations of ultrasound include operator dependency, a difficulty in interpretation of the peak systolic velocities in the presence of vessel tortuousity and kinking, a difficulty in detecting flow in the presence of heavily calcified plaques, and the inability to detect stenosis in the distal internal carotid artery. The sensitivity and specificity of ultrasound in detecting a stenosis of greater than 70% to near total occlusion varies from 91%–95% and 86%–97%, respectively.[53] In grading stenosis, color Doppler ultrasound and DSA are in agreement in at least 90% of the cases.

CT and MR imaging allow simultaneous visualization of the entire extent of the carotid artery and intracranial cerebral circulation. They are less operator dependent and provide information about the presence and extent of atherosclerotic plaques and the severity of luminal narrowing. Isotropic voxels, high spatial resolution, and the ability to perform various multiplanar, curved, and 3D reformations improved the sensitivity and specificity of multidetector CT in diagnosing carotid artery disease (**Fig. 10**). During CT examinations, care should be taken to avoid artifacts from dental fillings. Current 16- and 64-slice scanners allow scanning the entire 25 cm field of view in 4–7 seconds, with submillimeter (0.6–0.75 mm) detector collimation, a pitch of 1.3–1.5, and a gantry rotation time of 350–500 ms. Generally, the

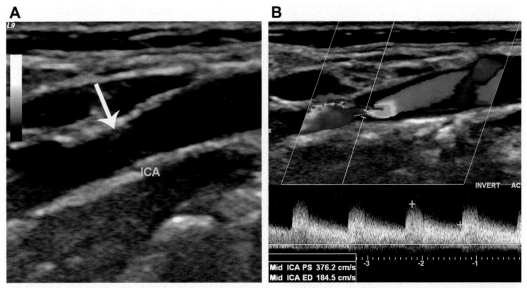

Fig. 9. (A) Gray-scale ultrasound and (B) color Doppler of the right internal carotid artery in a 65-year-old woman who has transient ischemic attack. (A) Gray scale ultrasound demonstrates an irregular, hypoechoic plaque (*arrow*) causing luminal narrowing. (B) Doppler evaluation demonstrates high velocities consistent with severe (greater than 70%–99%) stenosis at this location.

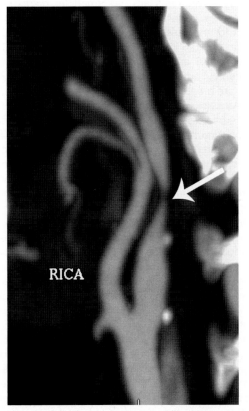

Fig. 10. Same patient as in Fig. 9. Sagittal oblique maximum intensity projection of CTAdata confirms high grade stenosis (*arrow*) of the right internal carotid artery.

entire extent of the carotid arteries in the neck and intracranial circle of Willis are included in the scan range, and some centers acquire images of the aortic arch at the end. 80–100 mL of iodinated contrast material is injected at a rate of 3–6 mL/sec, and scanning is started after a delay that is determined through bolus triggering or the test bolus method. Images are reconstructed at submillimeter slice thickness with 50% overlap, and reformations are obtained. All measurements are obtained perpendicular to the true longitudinal plane of the carotid artery. It is important to report the method used (North American Symptomatic Carotid Endarterectomy Trial [NASCET] versus European Carotid Surgery Trial [ECST] criteria) for estimating the stenosis. Overall, CTA has a sensitivity of 95% (91%–97% confidence interval [CI]) and specificity of 98% (96%–99% CI) for detecting severe (greater than 70%) carotid artery stenosis.[54] The sensitivity of CT approaches that of DSA in diagnosing near total occlusions. CT allows characterization of the plaque based on the attenuation of the plaque: soft plaque (Hounsfield units [HU] less than 50), intermediate plaque (HU 50–119), and calcified plaque (HU greater than 120). It also is possible to assess plaque ulceration and intra-plaque hemorrhage on CT.[55] CT is useful when assesing in-stent restenosis following revascularization (Fig. 11).

MRA with the TOF technique allows visualization of the entire extent of the carotid artery and intracranial circulation without the use of contrast material, and it is useful in patients who cannot

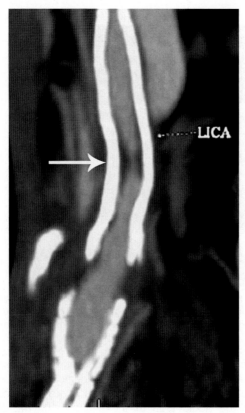

LICA

Fig. 11. CTA of the carotid artery 1 year after endovascular stent placement demonstrates instent restenosis (*arrow*).

receive contrast material. The sensitivity of TOF approaches that of CTA in detecting severe (greater than 70%) stenosis. The main disadvantages of the TOF technique are overestimation of stenosis and signal drop if the vessels run in the plane of acquisition. CE-MRA is more reliable than the TOF technique in determining the presence of stenosis and grading the stenosis. A recent meta-analysis of 41 studies comprising 2541 patients (4876 arteries) revealed that CE-MRA was more sensitive (0.94, 95% CI 0.88–0.97) and specific (0.93, 95% CI 0.89–0.96) for 70%–99% stenosis than Doppler ultrasound, non-contrast MRA, and CTA (sensitivities 0.89, 0.88, 0.76; specificities 0.84, 0.84, 0.94, respectively).[56]

Catheter based DSA still remains the gold standard for accurately grading the stenosis. It differentiates near total occlusion from total occlusion. It has the highest temporal resolution compared with any other imaging modality. It allows simultaneous visualization of tandem lesions and intracranial steno-occlusive disease, the presence of ulcerated plaques, patterns of collateral filling of intracranial vessels in the presence of severe

carotid artery disease, and it allows accurate diagnosis of recurrent disease. However, it does not provide information about the type and amount of atherosclerotic plaque.

Coronary Artery Disease

Coronary artery disease remains the leading cause of death in the western nations. Evaluation for presence of risk factors for atherosclerosis and a few noninvasive tests, including EKG, stress test, and echocardiography provide indirect evidence for the presence of coronary artery disease and allow a clinician to stratify patients into low, intermediate, and high risk for coronary artery disease. Though such stratification allows the clinician to act on risk factor modification in patients who have no or minimal symptoms, it is of less clinical use when a patient presents with acute chest pain. Catheter based coronary angiography provides information about the presence of steno-occlusive disease and allows planning of endovascular treatment or coronary bypass surgery; however, it is invasive and is not available at all centers. More than half of the catheter based coronary angiograms are performed for diagnostic purposes only, and thus, a reliable noninvasive test for the assessment of coronary arteries is of high clinical interest. Recent advances in CT technology allow the noninvasive assessment of coronary arteries. Technical details of coronary CT are omitted because of space restrictions.

As calcium in the coronary arteries represents atherosclerosis, its detection with CT provides the most direct evidence for atherosclerosis in the coronary arteries. CT has high sensitivity for detecting calcification in the coronary arteries, and absence of calcification on coronary CT has a high negative predictive value for ruling out atherosclerosis and significant coronary artery disease in patients who have acute chest pain.[57] Similarly, high calcium scores on CT calcium scoring studies suggest a moderately increased risk for hard cardiac events in high risk, asymptomatic patients. Calcium scoring CT also helps monitor changes in plaque burden following statin therapy. Though a high calcium score suggests the presence of severe atherosclerotic disease, it does not provide information about the location and degree of stenosis.

Coronary CTA with either prospective or retrospective EKG gating provides direct assessment of the coronary artery lumen (**Fig. 12**), atherosclerotic plaque burden (including noncalcified and calcified), and the presence of coronary artery anomalies. 64-slice coronary artery CTA has very high (greater than 95%) negative predictive value in ruling out significant (greater than 50% luminal

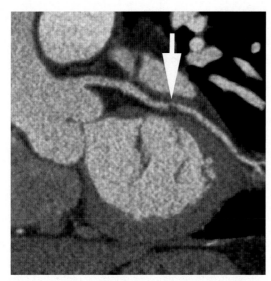

Fig. 12. A 55-year-old patient who has angina pectoris. Curved planar reformation along the left circumflex coronary artery demonstrates focal high grade stenosis (*arrow*) of greater than 50% luminal narrowing. CT allows direct visualization of the atherosclerotic plaque.

narrowing) coronary artery disease. Its sensitivity in detecting significant coronary artery stenosis exceeds 90% in all evaluable segments.[58] Sixty-four slice coronary artery CTA provides information for planning coronary artery bypass surgery and allows the evaluation of bypass grafts for occlusion or stenosis. It is also used to detect instent restenosis.

The role of MR imaging in the evaluation of coronary artery disease is emerging. At present, its precise role relates to the detection of infarcted myocardium, differentiating it from hibernating or stunned but viable myocardium, and providing prognostic information about functional recovery after revascularization following myocardial infarction.[59] MR imaging is also used to assess cardiac function and wall motion abnormalities.

Aortic Aneurysm

Aneurysm is defined as a localized or diffuse dilatation of more than 50% of the diameter of the aorta. Thoracic and abdominal aortic aneurysms occur more often with increasing age and are associated with atherosclerosis and hypertension. In general, aortic aneurysms are more common in men. Abdominal aortic aneurysms occur at a frequency of 5%–7% in the 60 year or older population, whereas thoracic aortic aneurysms occur at a frequency of 3%–4% in the 65 year or older population. Twenty five percent of patients who have a thoracic aortic aneurysm have an abdominal aortic aneurysm. Atherosclerotic aneurysms often

involve the arch and descending thoracic and abdominal aorta and less commonly involve the ascending aorta. Other causes of aortic aneurysm include infections (syphilis), trauma, and postoperative and genetic conditions (Ehler Danlos syndrome and Marfan's syndrome). The symptoms of aortic aneurysm depend on their location, size, pressure, effect on adjacent structures, involvement of branch vessels, and complications. The main dreaded complication of aortic aneurysm is rupture, which occurs with increasing frequency as the aneurysm size (the diameter) exceeds 5 cm.

Screening of the abdominal aortic aneurysm may be performed with ultrasound. Ultrasound can detect the presence of and estimate the size of the aneurysm. However, it is not useful for assessing the exact extent of and branch vessel involvement. In addition, it often is difficult to compare two serial examinations, because the aortic diameter measurements often are affected by the operator and changes in the shape or configuration of the aneurysm. Thoracic and abdominal aortic aneurysms are evaluated best with CT or MR imaging.[60] Both modalities provide information about the extent and size of the aneurysm, the presence of intraluminal thrombus, the involvement of branch vessels, the pressure effects on adjacent structures (such as the bones, veins, and other organs), and the relation of the aneurysm to branch vessels (**Fig. 13**). This information is important when planning surgical or endovascular therapy. In case of thoracic aortic aneurysms, it is important to diagnose aortic root or aortic valve

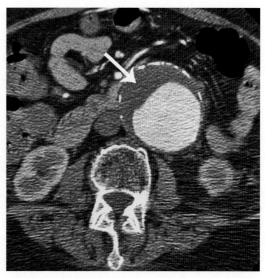

Fig. 13. A 70-year-old woman who has pulsatile abdominal swelling on routine physical examination. Axial contrast-enhanced CT scan shows abdominal aortic aneurysm with intraluminal thrombus (*arrow*).

involvement, because this will affect surgery planning. Though aortic root diameter can be assessed with ECG-gated CTA or MRA, the presence of aortic valve regurgitation is evaluated best with phase contrast MR imaging or transesophageal echocardiography. ECG-gated CTA is used to assess the presence of coronary artery disease and the relationship of the coronary ostia to the aneurysm. Following endovascular repair with stent-grafts, CT and MR imaging provide information about the presence of branch vessel occlusion, perianeurysmal fibrosis, aortoenteric fistula, infection, and endoleaks (persistent contrast-opacification of the aneurysm sac) and help characterize the type of endoleak. Plain radiography and CT provide information about the structural integrity, kinking, and migration of the stent-grafts. CT and MR imaging also are useful in evaluating postsurgical complications, such as anastomotic aneurysms, mycotic aneurysms, rupture, and branch vessel occlusions. DSA usually is reserved for unresolved issues on CT and is part of planned interventional procedures.

CT is the modality of choice to diagnose the rupture of the aortic aneurysm.[61] Unenhanced CT demonstrates periaortic high density material (hemorrhage) (**Fig. 14**), that may extend into the retroperitoneum (in case of abdominal aortic aneurysm) or into the mediastinum (in case of thoracic aortic aneurysm). Associated pleural and pericardial effusions may be seen. Contrast material enhanced CT may demonstrate a leak of contrast material in to the surrounding tissue, crescent shaped collection of contrast material in the wall of the aneurysm, a pseudoaneurysm (see **Fig. 14**), or "pointing" of the contrast material at a particular location.

Acute Aortic Syndromes: Penetrating Aortic Ulcer, Intramural Hematoma, and Dissection

These three conditions (penetrating aortic ulcer, intramural hematoma, and dissection) may be considered as one disease process, with each representing a different stage in evolution. Penetrating aortic ulcers may present as acute aortic syndrome or chronic asymptomatic condition. Intramural hematomas and dissections generally present with acute symptoms: chest pain or back pain. Often, the patients are elderly and have atherosclerosis and hypertension.

Penetrating aortic ulcer refers to ulcerated atherosclerotic plaque that has eroded the internal elastic lamina of the aortic wall and has resulted in a hematoma in the medial layer. These ulcers are common in the aortic arch and proximal descending aorta. Unenhanced CT may demonstrate hyperattenuating intramural hematoma, which is associated often with a penetrating aortic ulcer. Similarly, there may be inward displacement of intimal calcification. Contrast material enhanced CT demonstrates a collection of contrast material outside the aortic lumen with associated thickening of the aortic wall, which may show enhancement. Diffuse atherosclerotic changes in the entire aorta may be present. Penetrating ulcers

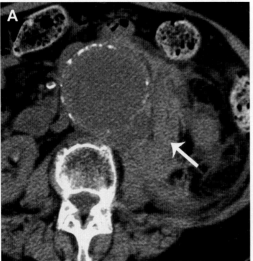 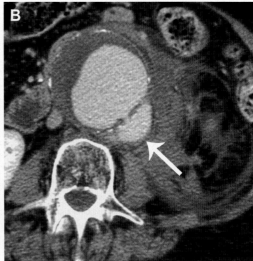

Fig. 14. A 70 year old woman who has known abdominal aortic aneurysm presented to the emergency room with hypotension and abdominal pain. (*A*) Noncontrast CT demonstrates retroperitoneal hemorrhage (*arrow*) adjacent to the aorta. (*B*) Contrast enhanced CT demonstrates a focal pseudoaneurysm (*arrow*) consistent with rupture of the aortic aneurysm.

may progress to intramural hematoma, dissection, or aneurysm or may completely resolve.

Aortic intramural hematoma is caused by a spontaneous hemorrhage from the rupture of vasa vasorum of the medial layer. On unenhanced CT, intramural hematoma is seen as a crescent shaped high attenuation within the aortic wall (**Fig. 15**). The intimal calcifications are displaced toward the lumen. MR imaging may demonstrate high signal on T1-weighted images, suggesting the presence of hemorrhage in the aortic wall. On contrast material enhanced CT or MR imaging, the crescent shaped intramural hematoma shows no enhancement. Findings that may suggest a progression of intramural hematoma to aortic dissection include, maximum aortic diameter of greater 50 mm, involvement of the ascending aorta, large intramural hematoma compressing the aortic lumen, and the presence of pericardial effusion.[62]

Aortic dissection results from intimal tear that allows blood to enter the aortic media leading to the formation of a false lumen in the aortic wall. Acute dissections refer to dissections that are less than 2 weeks old and are often symptomatic. Dissections are classified based on the involvement of the ascending aorta (type A involves the ascending aorta, whereas type B does not involve the ascending aorta). Dissections that involve the ascending aorta are associated often with high mortality and require immediate surgical intervention, because they may involve the aortic root and cause acute aortic regurgitation, dissection of the coronary arteries, and pericardial hemorrhage. CT and MR imaging are well suited for the diagnosis of aortic dissection, but in acute situations, CT may be preferable.[63] Unenhanced CT may show displacement of intimal calcification and high attenuation of the aortic wall if the false lumen is thrombosed. Contrast material enhanced CT or MR imaging demonstrate the intimal flap (**Fig. 16**), opacification of the true and false lumen, the extent of the dissection, involvement of the branch vessels, and end organ ischemia. MR imaging may be used to assess the aortic root involvement and presence of aortic regurgitation, but transesophageal echocardiography is preferred often. CT and MR imaging are useful when assesing postoperative complications following the repair of ascending aortic dissections.

NON-ATHEROSCLEROTIC ARTERIAL DISORDERS IN THE ELDERLY
Segmental Arterial Mediolysis

Segmental arterial mediolysis is a rare nonatherosclerotic noninflammatory vascular disease of

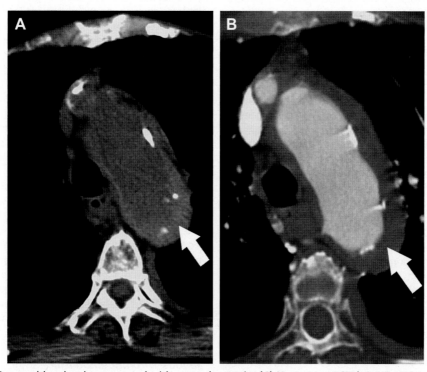

Fig. 15. A 60-year-old male who presented with acute chest pain. (*A*) Noncontrast CT shows crescent shaped high density (*arrow*) within the aortic wall. There is inward displacement of the intimal calcification. (*B*) On contrast material enhanced CT, there is enhancement (*arrow*) within the high density aortic wall.

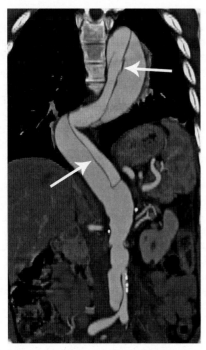

Fig. 16. Contrast enhanced CT demonstrates a spiral dissection flap (*arrows*) affecting the descending aorta.

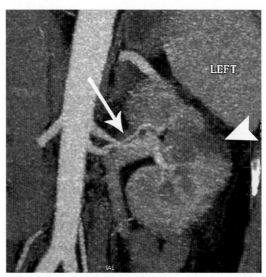

Fig. 17. A 65-year-old male who presented with acute left flank pain. Coronal subvolume maximum intensity projection shows irregular, wavy contour of the left renal artery (*arrow*), suggesting dissection. There is also an infarct (*arrowhead*) in the midpole of the left kidney. These features suggest segmental arterial mediolysis.

unknown origin affecting the visceral arteries. The elderly population between the ages of 50 years and 70 years are affected, with a male predominance.[64] Patients present with severe acute abdominal pain or hypotension caused by an intra-abdominal hemorrhage or bowel infarction. CT and MR may demonstrate infarcts in the bowel or kidneys with associated dissections (**Fig. 17**), saccular or fusiform aneurysms affecting the celiac, or mesenteric or renal arteries. The dissected false lumen may enlarge and form pseudoaneurysms. DSA is more definitive in demonstrating the dissections, aneurysms, and string of beads appearance. During follow-up these aneurysms and dissections may resolve completely. At present, there is no specific treatment available for this condition, but control of high blood pressure and antiplatelet therapy may be beneficial. Endovascular therapy is recommended if there is acute bleeding or endorgan ischemia.[65]

Giant Cell (Temporal) Arteritis

This is a type of large vessel vasculitis that affects the elderly population (exclusively aged 50 years or more). Three of the following five criteria must be present for diagnosis of giant cell arteritis[66]: aged 50 years or more, a new onset of localized headache, temporal artery tenderness or decreased pulse, an erythrocyte sedimentation rate of 50 or more, and positive histologic findings of mononuclear cell infiltration or granulomatous inflammation with or without giant cells. Women are affected more often. Jaw claudication, eye involvement, and upper limb involvement have been reported to occur with a frequency of 30%–40% in patients diagnosed with giant cell arteritis.[67] Ultrasound of the temporal artery with 8–10 MHz frequency probes demonstrates hypoechoic, circumferential thickening of the arterial wall, which may disappear following corticosteroid therapy. Color Doppler shows areas of stenosis as flow turbulence and increased (greater than 100% compared with the proximal segment) peak systolic velocities.[68] An occluded artery may be seen as a hypoechoic vessel with no demonstrable flow on the color Doppler. DSA, CTA, and MRA may help delineate characteristic patterns in large-vessel giant cell arteritis. The lesions often present with bilateral stenoses or occlusions with a smooth, tapered appearance in the subclavian, axillary and proximal brachial arteries.[69] PET is used to detect extra-cranial disease and may help to assess the disease activity.

VENOUS DISORDERS
Venous Thromboembolism

Venous thromboembolism consists of deep venous thrombosis and pulmonary embolism.

Venous thromboembolism occurs at a frequency of 100 cases per 100,000 population each year in the United States. The incidence of venous thromboembolism increases exponentially with age: from 30 cases per 100,000 in people aged 25–35 years to 300–500 cases per 100,000 in people aged 70–79 years.[70] The relative frequency of pulmonary embolism and deep venous thrombosis varies depending on the series; in autopsy series, the relative frequency of pulmonary embolism and deep venous thrombosis was 55% and 45%, respectively, whereas in nonautopsy series, it was 33% and 66%. Three pathophysiologic factors, classically described as Virchow's triad, are associated with venous thromboembolism—endothelial injury, stasis of blood flow, and hypercoagulable state. Various risk factors are associated with venous thromboembolism, including cancer, postoperative state, trauma, stroke, myocardial infarction, prolonged immobilization, atrial fibrillation, and smoking.

More than 90% of pulmonary emboli originate in the lower extremities. Currently, ultrasound is the imaging procedure of choice for the diagnosis of deep venous thrombosis. A normal, patent vein is compressible and demonstrates phasic respiratory variations on Doppler with augmentation of flow on distal compression. Acute thrombus appears hypoechoic with enlargement of the affected vein (**Fig. 18**). The vein is not compressible, and color Doppler shows no demonstrable flow (see **Fig. 18**). Subacute thrombus may appear hyperechoic with minimal enlargement of the vein, but the vein remains noncompressible. In chronic deep venous thrombosis, the vein appears small, with thickening or calcification of the vein wall and variable flow within the lumen caused by recanalization of the thrombus. The sensitivity and specificity of ultrasound varies from 89%–96% and 94%–99%, respectively, for the diagnosis of symptomatic deep venous thrombosis involving the femoropopliteal veins. In asymptomatic femoropopliteal deep venous thrombosis, the sensitivity of ultrasound varies from 47%–62%.[71]

Indirect CT venography is another method used to diagnose deep venous thrombosis. Generally, this is combined with CT pulmonary angiography when evaluating for pulmonary embolism. A CT scan of the pelvis and lower extremities, up to the level of the popliteal fossa, is performed 3 minutes following the administration of IV contrast material, at a slice thickness of 5–7.5 mm. A diagnosis of deep venous thrombosis is made if there is a filling defect in two consecutive slices with associated enlargement of the vein. There may be a rim enhancement of the wall with perivenous edema (**Fig. 19**). Chronic deep venous thrombosis is diagnosed when the vein appears small with calcification of

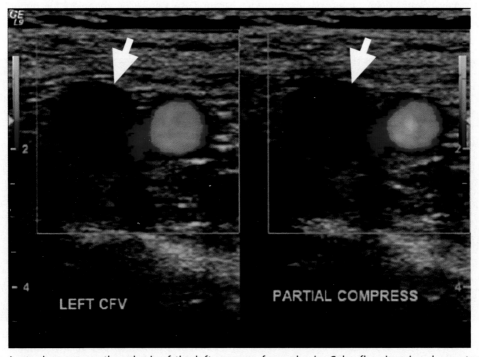

Fig. 18. Acute deep venous thrombosis of the left common femoral vein. Color flow imaging demonstrates an enlarged, hypoechoic, noncompressible (*arrows*) left common femoral vein with no color flow suggesting acute deep venous thrombosis.

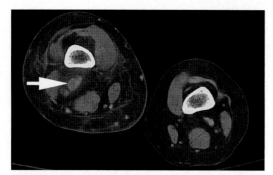

Fig. 19. Indirect CT venography following CT pulmonary angiography in a patient suspected of having pulmonary embolism. The right popliteal vein is enlarged, with intraluminal filling defect (*arrow*) and perivenous edema, consistent with an acute thrombus. The right leg is also swollen compared with the left leg.

the vein wall. The addition of CT venography to CT pulmonary angiography improves the sensitivity of CT in diagnosing venous thromboembolism. An incremental benefit of 20% has been reported in various studies. In addition, it allows detection of pelvic vein and inferior vena cava thrombosis.

MDCT is the preferred imaging test for the diagnosis of pulmonary embolism. Thin-section (1–1.5 mm) CT of the entire chest is performed after administering 100–120 cm^3 of contrast material intravenously. Scan delay may be estimated through bolus triggering or test bolus. A standard delay of 20–25 seconds may be sufficient in many patients, however, in elderly patients who have cardiac failure, this may result in inadequate pulmonary arterial opacification. Pulmonary emboli are seen as central, intravascular filling defects (**Fig. 20**) with peripheral enhancing lumen (which are often called "polo mint" signs on images obtained in the transaxial plane, and "tram-track" signs on images obtained in the longitudinal plane of the vessel in question). Pulmonary emboli preferentially lodge at vessel bifurcation points. CT also may demonstrate peripheral wedge shaped parenchymal consolidation and pleural effusion. The hemodynamic effects of the pulmonary emboli often can be seen on CT. The CT signs that suggest right ventricular strain include,[72] a dilated right ventricle (a ratio of greater than 1.5 between right and left ventricular diameters), leftward bowing of the interventricular septum (see **Fig. 20**), a dilated (greater than 30 mm) main pulmonary artery, and a reflux of contrast material in the inferior vena cava and hepatic veins.

Elderly patients who cannot tolerate CT contrast material because of renal failure or allergy may benefit from ventilation perfusion scintigraphy. The results are interpreted in conjunction with chest radiography findings and are correlated with pretest clinical probability of pulmonary embolism. The results are reported as low, intermediate, or high probability for pulmonary embolism. DSA usually is reserved for patients who have a high clinical probability of pulmonary

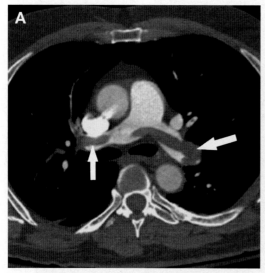
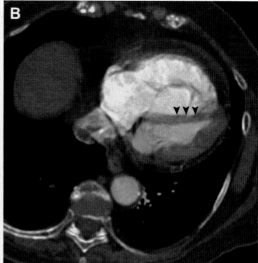

Fig. 20. (*A, B*) CT pulmonary angiography of a 65-year-old patient who developed tachycardia and shortness of breath following repair of a fractured femur shows central pulmonary emboli (*arrows* in *A*) affecting the right and left main pulmonary arteries. The right heart is dilated, and the interventricular septum (*arrowheads* in *B*) is deviated with convexity toward the left ventricle suggesting severe right heart strain secondary to the pulmonary emboli.

embolism but who have indeterminate or negative CT studies.

Varicose Veins and Chronic Venous Insufficiency

Chronic venous insufficiency refers to an abnormality in the peripheral venous system that reduces or impedes venous return. The symptoms of chronic venous insufficiency include asymptomatic and symptomatic varicose veins, leg edema, hyperpigmentation, lipodermosclerosis, and ulceration. Varicose veins appear because of primary or secondary valvular insufficiency and affect the truncal veins (the great and small saphenous veins and their first and second order branches), reticular veins, and intradermal veins. Varicose veins and chronic venous insufficiency are more common in the elderly, with a higher prevalence among women. The prevalence of varicose veins in people aged 30 or less is 1% in men and 10% in women, whereas it is 57% and 77%, respectively, among individuals aged 70 years or more.[73] The risk factors for varicose veins include familial history, obesity, hypertension, and history of previous venous thrombosis.

Ultrasound is the imaging test for evaluation of the varicose veins. The deep veins should be evaluated for the presence of deep venous thrombosis and valvular insufficiency. Valvular insufficiency is assessed by measuring the duration of flow reversal (the reflux) in the specified vein following Valsalva maneuver or distal calf compression and release. A reflux of less than 1 second is considered normal in deep veins. The great saphenous and small saphenous veins and their proximal tributaries are tested for venous reflux. A reflux of greater than 0.5 seconds is considered abnormal in superficial veins. It is important to assess the relationship of varicose veins to major truncal veins to plan proper therapy. The perforator veins also are evaluated for reflux and their contribution to the varicose veins. The current treatment options for symptomatic varicose veins are endovenous thermal ablation, sclerotherapy, ambulatory phlebectomy, and surgical stripping.

REFERENCES

1. Grundy SM. Cardiovascular and metabolic risk factors: how can we improve outcomes in the high-risk patient? Am J Med 2007;120(9 suppl 1):S3–8.
2. Ostchega Y, Paulose-Ram R, Dillon CF, et al. Prevalence of peripheral arterial disease and risk factors in persons aged 60 and older: data from the National Health and Nutrition Examination survey 1999–2004. J Am Geriatr Soc 2007;55(4):583–9.
3. Stein R, Hrljac I, Halperin JL, et al. Limitation of the resting ankle-brachial index in symptomatic patients with peripheral arterial disease. Vasc Med 2006;11(1):29–33.
4. Kohler TR, Nance DR, Cramer MM, et al. Duplex scanning for diagnosis of aortoiliac and femoropopliteal disease: a prospective study. Circulation 1987;76(5):1074–80.
5. Karacagil S, Lofberg AM, Almgren B, et al. Duplex ultrasound scanning for diagnosis of aortoiliac and femoropopliteal arterial disease. Vasa 1994;23(4):325–9.
6. Ramaswami G, Al-Kutoubi A, Nicolaides AN, et al. The role of duplex scanning in the diagnosis of lower limb arterial disease. Ann Vasc Surg 1999;13(5):494–500.
7. Whelan JF, Barry MH, Moir JD. Color flow doppler ultrasonography: comparison with peripheral arteriography for the investigation of peripheral vascular disease. J Clin Ultrasound 1992;20(6):369–74.
8. Elsman BH, Legemate DA, van der Heyden FW, et al. The use of color-coded duplex scanning in the selection of patients with lower extremity arterial disease for percutaneous transluminal angioplasty: a prospective study. Cardiovasc Intervent Radiol 1996;19(5):313–6.
9. Ascher E, Mazzariol F, Hingorani A, et al. The use of duplex ultrasound arterial mapping as an alternative to conventional arteriography for primary and secondary infrapopliteal bypasses. Am J Surg 1999;178(2):162–5.
10. Spijkerboer AM, Nass PC, de Valois JC, et al. Evaluation of femoropopliteal arteries with duplex ultrasound after angioplasty. Can we predict results at one year? Eur J Vasc Endovasc Surg 1996;12(4):418–23.
11. Stone PA, Armstrong PA, Bandyk DF, et al. Duplex ultrasound criteria for femorofemoral bypass revision. J Vasc Surg 2006;44(3):496–502.
12. Hiatt MD, Fleischmann D, Hellinger JC, et al. Angiographic imaging of the lower extremities with multidetector CT. Radiol Clin North Am 2005;43(6):1119–27.
13. Schoellnast H, Tillich M, Deutschmann MJ, et al. Aortoiliac enhancement during computed tomography angiography with reduced contrast material dose and saline solution flush: influence on magnitude and uniformity of the contrast column. Invest Radiol 2004;39(1):20–6.
14. Fleischmann D. Use of high concentration contrast media: principles and rationale-vascular district. Eur J Radiol 2003;45(Suppl 1):S88–93.
15. Heijenbrok-Kal MH, Kock MC, Hunink MG. Lower extremity arterial disease: multidetector CT angiography–meta-analysis. Radiology 2007;245(2):433–9.
16. Schernthaner R, Fleischmann D, Lomoschitz F, et al. Effect of MDCT angiographic findings on the

management of intermittent claudication. AJR Am J Roentgenol 2007;189(5):1215–22.

17. Willmann JK, Mayer D, Banyai M, et al. Evaluation of peripheral arterial bypass grafts with multi-detector row CT angiography: comparison with duplex US and digital subtraction angiography. Radiology 2003;229(2):465–74.

18. Kuo PH, Kanal E, Abu-Alfa AK, et al. Gadolinium-based MR contrast agents and nephrogenic systemic fibrosis. Radiology 2007;242(3):647–9.

19. Kramer H, Michaely HJ, Reiser MF, et al. Peripheral magnetic resonance angiography at 3.0 T. Top Magn Reson Imaging 2007;18(2):135–8.

20. Ho VB, Corse WR. MR angiography of the abdominal aorta and peripheral vessels. Radiol Clin North Am 2003;41(1):115–44.

21. Dellegrottaglie S, Sanz J, Macaluso F, et al. Technology insight: magnetic resonance angiography for the evaluation of patients with peripheral artery disease. Nat Clin Pract Cardiovasc Med 2007;4(12):677–87.

22. Tongdee R, Narra VR, McNeal G, et al. Hybrid peripheral 3D contrast-enhanced MR angiography of calf and foot vasculature. AJR Am J Roentgenol 2006;186(6):1746–53.

23. Zhang HL, Ho BY, Chao M, et al. Decreased venous contamination on 3D gadolinium-enhanced bolus chase peripheral mr angiography using thigh compression. AJR Am J Roentgenol 2004;183(4):1041–7.

24. Andreisek G, Pfammatter T, Goepfert K, et al. Peripheral arteries in diabetic patients: standard bolus-chase and time-resolved MR angiography. Radiology 2007;242(2):610–20.

25. Baum RA, Rutter CM, Sunshine JH, et al. Multicenter trial to evaluate vascular magnetic resonance angiography of the lower extremity. American College of Radiology Rapid Technology Assessment Group. JAMA 1995;274(11):875–80.

26. Yucel EK, Kaufman JA, Geller SC, et al. Atherosclerotic occlusive disease of the lower extremity: prospective evaluation with two-dimensional time-of-flight MR angiography. Radiology 1993;187(3):637–41.

27. Mell M, Tefera G, Thornton F, et al. Clinical utility of time-resolved imaging of contrast kinetics (TRICKS) magnetic resonance angiography for infrageniculate arterial occlusive disease. J Vasc Surg 2007;45(3):543–8.

28. Loewe C, Cejna M, Schoder M, et al. Contrast material-enhanced, moving-table MR angiography versus digital subtraction angiography for surveillance of peripheral arterial bypass grafts. J Vasc Interv Radiol 2003;14(9):1129–37.

29. Oliva VL, Denbow N, Thérasse E, et al. Digital subtraction angiography of the abdominal aorta and lower extremities: carbon dioxide versus iodinated contrast material. J Vasc Interv Radiol 1999;10(6):723–31.

30. Bloch MJ, Basile J. Clinical insights into the diagnosis and management of renovascular disease. An evidence-based review. Minerva Med 2004;95(5):357–73.

31. Soulez G, Oliva VL, Turpin S, et al. Imaging of renovascular hypertension: respective values of renal scintigraphy, renal Doppler US, and MR angiography. Radiographics 2000;20(5):1355–68.

32. Ripollés T, Aliaga R, Morote V, et al. Utility of intrarenal doppler ultrasound in the diagnosis of renal artery stenosis. Eur J Radiol 2001;40(1):54–63.

33. Riehl J, Schmitt H, Bongartz D, et al. Renal artery stenosis: evaluation with colour duplex ultrasonography. Nephrol Dial Transplant 1997;12(8):1608–14.

34. House MK, Dowling RJ, King P, et al. Using doppler sonography to reveal renal artery stenosis: an evaluation of optimal imaging parameters. AJR Am J Roentgenol 1999;173(3):761–5.

35. Mittai BR, Kumar P, Arora P, et al. Role of captopril renography in the diagnosis of renovascular hypertension. Am J Kidney Dis 1996;28(2):209–13.

36. Taylor AT, Fletcher JW, Nally JV, et al. Procedure guidelines for diagnosis of renovascular hypertension. J Nucl Med 1998;39(7):1297–302.

37. Johansson M, Jensen G, Aurell M, et al. Evaluation of duplex ultrasound and captopril renography for detection of renovascular hypertension. Kidney Int 2000;58(2):774–82.

38. van de Ven PJ, de Klerk JM, Mertens IJ, et al. Aspirin renography and captopril renography in the diagnosis of renal artery stenosis. J Nucl Med 2000;41(8):1337–42.

39. Fraioli F, Catalano C, Bertoletti L, et al. Multidetector-row CT angiography of renal artery stenosis in 50 consecutive patients: prospective interobserver comparison with DSA. Radiol Med (Torino) 2006;111(3):459–68.

40. Coulier B, Mailleux P, Joris JP. 64-row MDCT diagnosis of intimal hyperplasia causing restenosis of renal arterial stent. JBR-BTR 2007;90(3):228.

41. Maki JH, Wilson GJ, Eubank WB, et al. Steady-state free precession MRA of the renal arteries: breath-hold and navigator-gated techniques vs. CE-MRA. J Magn Reson Imaging 2007;26(4):966–73.

42. Tan KT, van Beek EJ, Brown PW, et al. Magnetic resonance angiography for the diagnosis of renal artery stenosis: a meta-analysis. Clin Radiol 2002;57(7):617–24.

43. Caridi JG, Stavropoulos SW, Hawkins IF Jr. CO2 digital subtraction angiography for renal artery angioplasty in high-risk patients. AJR Am J Roentgenol 1999;173(6):1551–6.

44. Thomas JH, Blake K, Pierce GE, et al. The clinical course of asymptomatic mesenteric arterial stenosis. J Vasc Surg 1998;27(5):840–4.

45. Hermsen K, Chong WK. Ultrasound evaluation of abdominal aortic and iliac aneurysms and mesenteric ischemia. Radiol Clin North Am 2004;42(2):365–81.

46. Horton KM, Fischman EK. Multidetector CT angiography in the diagnosis of mesenteric ischemia. Radiol Clin North Am 2007;45(2):275–88.

47. Meaney JF, Prince MR, Nostrant TT, et al. Gadolinium-enhanced MR angiography of visceral arteries in patients with suspected chronic mesenteric ischemia. J Magn Reson Imaging 1997;7(1):171–6.

48. Rothwell PM, Eliasziw M, Gutnikov SA, et al. Analysis of pooled data from the randomised controlled trials of endarterectomy for symptomatic carotid stenosis. Lancet 2003;361(9352):107–16.

49. Rothwell PM, Mehta Z, Howard SC, et al. From subgroups to individuals: general principles and the example of carotid endarterectomy. Lancet 2005;365(9455):256–65.

50. Young B, Moore WS, Robertson JT, et al. An analysis of perioperative surgical mortality and morbidity in the asymptomatic carotid atherosclerosis study. ACAS Investigators. Asymptomatic Carotid Arteriosclerosis Study. Stroke 1996;27(12):2216–24.

51. Thiele BL, Jones AM, Hobson RW, et al. Standards in noninvasive cerebrovascular testing. Report from the Committee on Standards for Noninvasive Vascular Testing of the Joint Council of the Society for Vascular Surgery and the North American Chapter of the International Society for Cardiovascular Surgery. J Vasc Surg 1992;15(3):495–503.

52. Grant EG, Benson CB, Moneta GL, et al. Carotid artery stenosis: gray-scale and doppler US diagnosis—Society of Radiologists in Ultrasound Consensus Conference. Radiology 2003;229(2):340–6.

53. Landwehr P, Schulte O, Voshage G. Ultrasound examination of carotid and vertebral arteries. Eur Radiol 2001;11(9):1521–34.

54. Hollingworth W, Nathens AB, Kanne JP, et al. The diagnostic accuracy of computed tomography angiography for traumatic or atherosclerotic lesions of the carotid and vertebral arteries: a systematic review. Eur J Radiol 2003;48(1):88–102.

55. Saba L, Sanfilippo R, Pirisi R, et al. Multidetector-row CT angiography in the study of atherosclerotic carotid arteries. Neuroradiology 2007;49(8):623–37.

56. Wardlaw JM, Chappell FM, Best JJ, et al. Noninvasive imaging compared with intra-arterial angiography in the diagnosis of symptomatic carotid stenosis: a meta-analysis. Lancet 2006;367(9521):1503–12.

57. Ohnesorge BM, Hofmann LK, Flohr TG, et al. CT for imaging coronary artery disease: defining the paradigm for its application. Int J Cardiovasc Imaging 2005;21(1):85–104.

58. Sun Z, Lin C, Davidson R, et al. Diagnostic value of 64-slice CT angiography in coronary artery disease: a systematic review. Eur J Radiol 2007;10.1016/j.ejrad.2007.07.014.

59. Sakuma H. Magnetic resonance imaging for ischemic heart disease. J Magn Reson Imaging 2007;26(1):3–13.

60. Hartnell GG. Imaging of aortic aneurysms and dissection: CT and MRI. J Thorac Imaging 2001;16(1):35–46.

61. Rakita D, Newatia A, Hines JJ, et al. Spectrum of CT findings in rupture and impending rupture of abdominal aortic aneurysms. Radiographics 2007;27(2):497–507.

62. Choi SH, Choi SJ, Kim JH, et al. Useful CT findings for predicting the progression of aortic intramural hematoma to overt aortic dissection. J Comput Assist Tomogr 2001;25(2):295–9.

63. Castañer E, Andreu M, Gallardo X, et al. CT in nontraumatic acute thoracic aortic disease: typical and atypical features and complications. Radiographics 2003;23:S93–110.

64. Michael M, Widmer U, Wildermuth S, et al. Segmental arterial mediolysis: CTA findings at presentation and follow-up. AJR Am J Roentgenol 2006;187(6):1463–9.

65. Soulen MC, Cohen DL, Itkin M, et al. Segmental arterial mediolysis: angioplasty of bilateral renal artery stenoses with 2-year imaging follow-up. J Vasc Interv Radiol 2004;15(7):763–7.

66. Hunder GG, Bloch DA, Michel BA, et al. The American College of Rheumatology 1990 criteria for the classification of giant cell arteritis. Arthritis Rheum 1990;33(8):1122–8.

67. Smetana GW, Shmerling RH. Does this patient have temporal arteritis? JAMA 2002;287(1):92–101.

68. Schmidt WA, Kraft HE, Vorpahl K, et al. Color duplex ultrasonography in the diagnosis of temporal arteritis. N Engl J Med 1997;337(19):1336–42.

69. Schmidt WA, Gromnica-Ihle E. What is the best approach to diagnosing large-vessel vasculitis? Best Pract Res Clin Rheumatol 2005;19(2):223–42.

70. White RH. The epidemiology of venous thromboembolism. Circulation 2003;107(23 suppl 1):I4–8.

71. Segal JB, Eng J, Tamariz LJ, et al. Review of the evidence on diagnosis of deep venous thrombosis and pulmonary embolism. Ann Fam Med 2007;5(1):63–73.

72. Ghaye B, Ghuysen A, Bruyere PJ, et al. Can CT pulmonary angiography allow assessment of severity and prognosis in patients presenting with pulmonary embolism? What the radiologist needs to know. Radiographics 2006;26(1):23–39.

73. Beebe-Dimmer JL, Pfeifer JR, Engle JS, et al. The epidemiology of chronic venous insufficiency and varicose veins. Ann Epidemiol 2005;15(3):175–84.

Aging and the Respiratory System

Lorenzo Bonomo, MD[a],*, Anna Rita Larici, MD[a], Fabio Maggi, MD[a],
Francesco Schiavon, MD[b], Riccardo Berletti, MD[b]

KEYWORDS
- Elderly • Respiratory system • Radiologic modifications

Radiologic tests are performed on elderly patients (conventionally defined as individuals 65 years of age and older) with increasing frequency because of the progressive increase in the average age, owing to better life conditions and to progress in medical, surgical, and anaesthesiologic knowledge.[1]

In the elderly, it is often difficult to establish what normality, or rather, what "compatibility," is, because of the numerous anatomic and physiologic modifications that occur during the aging process. As a result, the major problem in later life is to recognize the point to which aging is normal and the point at which the disease begins.[2]

The overall anatomic/radiologic modifications of the thorax that occur with advanced age are summarized in **Box 1**. The authors then discuss them in greater detail.

THORACIC FRAME

The thoracic frame may be subdivided into (1) the thoracic wall and (2) the diaphragm.

Thoracic wall

Reduction in wall thickness is constant and is well shown by computed tomography (CT), particularly when compared with younger individuals (**Fig. 1**). This reduction is one of the principal causes of hyperlucency in the elderly chest.[3]

Islands of compact matter and bony, costal reparatory calluses are common, as is calcification of the costal cartilage. In general, the cartilage calcifies according to the standard defined, that is, in the periphery in men and in the center in women, but sometimes, although not often, with nodular appearance.[2]

These alterations give rise to differential diagnosis problems with respect to nodular pulmonary lesions. Three factors need to be taken into consideration: first, in the elderly, radioscopy is not always reliable because of limited patient cooperation and possible reduction of respiratory excursions; second, lung cancer is most frequent between the ages of 60 and 70, often in the form of peripheral nodes (adenocarcinoma); third, postthoracotomy mortality in the elderly today is close to that of younger adults and the diagnostic commitment must therefore be the same.[4]

The principal modifications of the spinal column are osteoporosis, consistent with age if not associated with subjective disturbances ("elderly" osteoporosis), and osteophytosis, generally more pronounced on the right side of the vertebral column because of the protection of the aorta on the left side. This occurrence is also a source of problems of differential diagnosis with respect to posterior pulmonary nodules, along with costo/transversal arthrosis (it may be useful for diagnostic purposes to consider the side on which the doubtful image appears: if on the right side, degenerative alteration is more probable; if on the left side, the hypothesis of pulmonary lesion may be more consistent) (**Fig. 2**). Accentuation of the dorsal kyphosis, associated with the greater convexity of the sternum, contributes to the "barrel" thorax configuration (**Fig. 3**).

[a] Department of Bioimaging and Radiological Sciences, Catholic University of the Sacred Heart, Policlinico Agostino Gemelli, L.go F. Vito 8, 00168 Rome, Italy
[b] Department of Imaging Diagnostics and Radiological Sciences, San Martino Hospital, Viale Europa 22, 32100 Belluno, Italy
* Corresponding author.
E-mail address: lbonomo@rm.unicatt.it (L. Bonomo).

Radiol Clin N Am 46 (2008) 685–702
doi:10.1016/j.rcl.2008.04.012
0033-8389/08/$ – see front matter © 2008 Elsevier Inc. All rights reserved.

All of these parietal modifications lead to hardening of the thoracic cage, with unfavorable rebound on respiratory function.[5–7]

Diaphragm

Although nearly always in a normal position, the diaphragm often shows protuberances and is stippled because of muscular hypertrophy and dyskinesia, particularly on the right, probably caused by the increased effort by the hemidiaphragm in maintaining the anatomic relationship between the lung and the liver. The anatomic hiatuses are generally wider, and hernias are more frequently found and may resemble mediastinal and paramediastinal masses.[6]

The presumed "bulges" of the diaphragm may also constitute diagnostic traps, making differential diagnosis necessary with thoracic diseases that lower the diaphragm and with abdominal masses that raise it (**Fig. 4**). It is therefore important, when the position of the diaphragm is different from the norm, to determine its position precisely. Echography may be of use in this case and in suspected infrapulmonary effusion, frequent in the hemodynamically decompensated elderly (**Fig. 5**).

The lowering of the diaphragm may be due, in addition to pleural effusion, to cardiomegaly, which increases the weight of the heart on the diaphragm (see later discussion).

MEDIASTINUM

The modifications of most interest concern the heart, the aorta, and the trachea.

Heart

The anatomic/pathologic aspects of the "elderly heart" essentially refer to what is known as "primary" aging, that is, to a limited and fortunate percentage of healthy elderly (approximately 10%). These individuals are best suited for assessment of modifications caused by age only, whereas "secondary" aging, that is, the much more frequent situation influenced by basic pathologic conditions (arterial hypertension, atherosclerotic, pulmonary emphysema and chronic bronchitis, diabetes mellitus, renal insufficiency, and so forth) or by an unhealthy lifestyle (reduced physical activity, improper diet, abuse of alcohol and tobacco) is obviously excluded, being influenced by too many individual variables.[8,9]

The principal involutions that characterize the "elderly heart" are an increase in the cardiac mass and the thickness of the myocardium, of the left ventricle in particular, due to hypertrophy

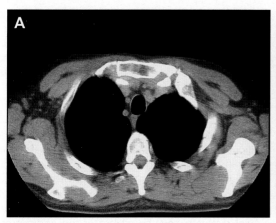 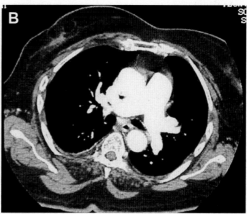

Fig. 1. With advanced age comes progressive atrophy of the muscles of the thoracic wall, responsible for a significant increase in thoracic radiotransparency when radiographic tests are performed, because of lower reduction of the radiogenic beam. It is a question of an apparent increase in pulmonary transparency, which can be attributed to lower contribution to the parietal opacity rather than an actual alteration of the pulmonary parenchyma (emphysema). (*A*) Axial CT scan of the chest of a young individual with good tropism of the parietal musculature. (*B*) Axial CT scan of the chest of an elderly patient who has evident muscular atrophy, particularly of the pectoral muscles and those of the posterior wall.

of the residual myocytes and to an increase in the matrix of connective tissue; thickening of the valvular margins (often mitral and aortic) due to the deposit of fats, collagen, and calcium salts, with initial wearing out of the valvular annulus which, at the mitral level, causes a slight insufficiency in 90% of those over the age of 80; coronary sclerosis, with possible alterations of the cardiac perfusion.[8–14]

In any case, apart from the involutions described in "primary" aging, every significant morphodimensional variation of the heart must be considered as a possible sign of alteration of the intrinsic or extrinsic hemodynamics.[10]

In most cases, the signs of right cardiac overload are due to an increase in the resistance of small pulmonary vessels, as in the case of obstructive or restrictive diseases and mitral defects,

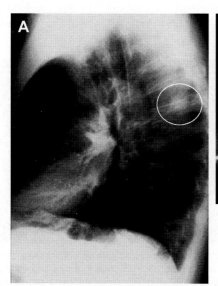 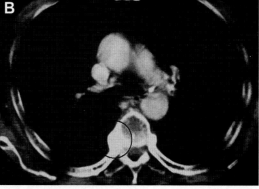

Fig. 2. Arthrosis of the costo-vertebral joint. The chest radiograph in lateral projection (*A*) shows the image of a doubtful pulmonary nodular lesion projecting against the spinal column (*circle*). The CT scan of the chest subsequently performed (*B*) reveals the degenerative nature of the radiographic finding (*circle*).

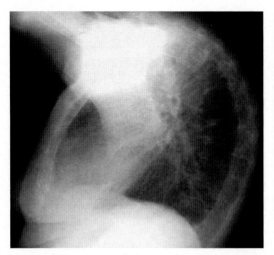

Fig. 3. Aging causes a reduction in the calcium content of the bones and involutive alterations that may result in fractures and deformations of thoracic cage structures. Radiograph of the chest in lateral projection: "barrel" chest, due to accentuation of the dorsal kyphosis and convexity of the sternum.

whereas the signs of left overload (ie, left ventricle hypertrophy) may partially be due to modifications of the "elderly heart."[11]

Calcification of the thoracic aorta, of the cardiac valves (margins and annulus), and of the coronary arteries (often of the descending left anterior branch) must be checked for, because they indicate, in the elderly, those individuals subject to a risk for cardiovascular pathology (**Fig. 6**).[2,13]

Thus, in addition to the coronary circulation, the "elderly heart" has two attack points: the myocardial structures and the cardiac valves.

Both can be assessed with imaging, producing two histopathologic and clinical aspects of particular importance: increase in the weight of the heart and double genesis of cardiac, systolic, and diastolic decompensation,[14] which are discussed in more detail below.

Aorta

Essentially, the aorta's anatomic/pathologic modifications can be added to those of the heart, and result in lengthening and dilation, factors principally responsible for enlargement of mediastinal contours in chest radiograph frontal projections.[15]

In general, the lengthening is greatest in the cranial direction and the calibre of the aortic arch, measurable, for example, on the transparency of the tracheal air column, may reach up to 4 cm or more (**Fig. 7**). But differential diagnosis must always be considered with intrinsic alterations, such as aneurysm, or with extrinsic alterations, such as masses of the contiguous mediastinal structures.[8]

The almost constant atheromatic calcification, often of the arch and of the descending section, do not always relate to the gravity of the clinical situation, and may be associated with various conditions (such as chronic renal insufficiency and so forth).[9,15]

Trachea

The trachea is an important anatomic reference in assessing the condition of the superior mediastinum. It is visibly deviated to the right from the aortic arch in 30% of cases, sometimes resembling mediastinal involvement.[6] In this case, locating the right paratracheal line and the normality of

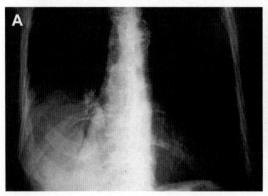

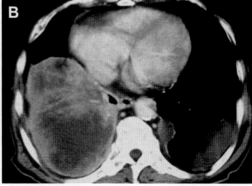

Fig. 4. In the elderly, it is not always easy to identify the exact position of the hemidiaphragms because of intrinsic modifications caused by aging and the presence of masses or liquids that can collect above and below the diaphragm. An example is given here: in the frontal radiograph (*A*), hyperelevation of the hemidiaphragm was first suggested, but the evidence of the homolateral inferior cardiac contour, caudal with respect to the presumed hemidiaphragm, resulted in the correct diagnosis, later confirmed by CT (*B*), which showed a basal pulmonary mass.

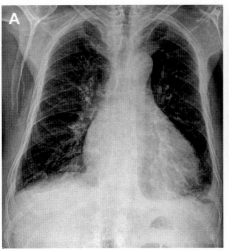

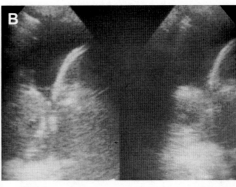

Fig. 5. Infrapulmonary pleural effusion. (*A*) Standard chest radiograph: signs of initial CD with infrapulmonary effusion, most visible on the left, due to an increase in the normal distance between the lung and the colic flexure, with involvement of the costal-phrenic sinus. (*B*) Echographic scans of the left hypochondrium, which confirmed the presence of infrapulmonary effusion.

the homolateral mediastinal space, corresponding to the innominate/caval axis, assists in correct assessment (**Fig. 8**). The frequent presence of catheters or pacemaker electrodes in the superior vena cava of elderly patients helps in the assessment of the vascular nature of the enlarged mediastinum.[4,6]

The trachea may present a "saber-like" appearance, often in a bronchitic/emphysematous context, because of parietal malacia that increases the tracheal antero-posterior diameter and tends to cause the collapse of the lateral walls (**Fig. 9**).[7,16]

LUNG

Parenchymal modifications are caused by reduced blood flow from the systemic circulation through the bronchial arteries and by the reduced

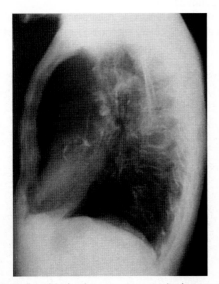

Fig. 6. In the elderly, the coronary arteries become tortuous and often present deposits of calcium salts and atherosclerotic plaque. The aorta undergoes similar alterations; the cardiac valvular apparatus also shows calcium deposits (particularly at the level of the aortic valve and the mitral annulus). Chest radiograph in lateral projection: vascular and valvular calcifications.

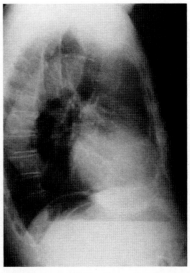

Fig. 7. Modifications of the thoracic aorta associated with aging. The chest radiograph in lateral projection shows an increase in the vessel's calibre and length.

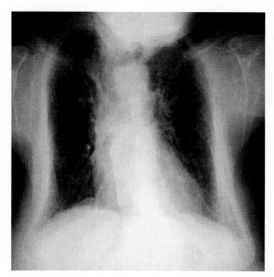

Fig. 8. In the elderly, tracheal deviations are frequently found: study of the relationships with contiguous anatomic structures and analysis of the mediastinal lines and spaces are of assistance in diagnosis. The chest radiograph taken of a supine patient shows a deviation to the right of the trachea due to ectasia of the aortic arch.

function of the cellular membranes, and result in quantitative/qualitative modifications to collagen and variations in the relationship between elastic tissue and support tissue, with progressive reduction of lung elasticity.[6,7]

The first physiopathologic consequence is proximal shifting of the closing point of the distal airways, with a progressive increase in residual volume. This mechanism is analogous to that of pulmonary emphysema, with two major differences: no signs of inflammation and no increase in total pulmonary capacity.[17,18]

At the same time, the ventilation/perfusion relationship is modified because of a reduction in the number of alveoli with optimal gas exchange, which has two physiopathologic consequences: an increase in the physiologic dead space and the "shunt effect," with a reduction of arterial oxygenation.[7,18]

From the radiologic point of view, these modifications translate into what is known as the "dirty chest," caused by the increase of supporting connective tissue (ie, of the interstitium), which becomes a normal component of the chest radiograph, adding to and becoming superimposed on vascular trauma (Fig. 10), and by the increase in the background transparency of the chest, caused by an increase in the pulmonary air content, a reduction in vascularization, and reduced thickness of the thoracic wall (Fig. 11).[6,7]

In addition, modest pulmonary hypertension (a clinical expression of vascular involution) may make occupation of the "reserve" vascular area common in the elderly, inhibiting use of redistribution of the pulmonary flow as a first radiologic sign of cardiac decompensation (CD). In such cases, left CD may be assessed only by later signs, such as the shaded appearance of hilar structures and vascular contours, which are an indication of interstitial edema.[19–21]

Although in younger adults the calibre of the principal pulmonary arteries is related to arterial

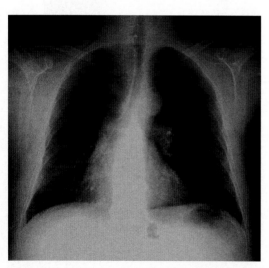

Fig. 9. "Saber-sheath" trachea. The standard chest radiograph shows pulmonary emphysema, with reduction of the tracheal calibre on the frontal plane.

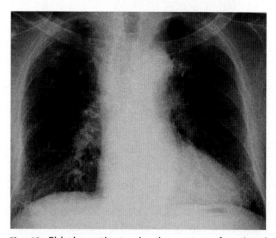

Fig. 10. Elderly patient who has severe functional obstruction detected with respiratory functional tests and evidenced by longstanding productive cough. The radiographic examination of the chest shows a "dirty lung," with significant accentuation of bronchovascular findings (increased markings).

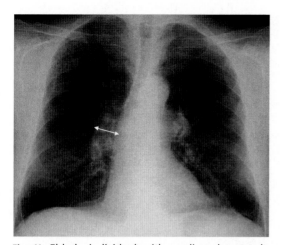

Fig. 11. Elderly individual with medium-degree obstruction detected with respiratory functional tests. Radiographic evidence of emphysema with pulmonary hyperinsufflation and reduction of the vasal picture (arterial deficiency) due to hypertension of the lesser circulation, documented by dilation of the descending branch of the right pulmonary artery (*arrow*).

pulmonary pressure, in the elderly this may no longer be the case, because a certain degree of pulmonary atherosclerosis and sometimes emphysema (confirmed by anatomic/pathologic findings), is always present. For this reason, atherosclerosis and pulmonary hypertension form a closed circle, each contributing to the other, as is found paraphysiologically in the elderly.[20,21]

The role of multiple and repeated episodes of pulmonary embolism, fibrosis, and mitral stenosis must also be taken into consideration in the genesis of pulmonary hypertension in the elderly, among whom all of the foregoing are frequent pathologic and clinically silent conditions.[18,19]

Enlargement of the distal airspaces (see later discussion) may provoke compression and reduction of the capillary arterial bed, which might explain any peripheral hypoperfusion.[17,20] This finding is common among bedridden, inactive elderly patients, probably also because of a decrease in the cardiac output. In fact, because the chest radiographs of physically active and healthy elderly individuals show no signs of hypoperfusion, it may be deduced that the more inactive the elderly individual is, the lower effective perfusion present.[21]

Involution of respiratory function begins as early as 30 years of age, as shown by spirometric tests. The curve of forced expiratory volume in 1 second falls slowly and inexorably until reaching, at advanced age, values at the limits of survival.[18]

In addition to involution of the parietal thoracic component with aging is a significant restructuring of the pulmonary architecture, due particularly to an increase in the collagen and elastin of the bronchial walls and interstitium, expressed radiologically with the picture of the "dirty chest," mentioned previously.

These modifications to the pulmonary architecture result in enlargement of the distal airspaces and a reduction of the extension of the intra-alveolar septa.[16,22]

The internal surface of the lung thus diminishes from an average of 70 m^2 at 30 years of age to 60 m^2 at 70 years. In other words, in the third decade of life, in step with the decreased expiratory flow comes a loss of pulmonary alveolar surface, amounting to 4% per decade, which is known as reduction of the ventilatory surface.[23,24]

The ensuing radiologic aspects (also taking into consideration the increase in residual volume) are the following: bronchial and bronchiolar expiratory collapse, often posterior/basal; small dependent gravitational thickening; and dependent subpleural linear atelectasis.[17]

In particular, CT regularly shows a slight halo of hyperdensity in the dependent subpleural areas, which disappears when the position of the patient is changed (**Fig. 12**). This picture is essentially a representation of the radiologic aspects previously listed.[17,25]

The slight hyperdistension of the alveoli, with dilation of the respiratory bronchioles and concomitant reduction of the alveolar capillaries, could result in a picture of centrilobular emphysema. In reality, the signs and symptoms of true emphysema (dyspnea, cough, and so forth) are absent in the "elderly lung." In addition, even if the elderly person becomes polypneic at rest and under stress, and the current volume diminishes (that is, the quantity of air ventilated with each respiratory act), the inflammatory aspects and increase in the total pulmonary capacity, typical of pulmonary emphysema, are absent. For these reasons, "elderly emphysema" does not exist as a distinct clinical/radiologic entity.[23]

It is, however, true that the progressive "reduction" of the parietal/alveolar tissue may result in alveolar ruptures and hence in the formation of 2 to 3 cm blisters, located particularly in the upper and anterior part of the lung. Furthermore, the terminal bronchioles often show an acute or chronic inflammatory process, particularly in the elderly with a history of smoking. But, in general, emphysema, when radiographically demonstrable, is an advanced process from anatomic and physiopathologic points of view, insofar as its early phase is confused, or rather, is consistent, with the normal elderly chest.[23,24]

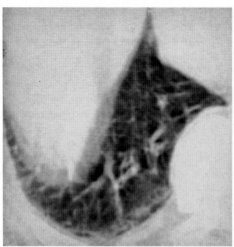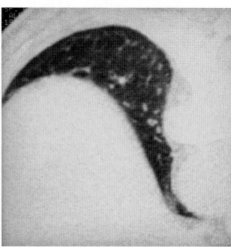

Fig. 12. Dependent parenchymal hyperdensity is a frequent CT finding, particularly in the elderly. The cause seems to be a diminishing of the closing pressure of the most distal airways, which facilitates bronchial collapse, associated with lines of parenchymal dysventilation with analogous physiopathologic significance. This aspect is reversible by varying the body position. The CT scan performed in a supine position (*left*) shows "ground glass" dependent hyperdensity of the pulmonary base, which disappears when the patient is placed in a prone position (*right*) because of a variation in blood pressure conditions.

PRINCIPAL PHYSIOPATHOLOGIC MODELS

Once the principal involutions of thoracic structures have been described, one can observe two physiopathologic models most common in the elderly: the "cardiac lung" (CL) and the "pulmonary heart" (PH), the clinical expressions of which are, respectively, cardiogenic pulmonary edema (ie, CD) and chronic obstructive pulmonary disease (COPD).

"Cardiac Lung"

The numerous epidemiologic studies now available agree on the fact that CD is the cause of death in approximately 80% of subjects over the age of 80 and is the most frequent pulmonary and, more generally, internal medical reason for hospitalization.[26] The symptom at the basis of all the pictures attributable to CD is dyspnea and the corresponding clinical picture is that of pulmonary edema.[27–32]

The physiopathologic model at the basis of CD, as explained by the clinical presentation, is the CL.[30]

The definition of the CL derives from a simple consideration: the two pumps in the chest, the cardiac and the pulmonary, are vital and must be in perfect balance for optimal functioning. The functional insufficiency of one inevitably has consequences for the other.[28] This consideration concerns the impact of primitive pulmonary pathology on the heart, known as the PH, which the

authors discuss below, and the impact of primitive cardiac diseases on the lung that is, the CL.[29–31]

In the CL, the situation reproduced in **Fig. 13** is created. The enlarged heart occupies more space in the thoracic cavity (which is nonexpandable) than it should, to the detriment of the lungs, which reduce their respiratory excursions. Imbalance is thus created between the pumps, with the cardiac pump dominating the pulmonary pump.[28]

The authors discussed the "elderly heart" earlier. Two factors result: an increase in the weight of the heart and the double genesis of systolic and diastolic CD.

An increase in the weight of the heart is easily visible in a patient equipped with a pacemaker and in whom the position of the stimulating probe in the right ventricle shows a lowering of the diaphragm, due to the weight of the heart (**Fig. 14**). This aspect is a further cause of dyspnea (and hence of respiratory insufficiency) in patients who have CD, because it has an unfavorable effect on the work of the diaphragm, which is the principal inspiratory muscle. Thus, correction of the cardiopathy is positively reflected in respiratory performance.[30]

The distinction between systolic and diastolic CD represents a significant challenge for the radiologist because the clinical contexts are different and important: ischemic cardiopathy for the former, systemic arterial hypertension for the latter. In particular, it has been shown that, in those older than 65, 40% of CD has diastolic causes, which

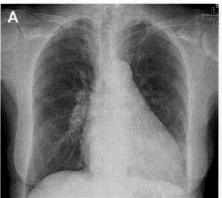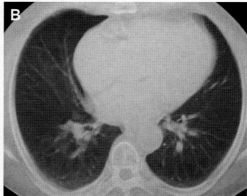

Fig.13. The principal physiopathologic characteristic of the CL is the imbalance created between the cardiac pump and the respiratory pump because of enlargement of the heart, which occupies a large part of the chest to the detriment of the lungs, with reduction of respiratory excursions and alteration of the ventilation/perfusion dynamics. Standard radiograph (*A*) and CT (*B*) of the chest: enlargement of the heart, particularly of the left cavity, with signs of redistribution of the pulmonary circulation, due to recruitment of the "reserve" area.

constitute a significant practical problem, because the therapeutic approach is different.[33–38]

The physiopathology of systolic CD involves the dilation of the left ventricle, without alteration in wall thickness, and a reduction of the ejection fraction. For diastolic CD, parietal thickening of the left ventricle occurs without dilation, with a negative effect on the rates of diastolic refilling and normal state of the ejection fraction.[36–38]

Chest radiograph is fundamental for distinguishing between the two types of failure and is closely related to the physiopathology. In both forms, the

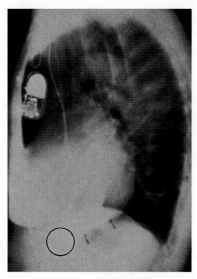

Fig.14. Chest radiograph in lateral projection. Increase in the weight of the heart in a patient fitted with a pacemaker is shown by the extreme distal position of the stimulating electrode (*circle*), providing evidence of the lowering of the left hemidiaphragm.

appearance of pulmonary circulation, that typical of CD and described later, is similar, whereas that of the heart is different: enlarged in systolic CD, within the limits in diastolic CD (**Fig. 15**).[33,39]

The authors now describe the principal, associated, and subsequent radiologic pictures of the CL, relating them to the physiopathologic events, while bearing in mind that such a representation is of explanatory use only (**Fig. 16**).[28,31] The entire process is summarized in **Table 1**.

Picture I: reduction of the cardiac range, with venous stasis and increase in the intravascular pulmonary liquid

The increase in pulmonary haematic volume (ie, the venous stasis) is first of all expressed by redistribution of the vessels in the caudal/cranial direction, as an expression of recruitment of the "reserve" area, and hence by an increase in their calibre. They thus maintain clear contours. The heart may, although not necessarily, have signs of moderate enlargement of the left atrium. The lungs and heart increase in weight because of the venous stasis, resulting in insufficient pump function, which provokes further lowering of the left hemidiaphragm; in normal condition the right hemidiaphragm is higher than the left not because of the pressure from the liver but because of the weight of the heart (in particular ventricles) on the left hemidiaphragm.

Picture II: increase in extravascular pulmonary liquid

Signs of liquid effusion, that is, of interstitial edema, appear in the interstitium. They include shading of the vascular picture and of the hilar structures, the Kerley lines, particularly type B,

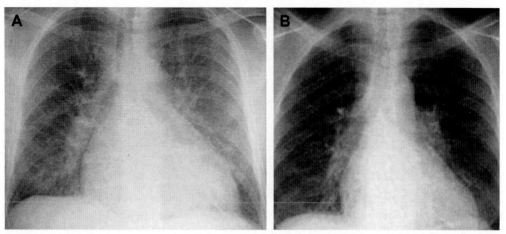

Fig. 15. Systolic versus diastolic CD. (*A*) Standard chest radiograph: systolic CD is characterized by signs of pulmonary stasis and by enlargement of the heart, particularly of the left sections, due to deficit in the systolic function of the left ventricle. (*B*) Standard chest radiograph: in diastolic CD, the signs of pulmonary circulation overload are associated with concentric hypertrophy of the left ventricle, without significant increase in its size. This condition is, in fact, characterized by a reduction of the ventricular telediastolic volume without deficit of systolic function (election fraction >45%). Other causes of failure, such as anemia, thyrotoxicosis, valvular diseases, and so forth, are, in any case, excluded.

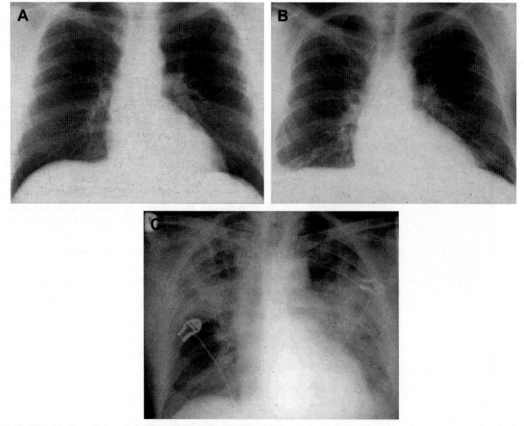

Fig. 16. Phases of cardiogenic failure. Chest radiographs of the same patient, from simple venous overload to evident pulmonary edema. (*A*) The CL in relative hemodynamic compensation. (*B*) Signs of interstitial edema with pleural effusion and enlargement of the cardiac image. (*C*) Alveolar edema with extended parenchymal opacities, increase in pleural effusion, and further enlargement of the heart.

Table 1
Main radiologic, clinical, and instrumental characteristics of the "cardiac lung"

	Clinical/Instrumental Characteristics	Radiologic Characteristics
Stage I	↓ Clinical range ↑ Pulmonary hematic volume	Caudal/cranial redistribution of the pulmonary picture ("reversed" distribution)1/1 relationship between superior/inferior vessel calibres ("balanced distribution")
Stage II	Dyspnea ↑ Extravascular liquid↑ HGA + − (under stress)	Interstitial edema (Kerley lines, shaded hila, pleural effusion) Heart + Pulmonary volume ↓
Stage III	As in stage II	As in stage II, with gravitational distribution, often bilateral pleural effusion
Stage IV	Dyspnea ↑↑ Obligatory seated position	Heart ++ Lowering of diaphragm ↑↑
Stage V	Dyspnea ↑↑↑ HGA − −	Lowering of diaphragm ↑↑↑ Thickening of thoracic wall ↑↑
Stage VI	Dyspnea ↑↑↑↑ HGA − − − −	Gravitational, confluent and shaded parenchymal opacities. Bilateral pleural effusion Heart ++++ Lowering of the diaphragm ↑↑↑

Abbreviations: 0, normal; +, enlarged; −, reduced; ↑, increased; ↓, reduced; HGA, hemogas analysis.

moderate subpleural parenchymal thickening, enlargement of the diameters of the heart with more evident enlargement of the left cavities, and possible limited pleural effusion. A reduction in respiratory volume begins, with minor expansion of the thorax as detected by radiograph, plus reduction of respiratory excursions.

Picture III: pleural effusion
When present (most typically bilaterally), the signs of gravitational edema will already have appeared. Pleural effusion is therefore part of a picture of medium-advanced interstitial edema.

Picture IV: evident cardiomegaly
The signs of cardiomegaly and the lowering of the diaphragm predominate, both clearly seen by chest radiograph. The supine hypoxia, typical of this phase, is well explained by CT (see later discussion).

Picture V: involvement of the respiratory muscles and the soft tissues
The authors have already referred to the lowering of the diaphragm. Imbibition on the wall (typical of pulmonary edema due to hyperhydration as well as nephrogenic edema) is, however, of

significance in cardiogenic edema on functional level, because respiratory muscles become more viscous and less efficient, making an increase in the force they use to move the thoracic cage necessary. It is therefore necessary that radiograph examination of the chest also allow assessment of wall thickness.

Picture VI: appearance of alveolar edema
This picture is well known, referred to only in the interests of completeness.

To better understand the mechanisms that govern the process described earlier, a few references to functional anatomy are necessary concerning the diaphragm, pulmonary arteries, alveolar compartment, lymphatics, and interstitium.[20,21]

Regarding the diaphragm (the principal inspiratory muscle), the normal anatomic position and its maintenance are important.

Regarding the pulmonary arteries, the smooth parietal musculature is considerably less represented at all ages, with respect to the systemic circulation, which in physiologic terms, means that the vessels are more distensive and therefore more prone to increasing rather than reducing their capacity.

Regarding the alveoli, the connective tissue between type I alveolocytes (ie, the cells that cover almost the entire alveolar surface) is closed and impermeable, as opposed to that between the endothelial cells of the capillaries, which easily allow the passage of liquid. The surfactant (a phospholipoprotein secreted by type II alveolocytes) covers the alveolar wall with water-repellent action, enabling ventilation and inhibiting atelectasis.

The alveolar septa (represented by the interstitial tissue between the epithelium and endothelium) are formed by two functionally distinct areas, one of which is thin, to allow gas exchange, and the other thick, for liquid exchange.

The capillary lymphatics are found at the level of the alveolar ducts and the respiratory bronchioles. The interstitial liquid runs from the alveolar walls to the capillary lymphatics, driven by the "pump" action of the ventilation, which is more efficient in the pulmonary mantle, as shown by the "butterfly wing" distribution often observed in cardiogenic alveolar edema (**Fig. 17**). The lymph moves from the capillaries through the lymphatic ducts with the help of valves at a distance of 1 to 2 mm.

The interstitium may be subdivided into two components: a peripheral, parietal, and subpleural component, thin and radiologically invisible; and another component found around the bronchi and the vessels (peribronchovascular cuffing), visible with chest radiograph as a small opaque circle of the bronchial walls taken tangentially. Both are connected to a thick reticule made up of the connective tissue of the alveolar septa.

The extravascular liquid is first collected in the large interstitium because of the more efficient peripheral ventilation and the greater compliance of the large interstitium, and, only if insufficient, in the alveolar septa. In fact, the interstitium is the natural site for liquid exchange and, when necessary, the peribronchovascular connective tissue up to the thickest part of the alveolar septa becomes a large reserve of "extravascular water," which inhibits alveolar flooding, preserving the gas exchanges.[29]

The lymphatic vessels have an aspiration pressure of 20 to 30 cm of H_2O on the fluids and solutes in the interstitium, guaranteed by the excursions transmitted to them by the transpulmonary respiratory pressure. Although able to increase the level of drainage considerably, the capacity of the lymphatic vessels is limited to the level of which the liquid passes at the extravascular site, even in consideration of their significantly disproportionate development with respect to the capillary network.[29]

A note on the circulation of the visceral pleura: disagreement exists as to its origin, deriving wholly or partially from the pulmonary arteries according to some investigators, or from the bronchial arteries according to others. In any case, its venous draining occurs through the pulmonary veins.[40]

The argument presented up to this point regarding functional anatomy raises several interesting radiologic observations.[41–43]

The first sign of venous stasis (phase I), is the "reversed" distribution of the flow (ie, with recruitment of the reserve vascular area of the superior lobes) and with "balanced" distribution (ie, with an increase in the calibre of the vessels recruited) (see **Fig. 13**).

A reduction in the pulmonary compliance (ie, increased rigidity of the lung due to an increase in the interstitial fluid [phase II]) and a rapidly worsening restrictive syndrome result in decreased lung expansion in the chest radiograph taken in inspiratory apnea and in a reduction of respiratory excursions, if the radiograph is also taken in expiratory apnea.

The work of the lymphatics at "low rate" to dispose of the extravascular liquid is also performed when the clinical picture is regressed and the hemodynamic picture is in the process of rebalancing, thus explaining the dissociation between clinical and radiologic resolution. In other words, accentuation of the texture, in addition to the clinical resolution, is an expression of the involvement of the lymphatics.

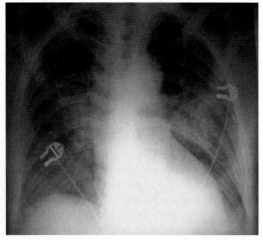

Fig. 17. CD with evident pulmonary edema. The chest radiograph of the supine patient shows characteristic "butterfly wing" edema caused by more effective lymphatic draining of the pulmonary mantle.

Pleural effusion concerns the systemic circulation and requires the failure of the right heart, different from pulmonary edema. This means that the mechanism of formation of pleural effusion hemodynamically requires conditions different from those for pulmonary edema and therefore, although nearly always present, is a complimentary sign of it (**Fig. 16B**) (phase III).

From phase IV, dyspnea appears with minimum effort, with a tendency to hypoxia at rest. The patient is therefore not able to lie in a supine position but tends to be seated to facilitate the activity of the respiratory muscles. CT clarifies dyspnea and postural worsening of hypoxia: if, in the non-compensated cardiopathic patient, a densitometric measurement is made of the pulmonary parenchyma, with the placement of a region of interest (ROI) at the level of the pulmonary mantle dorsally and ventrally, the densitometric gradient is reduced or eliminated (**Fig. 18**). This occurs because perfusion does not prevail in the lung's dorsal areas, as normally occurs in individuals in a supine position, but is increased, also ventrally, where ventilation should prevail, because of recruitment of the "reserve" pulmonary vascular area. This results in elimination of the densitometric gradient or, in physiopathologic terms, in the creation of a ventilation/perfusion discrepancy, the cause of hypoxia and dyspnea. In conclusion, the patient who has cardiogenic failure needs to assume an orthopneic position to restore the densitometric gradient, and an acceptable ventilation/perfusion relationship.[28]

"Pulmonary Heart"

COPD is the second most frequent cause of invalidity, hospitalization, and death of the elderly in the pneumologic context, and is three to five times more frequent at this age than at other ages.[44]

In such cases, the involutive aspects of the lung, as described previously, prevail and result in greater air content and hence, hyperdistension. The hyperexpanded lungs reduce the space available to the heart, particularly in the diastole, and almost "imprison" it, giving it a median or a vertical "drop" appearance (**Fig. 19**), which is the model of the PH.[16,22]

"Cardiac lung" versus "pulmonary heart"

The CL and PH physiopathologic models are opposites and specular images, equidistant from the normal. Comparison is therefore useful for better understanding. In **Table 2**, the radiologic, physiopathologic, and clinical aspects of the two models are listed.

The CL begins with left cardiopathy, including, in rapid succession, cardiomegaly, pulmonary venous hypertension, non-compensated left cardiopathy, and reduction of pulmonary volumes due to the cardiomegaly.[41,42] The PH almost always begins with COPD, which results in an increase in vascular resistance (ie, peripheral pulmonary oligemia), pulmonary arterial hypertension, the "involvement" of the right heart, and the limitation of heart expansion by the hyperexpanded lungs.[16,45–53]

Thus, from the physiopathologic point of view, in the case of the CL, the cardiomegaly results in the progressive reduction of pulmonary volume, with a restrictive spirometric pattern (see **Fig. 13**). In the PH, the alterations of the airways result in pulmonary hyperdistension with an obstructive-type spirometric picture (see **Fig. 19**).

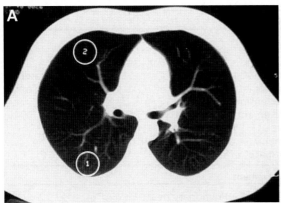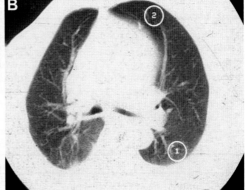

Fig. 18. Dorsal/ventral pulmonary densitometric gradient with CT. (*A*) Normal individual with densitometric gradient of approximately 50 UH between region of interest (ROI) 1 and 2. (*B*) Individuals with CD underway do not show a densitometric gradient between the two ROIs due to the presence of perfusion in the nondependent areas.

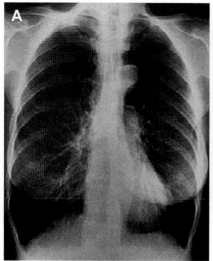 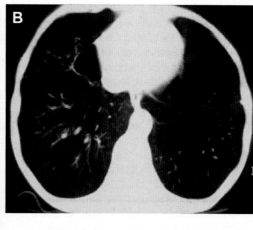

Fig. 19. Pulmonary heart. (*A*) Chest radiograph; (*B*) CT scan at the level of the pulmonary bases: the hyperexpanded lungs occupy more space than normal, limiting heart expansion, particularly in the diastolic refilling phase (clinical sign: tachycardia).

The specular aspect of the densitometric measurements that can be obtained on CT examination of the chest, as referred to earlier, should also be noted. In both cases, the densitometric gradient is eliminated. In the CL, this elimination is produced by an abnormal increase of perfusion in the lung's ventral areas, whereas in the PH, it is attributable to an abnormal increase in

Table 2
Radiologic, physiopathologic, and clinical characteristics of the "pulmonary heart" versus the "cardiac lung"

Cardiac Lung		
Pulmonary edema		
Radiology	Physiopathology	Clinically
Left cardiomegaly	Left cardiac insufficiency	Tachypnea
↓Pulmonary volumes	Pulmonary venous hypertension	Acute onset
CT: elimination of the dorsal/ventral gradient due to perfusion prevalence	Spirometry → restrictive pattern → Shunt effect	
Pulmonary Heart		
COPD		
Peripheral oligemia		
↑ Pulmonary volumes	↑ Vascular resistance	Tachycardia
Transverse cardiac diameter ↓	Pulmonary arterial hypertension and involvement of the right heart	Chronic onset
CT: elimination of the dorsal/ventral gradient due to ventilation prevalence	Spirometry → obstructive pattern "Dead space" effect	
Development		
Cardiac lung		Pulmonary heart
Almost rapid		Slow or stable
Reversible anatomic/pathologic alterations		Irreversible anatomic/pathologic alterations

ventilation of the dorsal areas. Thus, in the CL, the density moves toward higher values, whereas in the PH, it moves toward lower values. In both cases, a ventilation/perfusion deficit is created, responsible for hypoxemia and postural dyspnea.[28,46]

The foregoing correlates perfectly with the physiopathologic concepts according to which, when perfusion prevails, as in the case of the CL, there is a "shunt" effect, whereas, when ventilation prevails, as in the case of the PH, there is a "dead space" effect.[46,47]

From the clinical point of view, the distinctive sign of the CL is tachypnea, whereas that of the PH is tachycardia, both of which may progress to dyspnea. In the first case, a reduction of pulmonary volume subsequent to cardiomegaly results in the need to compensate for the deficit with an increased number of respiratory acts; in the second case, the pulmonary hyperexpansion hinders particularly the cardiac diastole (ie, ventricular refilling, often of the left ventricle) and results in an increased number of cycles.[46]

Separating the left and right sections of the heart and arterial and venous microcirculation of the lungs makes it easier to understand the specular physiopathology of the two models. The CL, originating in the left cardiac cavity, involves, in a retrograde manner, the pulmonary venous circulation; the PH, beginning in the arterial section of pulmonary microcirculation, involves the right cardiac cavity.[22,28]

The temporal aspect (ie, the time necessary for the conditions to become manifest) also emphasizes the mirror-like aspect of the two models. The CL, clinically expressed by pulmonary edema, establishes itself and develops rapidly, tumultuously, and sometimes dramatically, showing extremely variable radiologic pictures from day to day, insofar as the pathology is acute and the anatomic/pathologic aspects are reversible. The PH, clinically expressed by COPD, develops slowly, with essentially stabilized radiologic pictures (apart from superimposed acute episodes) because the disease is chronic and the anatomic/pathologic alterations are irreversible.[47]

The symptom common to the CL and the PH (dyspnea) also unites them in an significant aspect of the chest radiograph: the radiographs are taken in shallow inspiratory apnea, not because of insufficient patient cooperation or poor test quality, but because of reduced inspiratory capacity, as generally occurs in the elderly (above and beyond the two models proposed) because of the involution of the osteomuscular portion of the thoracic cage.[4,6]

TECHNICAL AND METHODOLOGIC CONSIDERATIONS

No single technique perfectly reveals all the chest components, but techniques exist that, together, constitute the best possible compromise, given the various, often contrasting, requirements. The latitude of the system, however broad, does not enable optimal simultaneous visualization of those areas with low radiant beam absorption, the lungs, and those with high absorption, the mediastinum.[4]

In the young and the adult, a complete visualization of the pulmonary fields, showing the "blind areas," is a priority because of the predominant clinical need to detect focal pulmonary lesions. In the elderly, on the other hand, it is above all important to assess the pulmonary and cardiac circulation because the principal causes of invalidity, hospitalization, and death are cardiovascular diseases.

Performing chest radiographs and preoperative tests in young, apparently healthy, individuals may give rise to doubts about use and costs; conversely they are essential in geriatric age, insofar as they immediately and reliably study vital, fundamental parameters in individuals often affected by multiple pathologies characterized by largely unresolved clinical semiotics.[2]

Given that the earliest radiologic sign of pulmonary circulation overload (ie, redistribution of the flow, which makes it possible to detect this hemodynamic anomaly in the preclinical phase) may not be visible in the elderly patient because of the frequent presentation of the "dirty chest," it becomes indispensable to increase to the maximum the value of the second sign, that is, the shaded aspect of the pulmonary picture caused by an increase in extravascular fluid, particularly if the chest radiograph has not been performed under standard conditions.[31]

If this second sign was not accessible or proved equivocal, it would present a risk for further delay in the radiologic diagnosis or, even worse, of referring it to the clinician in a phase of evident decompensation.[20]

The technique performed must therefore give priority to the gray pulmonary background, an expression of the extravascular interstitial compartment, and the contrast must not be compromised.[4]

High-voltage techniques compromise the contrast, because their purpose is to identify better the "blind" pulmonary areas (retrocardiac, paravertebral, and so forth). Medium-voltage techniques, on the other hand, are better suited to the clinical necessities of the elderly. Having less recording latitude, they may not identify small focal lesions but, instead, valorize all aspects of the pulmonary circulation, which is of greater interest.

In the elderly, technically limited radiologic examinations are the norm (ie, those done with a single anterior/posterior projection with the patient seated or supine) precisely because the signs of cardiovascular disease that must be examined with radiograph are also the primary cause of invalidity. For this reason, it is essential to valorize those few most meaningful aspects that chest radiographs done under these conditions, particularly the shaded aspect of the hilar/pulmonary vascular structure contours, make possible to evaluate.[2,11]

THE RADIOLOGIC REPORT

Although the acquisition of images is delegated, for the most part, to the radiology technician, the writing of the report is the sole responsibility of the radiologist who, in so doing, performs the clinical role of specialist.[54]

The report is the main means of communication with the requesting physician and its effectiveness is measured on the basis of its usefulness in clarifying the patient's clinical problems. The more a report influences diagnosis and treatment, the more it will be truly useful and the more the radiologist will have been able to act professionally.

To formulate a good report, the radiologist must have a good understanding of the clinical question and must adhere to certain basic rules of communication, summarized by Bonmati and colleagues as the six "c's": clear, correct, concise, complete, coherent, and competent, to which a further "c" should be added: common (in the sense of "shared").[55,56]

In fact, if the radiologist is not on the same wavelength as the person requesting the report (ie, if he/she does not take into consideration what the latter wants and whether or not the language used in the report will be understood), then this is a failure of communication. Thus, if the report on the chest radiograph in **Fig. 13** uses the expression "type 1:1 vascular distribution" without explaining the clinical meaning (occupation of the "reserve" vascular area as the first sign of venous overload of the pulmonary circulation), it may well be technically exemplary but clinically ineffective, because it is not a given that this expression will be understood by the requesting physician.

Further, in a study of the heart by means of chest radiograph, the signs may be numerous and should be listed in the report, because they are part of classic radiologic semeiotics. If they are not translated into clinical terms, however, a comprehensive picture is not provided, which

presents a risk that the report will be nothing more than a useless academic exercise. Thus, a competent report is produced but it is neither clear nor clinically effective.

A great deal has been, and is still being, discussed regarding the conciseness of the report, even more today, with the availability of tests replete with images, such as multidetector CT, and with details, such as chest radiograph with digital technique. The radiologist must not merely describe the findings but must also interpret them, expressing a professional opinion in the form of a diagnostic conclusion, if the intent is to have an influence on the patient's clinical course.

Thus, in conclusion, the report must be complete and must have a precise structure: clinical question, description of findings, diagnostic judgment, any indications for the performing of the diagnostic procedure, and so forth.[57]

In the elderly, then, basic knowledge of cardiorespiratory physiopathology is essential. For example, if, in the initial CD, pulmonary fields are underexpanded on inspiration, this is not because the patient is less cooperative but because the lungs are less compliant, which must be pointed out in the report.

The radiologist must always bear in mind the clinical requirements and, given the possibility of cardiopathy (above and beyond the presence or absence of focal lesions), must describe the conditions of the pulmonary circulation, particularly in the initial stages of CD, because this is the most important information for the clinician and, in these phases, the diagnosis of CD may be radiologic only. In subsequent phases, when CD becomes clinically evident, the radiologist need only monitor the clinical picture, particularly the extravascular pulmonary water and the cardiomegaly.

Hence, to be effective, the radiologist must give the chest radiograph examination a hemodynamic reading, always describing in the report the conditions of the pulmonary circulation, particularly if it is altered. A description of the normality of distribution and clarity of the contours and assessment of the appearance of the pulmonary circulation in relationship to the cardiac morphology should also be included. If the heart is large, it is more likely that the pulmonary circulation will not be altered.[57]

SUMMARY

In the elderly, the chest without evident pathology is characterized by findings that occupy a sort of "no man's land" between the normal and the pathologic. Aging results in physiologic modifications that must be recognized so as not to be interpreted erroneously as pathologies. On the other hand, the elderly tend to become ill more frequently and multipathologies are more frequent. Image diagnostics is a key element in the clarification of often blurry clinical pictures, which may make early diagnosis possible, a great advantage to timely treatment. In this sense, knowledge of heart/lung interactions makes it possible to obtain, from the onset, radiologic and clinical signs of the two physiopathologic models prevalent in the elderly, the "cardiac lung" and the "pulmonary heart."

REFERENCES

1. Maggi S, Marzari C, Crepaldi G. Epidemilogia dell'invecchiamento. In: Guglielmi G, Schiavon F, Cammarota T, editors. Radiologia geriatrica. Milano (Italy): Springer Verlag; 2006. p. 13–20.

2. Schiavon F, Cardini S, Favat M, et al. La radiologia delle strutture toraciche normali nel paziente anziano. Radiol Med 1993;86:418–31.

3. Huchon G. [Pulmonary aging]. Rev Prat 2001;51(7): 701–2 [in French].

4. Schiavon F, Nardini S, Tregnaghi P, et al. L'esame radiologico del torace nell'anziano: considerazioni tecniche e metodologiche. Radiol Med 1997;94: 193–7 [in Italian].

5. Muiesan G, Sorbini CA, Grassi V. Respiratory function in the aged. Bull Physiopathol Respir 1971;7: 973–1009.

6. Bernadac P. Le poumon du troisième age, Paris Encycl Med Chir. Radiodiagnostic 1991; 4.02,05 324980–10.

7. Zeleznik J. Normative aging of the respiratory system. Clin Geriatr Med 2003;180(2):513–8.

8. Badano L, Carratino L, Giunta L, et al. Modificazioni del sistema cardiovascolare indotte dall'età in soggetti normali. G Ital Cardiol 1992;22:1023–34 [in Italian].

9. Midiri M. L'esame del torace nell'invecchiamento cardiaco. In: Schiavon F, Berletti R, Guglielmi G, Cammarota T, editors. Diagnostica per immagini nell'invecchiamento. Radiol Med 2003;50–3 suppl 1 al N. 3.

10. Di Guglielmo L, Dore R, Raisario A, et al. L'imaging toracico nell'anziano: il cuore. In: Schiavon F, Nardini S, Feltrin GP, editors. Apparato respiratorio e invecchiamento. Pisa (Italy): Pacini Editore; 1999.

11. Di Guglielmo L, Dore R, Raisario A, et al. La diagnostica per immagini nello studio dell'invecchiamento cardiaco. Il "cuore senile" è una realtà? Radiol Med 1999;97:449–60 [in Italian].

12. Beker CR, Ohnesorge BM, Schoepf UJ, et al. Current development of cardiac imaging with multidetector row CT. Eur J Radiol 2000;36:97–103.

13. Mc Laughlin MA. The aging heart. State-of-the-art, prevention and management of cardiac disease. Geriatrics 2001;56(6):45–9.

14. Badano L, Caratino L, Giunta L, et al. L'invecchiamento fisiologico del sistema cardiovascolare. G Ital Cardiol 1992;23:619–28 [in Italian].

15. Di Cesare E. Lo studio radiologico nell'invecchiamento dell'aorta e delle arterie coronarie. In: Schiavon F, Berletti R, Guglielmi G, Cammarota T, editors. Diagnostica per immagini nell'invecchiamento. Radiol Med 2003;57–9 3suppl 1 al N.3.

16. Comino E, Cortese G, Nespoli P. Imaging delle bronco pneumopatie croniche ostruttive. In: Guglielmi G, Schiavon F, Cammarota T, editors. Radiologia geriatrica. Milano (Italy): Springer-Verlag; 2006. p. 179–87.

17. Gillody M, Lamb D. Airspace size in lungs of lifelong non smokers: effects of the age and sex. Thorax 1993;48:39–43.

18. Sharma G, Goodwin J. Effect of aging on respiratory system physiology and immunology. Clin Interv Aging 2006;1(3):253–60.

19. Freundlich IM. Redistribution of pulmonary blood flow. AJR Am J Roentgenol 1988;145(6): 1315–6.

20. Marano P, Cecconi L, Danza F. Studio radiologico del circolo polmonare nell'anziano e sue possibilità funzionali. G Gerontol 1975;23:761–73.

21. Marano P. La radiologia funzionale del torace. Verona (Italy): Cortina Editore; 1986.

22. Anglesio A, Marchisio U, Comino E. Le broncopneumopatie croniche ostruttive. In: Comino E, Cammarota T, editors. Diagnostica per immagini in geriatria. Torino (Italy): Edizioni Minerva Medica; 1995. p. 41–50.

23. Stolk J, Putter H, Bakker EM. Progression parameters for emphysema: a clinical investigation. Respir Med 2007;101(9):1924–30.

24. Aziz ZA, Wells AU, Desai SR, et al. Functional impairment in emphysema: contribution of airway abnormalities and distribution of parenchymal disease. AJR Am J Roentgenol 2005;185(6): 1509–15.

25. Matsuoka S, Uchiyama K, Shima H, et al. Bronchoarterial ratio and bronchial wall thickness on high-resolution CT in asymptomatic subjects: correlation with age and smoking. AJR Am J Roentgenol 2003;180(2):513–8.

26. Vettorazzi M. Epidemiologia dell'età senile. In: Schiavon F, Berletti R, Guglielmi G, Cammarota T, editors. Diagnostica per immagini nell'invecchiamento. Radiol Med 2003;7–9 suppl 1 al N.3.

27. Schiavon F, Berletti R, Cavagna E, et al. Lo studio radiologico dello scompenso cardiaco dell'anziano. In: Guglielmi G, Schiavon F, Cammarota T, editors. Radiologia geriatrica. Milano (Italy): Springer-Verlag; 2006. p. 139–44.

28. Schiavon F, Nardini S, Pesce L, et al. Il "polmone cardiaco": la radiologia correlata alla fisiopatologia respiratoria e alla clinica. Radiol Med 1996;91: 526–36 [in Italian].

29. Lloyd TC. Mechanical heart-lung interactions. In: Shaw SM, Cassidy SS, editors. Heart-lung interactions in health and disease. New York: Marcel Dekker Inc.; 1993.

30. Di Guglielmo L, Montemartini C. L'esame radiologico del torace nello studio del cuore. Radiol Med 1985; 71:816–35 [in Italian].

31. Milne E, Pistolesi M. Reading the chest radiograph. St Louis (MO): Mosby-Year Book; 1993.

32. Rusconi C, Faggiano P, Gardini A. Fisiopatologia della diastole dalle basi cellulari alle implicazioni cliniche. Milano (Italy): Ghedini Editore; 1992.

33. Dore R. La moderna diagnostica per immagini nell'invecchiamento cardiaco. In: Schiavon F, Berletti R, Guglielmi G, Cammarota T, editors. Diagnostica per immagini nell'invecchiamento. Radiol Med 2003;54–6 suppl 1 al N.3.

34. Boo JF. Understanding heart failure. Arch Cardiol Mex 2006;76(4):431–47.

35. Gehlbach BK, Geppert E. The pulmonary manifestations of left heart failure. Chest 2004;125(2):669–82.

36. Peperstraete B. Particular aspects of heart failure in elderly patients. Rev Med Brux 2006;27(5):430–6.

37. Kitzman DW. Diastolic heart failure in the elderly. Heart Fail Rev 2002;7(1):17–27.

38. Kitzman DW. Heart failure with normal systolic function. Clin Geriatr Med 2000;16(3):489–512.

39. Marcus M, Schelbert HR, Skorton DJ. Cardiac imaging. Philadelphia: WB Saunders; 1991.

40. Agostoni E. Mechanism of the pleural space. Physiol Rev 1972;52:57–64.

41. Cortese G, Sclavo MG, Comino E. Lo scompenso cardiaco. In: Comino E, Cammarota T, editors. Lezioni di diagnostica per immagini in geriatria. Torino (Italy): Edizioni Minerva Medica; 1995. p. 61–9.

42. Slutsky RA, Brown JJ. Chest radiographs in congestive heart failure. Difference between patients with acute and chronic myocardial disease. Radiology 1983;153(3):577–80.

43. Westcott JL, Rudick MG. Cardiopulmonary effects of intravenous fluid overload: radiologic manifestations. Radiology 1978;129(3):577–85.

44. The ILSA Working Group. Prevalence of chronic diseases in older Italians: comparing self reported and clinical diagnosis. Int J Epidemiol 1997;26: 995–1002.

45. Grosse C, Bankier A. [Imaging of emphysema]. Radiologe 2007;47(5):401–6 [in German].

46. Bellia V, Scichilone N, Ribella F, et al. Aging lung: dalla fisiologia alla clinica. Firenze (Italy): Scientific Press; 1997.

47. Antonelli Incalzi R. Caratteristiche cliniche della BPCO. G Gerontol 2002;50:440–6.

48. Mahler DA, Fierro-Carrion D, Briard TC. Evaluation of dyspnea in the elderly. Clin Geriatr Med 2003;19:19–33.

49. Ray P, Birolleau S, Riou B. La dyspnée aigue du sujet agé. Rev Mal Respir 2002;19:491–503 [in French].

50. Radenne F, Verkindre C, Tunnel PB. L'asthme du suyet agé. Rev Mal Respir 2003;20:95–103.

51. Calverley PM, Walker P. Chronic obstructive pulmonary disease. Lancet 2003;362:1053–61.

52. Pietila MP, Thomas C. Inflammation and infection in exacerbations of chronic obstructive pulmonary disease. Semin Respir Infect 2003;18:9–16.

53. White AJ, Gompertz S, Tockley RA. Chronic obstructive pulmonary disease: the aetiology of exacerbations. Thorax 2003;58:73–80.

54. Schiavon F, Berletti R. Il radiologo e la refertazione. Suggerimenti per una corretta comunicazione. Torino (Italy): Edizioni Minerva Medica; 2006.

55. Tardáguila F, Martí-Bonmatí L, Bonmatí J. El informe radiologico: filosofía general (I). Radiologia 2004; 46(4):195–8.

56. Tardáguila F, Martí-Bonmatí L, Bonmatí J. El informe radiologico: estylo y contenido (II). Radiologia 2004; 46(4):199–204.

57. Schiavon F, Grigenti G. Radiological reporting in clinical practice. Milano (Italy): Springer-Verlag; 2007.

Imaging of Diseases of the Axial and Peripheral Skeleton

Hsueh Wen Cheong, MBBS, MMed, FRCR[a],
Wilfred C.G. Peh, MBBS, MHSM, MD, FRCPE, FRCPG, FRCR[b],*,
Giuseppe Guglielmi, MD[c]

KEYWORDS

- Elderly skeletal diseases • Geriatric skeletal diseases
- Musculoskeletal imaging • Orthopedic imaging
- Peripheral skeletal diseases

The worldwide proportion of older people continues to increase, growing from 8% in 1950 to 10% in 2000, and is projected to reach 21% in 2050. In 2000, there were 35 million Americans over the age of 65 years. By 2050, the geriatric population will represent approximately 20% (or 70 million) of the American population.[1] Associated with this graying of population will be a significant increase in musculoskeletal injuries and disorders. Musculoskeletal disorders pose a particular burden for the elderly. The loss of mobility and physical independence resulting from fractures, arthritis, and osteoporosis can be devastating, both physically and psychologically. Trauma and fractures are also associated with increased mortality in the elderly. A current increase in geriatric imaging is likely to persist into the near future and requires radiologists to be more aware of musculoskeletal complaints and conditions pertaining to the geriatric population (**Table 1**). The main concerns in geriatric orthopedics are the increased incidence of trauma, degeneration, and malignancy, commonly compounded by comorbidities and the effects of ageing.

TRAUMA AND FRACTURES

Trauma is the fifth leading cause of death in patients over 65 years of age.[2] Although representing only 12% of the overall trauma population, the elderly sustain a disproportionate share of fractures and serious injury, accounting for approximately 28% of deaths. The frequency of fractures in the elderly results from the effects of osteoporosis and the tendency to fall. A combination of increased comorbidities, medications, and loss of muscle strength with ageing predisposes to falls. The most common reason for trauma in the elderly is falls.[3,4] Low-impact falls (from a standing height) are the most common reason for injury in geriatric patients. Insufficiency fractures are a subgroup of stress fractures, which develop from the effects of normal or physiologic stress on abnormal weakened bone, in which the elastic resistance is reduced[5] and in the case of elderly people is usually caused by osteoporosis. Osteoporosis is characterized by qualitatively normal, but quantitatively deficient, bone (ie, decrease in bone mass within otherwise normal bone), leading to enhanced bone fragility and a consequent increase in fracture risk.[6] Primary osteoporosis is predominant in the elderly and can be classified into types 1 and II. Type I (menopausal) osteoporosis commonly occurs in women aged 51 to 75 years. Type II (senescent) osteoporosis occurs in people more than 60 years of age, with women comprising the majority. Overlap between types I

[a] Department of Diagnostic Radiology, Changi General Hospital, 2 Simei Street 3, Singapore 529889, Republic of Singapore
[b] Department of Diagnostic Radiology, Alexandra Hospital, 378 Alexandra Road, Singapore 159964, Republic of Singapore
[c] University of Foggia, Scientific Institute Hospital, "Casa Sollievo della Sofferenza," Viale Cappuccini 1, 71013 San Giovanni Rotondo, Italy
* Corresponding author.
E-mail address: wilfred@pehfamily.per.sg (W.C.G. Peh).

Radiol Clin N Am 46 (2008) 703–733
doi:10.1016/j.rcl.2008.04.007

Table 1
Some more frequently encountered and typical skeletal conditions of the elderly

Fracture	Insufficiency fracture
	Pathologic fracture from malignancy
Degeneration	Osteoarthritis
	Rotator cuff and other tendon tears
	Spondylosis
	Diffuse idiopathic skeletal hyperostosis
Metabolic	Osteoporosis
	Gout
	Calcium pyrophosphate arthropathy
Neoplasm	Metastasis
	Myeloma
	Lymphoma
	Chondrosarcoma
	Chordoma
Infection	Osteomyelitis
	Septic arthritis
	Infected prosthesis
Others	Rheumatoid arthritis (advanced)
	Neuropathic arthropathy
	Paget's disease

and II is substantial, so this classification is of limited clinical use. Primary osteoporosis is thought to result mainly from the hormonal changes that occur with ageing, particularly decreasing levels of estrogen in women, and decreasing levels of both testosterone and estrogen in men.

There are many risk factors for osteoporosis. The major risk factors include history of fracture as an adult; older age; female gender; white or Asian race; family history (specifically in a first-degree relative) of osteoporosis or a fragility fracture; and thin body habitus. Other risk factors include low calcium or vitamin D intake; decreased lifelong exposure to estrogen or testosterone; inadequate weight-bearing exercise; use of certain drugs (eg, glucocorticoid for ≥3 months); current cigarette smoking; and excessive caffeine or alcohol intake. Diagnosis is best made by dual-energy x-ray absorptiometry. Bone loss in the elderly is considered normal if the bone mineral density is within 1 standard deviation of the mean density in young adults of the same gender and race, osteopenic if bone density is between 1 standard deviation and

2.5 standard deviation below the young adult mean, or osteoporotic if bone density is greater than 2.5 standard deviation below the young adult mean. The main radiographic features of generalized osteoporosis are increased radiolucency and cortical thinning. Early radiographic changes of osteopenia are subtle and may not be easy to appreciate, because a substantial amount (approximately 30%) of bone loss must occur before it can be detected radiographically.[7] Although usually generalized, the osseous manifestations are most obvious in the axial skeleton and proximal ends of long bones.[8] In the spine, cortical loss can give rise to a well-demarcated outline of the vertebral body, which has been aptly described as "picture-framing." Invagination of the disk into the vertebral body (which is weakened by bone loss), causes concavity of the end plates and produces a "fish" vertebra deformity. Vertebral compression fracture, often multiple, is a common and painful feature of osteoporosis.

Fractures of the Hip

Fractures of the hip are the second most common fractures (after the wrist) in elderly patients who fall.[9] The number of elderly persons who sustain hip fractures is estimated to double to 2.6 million by year 2025.[10] Almost half of all hip fractures occur in patients aged 80 years or over, with 18% to 28% expected to die within 1 year of their hip fracture.[11] Typically, these fractures are caused by a fall directly on the greater trochanter from a standing height, resulting in an impact force up to three times greater than the fracture strength of the femoral neck and trochanteric region. Fractures of the proximal femur occur through the intracapsular femoral neck or within the extracapsular intertrochanteric region. The key concern about a femoral neck fracture is the likelihood of proximal femoral circulation disruption by fracture displacement. Most of the vascular supply to the femoral head originates from the medial and lateral femoral circumflex arteries, which form an extracapsular ring around the femoral neck. Ascending cervical branches pass the femoral neck proximally and enter the capsule at its insertion. The damage to this circulation is in proportion to the degree of fracture displacement. Urgent anatomic reduction and internal fixation of displaced femoral neck fractures is advocated to restore the integrity of blood vessels.

The Garden classification of femoral neck fractures is based on the amount of fracture displacement evident on anteroposterior radiographs of the hip. This classification correlates with the prognosis for healing and the rates of avascular necrosis and nonunion. Significant fracture displacement may be apparent, however, on lateral radiographs and not seen on anteroposterior radiographs. Garden I and II fractures refer to undisplaced fractures that are incomplete and complete, respectively (**Fig. 1**). They have a good prognosis, and complete union is expected. Garden III fractures are complete fractures with partial displacement (**Fig. 2**), whereas Garden IV fractures show complete displacement (**Fig. 3**). These fractures are associated with a poor prognosis, with compete union in 93% of Garden III but only 57% of Garden IV fractures. There is a higher rate of osteonecrosis than in nondisplaced fractures, occurring in up to 30% of Garden III and IV fractures.[12] Nondisplaced fractures are typically treated by closed reduction and screw fixation. For displaced fractures, the poor outcome dictates the current approach of prosthetic replacement of the femoral head by hemiarthroplasty or total hip replacement. The major fracture line of the intertrochanteric fracture extends from the greater to the lesser trochanter, and is usually comminuted. Comminution of the posterior and medial cortices is an important prognostic feature and if present, indicates that the fracture is unstable and may require a displacement osteotomy. Otherwise, the fracture is stable and can be fixed with a compression screw (see **Fig. 2**). Most fractures of the proximal femur are easily diagnosed by conventional radiography. Undisplaced

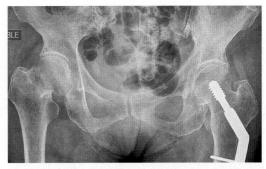

Fig. 2. Femoral neck fracture (Garden III). Anteroposterior radiograph of the pelvis shows a partially displaced complete subcapital fracture of the right femoral neck and a left dynamic hip screw. The patient had a previous left femoral neck fracture, now healed.

fractures may be negative or equivocal, however, and if a clinical suspicion of fracture persists, MR imaging is advocated.[13,14] MR imaging is both sensitive and specific for the detection of femoral neck fractures. This modality can show both the actual fracture line as linear area of hypointensity, surrounded by bone marrow edema, which is hypointense relative to normal marrow on T1-weighted and hyperintense on T2-weighted images (**Fig. 4**).

Insufficiency fractures may occur in the subcapital and intertrochanteric regions. Radiographic findings are often subtle, and bone scintiscans or MR imaging is often needed for diagnosis. MR imaging is the modality of choice in the setting of

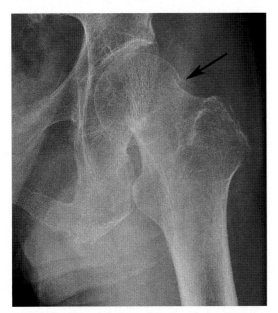

Fig. 1. Femoral neck fracture (Garden II). Anteroposterior radiograph shows an undisplaced but complete subcapital fracture (*arrow*) of the left femoral neck.

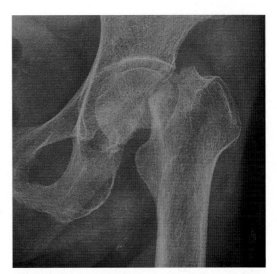

Fig. 3. Femoral neck fracture (Garden IV). Anteroposterior radiograph shows a completely displaced subcapital fracture of the left femoral neck.

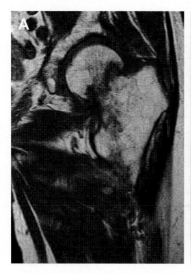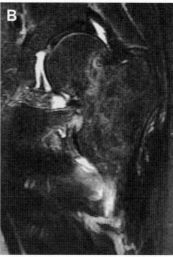

Fig. 4. MR image of femoral neck fracture (Garden II). Coronal (*A*) T1-weighted and (*B*) fat-saturated T2-weighted MR images show an undisplaced complete subcapital fracture of the left femoral neck of femur. The T2-weighted image shows adjacent bone marrow and surrounding soft tissue edema, and a hip joint effusion.

subchondral insufficiency fractures, which can appear normal on initial radiographs.[15] A recently recognized entity, subchondral insufficiency fracture typically occurs in osteoporotic elderly women. It is easily misdiagnosed as osteonecrosis because of its very similar clinical presentation and imaging appearance. On MR images, a hypointense line in the subcapital region, representing the fracture, is surrounded by an area of variable size producing T1-hypointense and T2-hyperintense signal, which enhances after intravenous gadolinium–diethylenetriamine pentaacetic acid administration.[16] In contrast, circumscribed lesions are commonly seen, with no enhancement within the circumscribed area (representing the necrotic segment), in osteonecrosis.[16]

Pelvic Fractures

Pelvic fractures occur commonly in the elderly and result from falls. As opposed to the lateral falls leading to fractures of the hip, pelvic fractures usually occur during a forward or backward fall. Because it is a rigid ringlike structure, a fracture in the anterior pelvis is almost always accompanied by an accompanying posterior fracture in the sacrum. In one study of elderly patients, pubic rami fractures were the most common (56%), followed by acetabular fractures (19%) and ischial fractures (11%).[17] Mortality in patients suffering from pelvic fractures has been reported to be 12% to 21%.[18] Spontaneous osteoporotic insufficiency fractures are common and not necessarily associated with trauma. They usually occur in the sacrum and pubic rami (**Fig. 5**), making up to 90% of fractures.[19] Fractures in the sacrum, and less commonly in the supra-acetabulum and ilium, are frequently occult. They are often either obscured by overlying bowel

or simply not demonstrable on conventional radiography.

Bone scintiscans are often diagnostic, with the classic H-shaped area of increased uptake corresponding to the alae and body of the sacrum; this finding is best appreciated on posterior views. Although the H-shaped pattern is considered diagnostic for insufficiency fractures, various incomplete sacral patterns, such as bilateral alar uptake with a partial horizontal bar and bilateral alar uptake, are regarded as sufficiently distinctive to differentiate these fractures from metastases or infection.[20,21] CT is also useful in detection of sacral insufficiency fractures, particularly for fractures that have an atypical appearance on bone

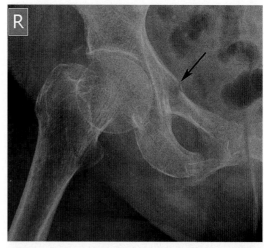

Fig. 5. Insufficiency fractures. Anteroposterior radiograph of the right hip shows mildly displaced insufficiency fractures of the superior (*arrow*) and inferior pubic rami.

scintiscans or MR imaging.[22] CT is also useful for demonstration of soft tissue masses that may be associated with a malignant lesion but is not seen in insufficiency fractures. On MR imaging, the fracture line is represented by a linear low-signal intensity on T1-weighted images, surrounded by bone edema that is moderately high signal intensity on T2-weighted and short tau inversion recovery sequences (**Fig. 6**).[22,23] They are typically located in the sacral ala parallel to the sacroiliac joint (**Fig. 7**). Unless the fracture is bilateral, the edema is usually confined to the sacral ala, not extending across the midline. In the supra-acetabulum, the characteristic curvilinear low-signal fracture line parallels the roof of the acetabulum (see **Fig. 7**). Insufficiency fractures may mimic metastatic disease and infection if the linear component of the fracture is not evident. If present, T2-hyperintense intrafracture fluid helps to differentiate fracture from metastatic disease. This sign is highly suggestive of insufficiency fractures, especially if they coexist with concomitant fractures of the pubis and ilium.[24] It is postulated that the fluid is caused by motion or nonunion at the fracture site and is unlikely to be present in malignant lesions. Otherwise, sequential MR imaging may be helpful, because resolution of marrow edema suggests a fracture rather than metastasis.[25]

Vertebral Compression Fractures

Vertebral compression fractures are often multiple, and are a common and painful feature of osteoporosis, affecting 25% of women aged 70 years and older and 40% of women aged 80 years and older.[26] The typical appearance is anterior wedging of vertebral bodies in the mid thoracic, lower thoracic, and upper lumbar region. Deformity is considered to be significant when the anterior height is less than 80% of the posterior height. In contrast to fractures of the long bones, osteoporotic vertebral fractures are rarely associated with a demonstrable break in the cortex or significant callus formation. Involvement of multiple vertebral bodies leads to kyphosis, which can cause a severely deformed posture known as the "dowager's hump" (**Fig. 8**). This in turn commonly leads to reduction in pulmonary capacity and decreased physical mobility. These fractures typically result from very minimal trauma, such as sneezing, lifting, bending, or coughing. Conservative treatment is generally indicated, although persistent neurologic symptoms from spinal compression may be present, requiring surgical decompression in a small minority of cases.[27] A common diagnostic dilemma is distinguishing between fractures caused by osteoporosis from those caused by malignancy.

Vertebroplasty is a technique in which polymethylmethacrylate, quick-setting bone cement, is percutaneously injected into a collapsed vertebral body under imaging guidance (**Fig. 9**). The primary purpose of vertebroplasty is to relieve pain and to strengthen and stabilize the vertebrae. Vertebroplasty is most often performed to treat osteoporotic fractures; however, other major indications include the treatment of myeloma and bone metastases, particularly in patients who are considered to be poor surgical candidates for vertebrectomy or other major surgical procedures.

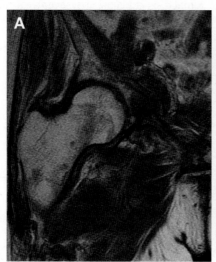
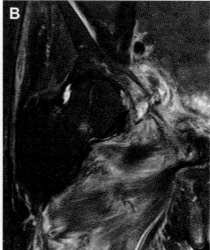

Fig. 6. Insufficiency fracture. Coronal (*A*) T1-weighted and (*B*) short tau inversion recovery (STIR) images show an insufficiency fracture (*arrow*) of the right superior pubic ramus.

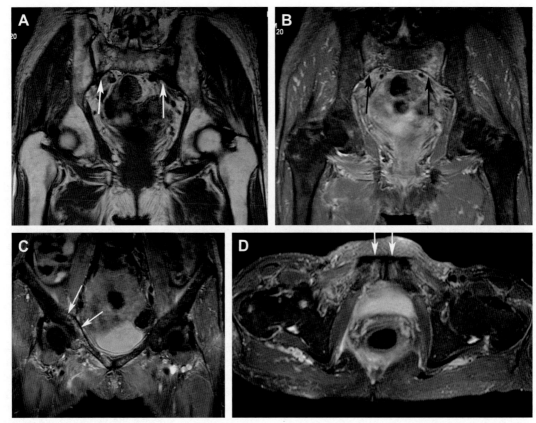

Fig. 7. Multiple insufficiency fractures of the sacrum and pelvic ring. Coronal (A) T1-weighted and (B) STIR images show bilateral sacral fractures (*arrows*) as T1-hypointense and T2-hyperintense alar bands that are parallel to the sacroiliac joints. (C) Coronal STIR image shows a right supra-acetabular insufficiency fracture (*arrows*). (D) Axial fat-saturated T2-weighted images of the pubic rami show concomitant bilateral parasymphyseal fractures (*arrows*).

Significant pain relief is expected in more than 70% of patients with vertebral malignancies and more than 90% of patients with osteoporotic fractures.[28] Complications include permanent neurologic damage and pulmonary embolization of the polymethylmethacrylate, but are rare if a meticulous technique is used.

Other Fractures

Elderly patients are at risk for various other long bone fractures that can result from simple falls or low impact trauma. Fractures of the distal radius, surgical neck of humerus, and ankle are among the most common fractures.

DEGENERATIVE JOINT DISEASE

Osteoarthritis or degenerative joint disease is the most common articular disease among persons aged 65 years and older. It may be primary (idiopathic) or secondary to preceding or pre-existing injury or arthropathy, and tends to affect women more commonly. It frequently leads to decreased function and loss of independence. Although the joints of the hand are the most commonly affected, they are less likely than the knee or hip to be symptomatic. In addition, the severity of radiographic changes does not always correlate with clinical symptoms.

The cardinal radiographic features of degenerative joint disease are

1. Narrowing of joint space from articular cartilage thinning at those areas subjected to the greatest pressures; this effect is in contrast to that of inflammatory arthritides, where there is uniform joint-space narrowing
2. Subchondral sclerosis
3. Osteophyte formation, which are usually marginal in location
4. Cyst or pseudocyst formation, resulting from microfractures and synovial fluid intrusion into subchondral bone

The main advantage of MR imaging is its ability to depict articular cartilage directly. This is useful in early disease where radiography is often negative.

spoiled gradient-recalled echo sequences display the hyaline cartilage as hyperintense tissue relative to bone, fat, and fluid. Abnormalities are seen as alterations of morphology of the hyperintense cartilage (eg, fissuring or thinning.) With intermediate or T2-weighted fast spin-echo images, normal articular cartilage is of intermediate signal intensity. Cartilage abnormalities are seen as regions of relatively increased intrasubstance signal intensity or as morphologic defects, such as fissuring or thinning. Although subchondral sclerosis often has low signal intensity on both T1- and T2-weighted images, a marrow edema pattern (T1-hypointense and T2-hyperintense) may also be seen.

Degenerative Disease of the Hip

The hallmarks of degenerative joint disease can be readily demonstrated on standard radiographic projections of the hip. In addition, migration of the femoral head with respect to the acetabulum can be observed, most commonly superolaterally (**Fig. 10**). CT may further delineate the characteristic features of osteoarthritis. Rapid destructive coxarthropathy of the hip or Postel coxarthropathy is an unusual and poorly recognized destructive osteoarthritis, occurring predominantly in women, with age onset at 60 to 70 years. Radiographic

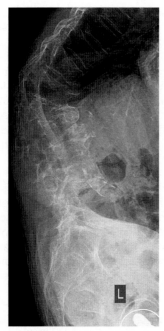

Fig. 8. Osteoporotic vertebral fracture. Lateral radiograph of the lumbar spine shows a kyphotic "dowager's hump." This was caused by anterior wedge compression vertebral body fractures developing at the thoracolumbar junction. Prominent osteophytes are present, indicating chronicity.

A variety of pulse sequences have been described, with the three-dimensional spoiled gradient-recalled echo and fast spin-echo imaging being the most widely used. The three-dimensional

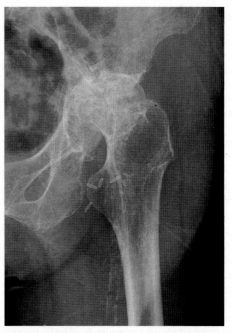

Fig. 10. Severe osteoarthritis. Anteroposterior radiograph of the left hip shows severe joint space narrowing, prominent subchondral cysts and sclerosis, protusio acetabuli, and superolateral migration of the femoral head.

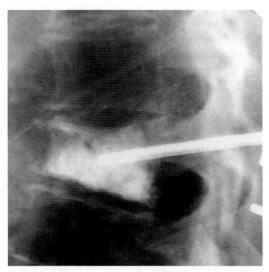

Fig. 9. Vertebroplasty for osteoporotic vertebral fracture. Lateral radiograph shows injection of polymethylmethacrylate into the compressed vertebral body through a large-bore needle that had been placed transpedicularly.

findings mimic those of disorders, such as septic arthritis, rheumatoid and seronegative arthritis, primary osteonecrosis with secondary osteoarthritis, or neuropathic osteoarthropathy, but affected patients do not have clinical, pathologic, or laboratory evidence of these entities. On histology, the findings are those of conventional osteoarthritis with severe degeneration in the cartilage. Osteophyte formation, however, is absent or minimal.

Degenerative Disease of Knee

In addition to the radiographic hallmarks of osteoarthritis, formation of intra-articular osteochondral bodies is a frequent complication. These may arise from synovial metaplasia, transchondral fractures, or articular degeneration. These intra-articular loose bodies cause further deterioration of the cartilage and other structures. The "tooth" sign describes the vertical ridges resembling teeth seen on axial view of the patella.[29] It represents an enthesopathy, probably related to stress at the attachment of the quadriceps. Degeneration affects the medial compartment more than the lateral or patellofemoral compartments early in the disease. As disease progresses, tricompartmental disease develops. Joint replacement may be required for severely arthritic joints. Similar complications, such as infection, periprosthetic fracture, and prosthesis failure, may occur.

Degenerative Disease of the Shoulder

Degenerative disease of the shoulder is fairly common. In a study of elderly subjects, 34% were found to have significant shoulder pain and 30% had disability related to decreased shoulder movement.[30] Rotator cuff disease is the major cause of shoulder disability. Rotator cuff degeneration occurs as a result of overuse, and can lead to a tear with minimal trauma. Large tears in the rotator cuff are more common in the older population.[31] It is also important to differentiate between degeneration and other causes, especially rheumatoid arthritis. Tears of the rotator cuff may result in the loss of the primary stabilizers of the glenohumeral joint, leading to articular wear and arthritis. The hallmarks of osteoarthritis are well depicted on radiography, and subacromial spurs that predispose to supraspinatus tears can also be seen. A supraspinatus tear is usually located distally, either near its attachment to the greater tuberosity or in the critical zone of the tendon located about 1 cm proximal to its insertion.

High-resolution ultrasound (US) is a noninvasive, sensitive, specific, and cost-effective method for examination of the rotator cuff tendons. As a dynamic study, US has the advantage of enabling examination of the rotator cuff during patient motion, with real-time evaluation of impingement being possible. Full-thickness tears are also well depicted on US. US is highly operator-dependent, however, with a relatively long learning curve. In addition, US examination is only limited to the distal rotator cuff tendons. The normal rotator cuff shows an anterior echogenic arch of subdeltoid fascia and peritendinous fat. Tears are seen as hypoechoic areas, with full-thickness tears extending through the entire substance or with complete loss of rotator substance with visualization of tear margins (**Fig. 11**). A tear is massive when there is nonvisualization of the rotator cuff with approximation of the deltoid muscle to the surface of the humeral head.[32] Although partial-thickness tears are not as well depicted on US, its diagnosis has minimal initial therapeutic impact because it is usually managed conservatively initially.

MR imaging is an excellent imaging modality for assessment of the soft tissues of the shoulder. Its sensitivity and specificity is further improved by use of intra-articular gadolinium–diethylenetriamine pentaacetic acid injection. Conventional MR imaging has a sensitivity of 91% to 100% and specificity of 81% to 95% in the detection of rotator cuff tears.[33,34] The sensitivity and specificity of MR arthrography in the diagnosis of full-thickness tears approaches 100%.[35] On conventional MR imaging, full-thickness tear are seen as areas of fluid intensity that extends across the full thickness of the tendon (**Fig. 12**). On MR arthrography, intra-articular contrast agent outlines the inferior rotator cuff surface, fills cuff tears, and leaks into the subacromial and subdeltoid bursa through the tear. With fat-suppression MR arthrography, full-thickness and partial-thickness

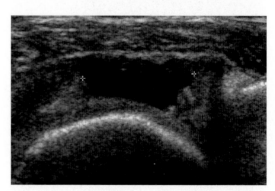

Fig. 11. US of supraspinatus tear. US image (longitudinal view) of the right supraspinatus tendon shows a full-thickness tear (*between cursors*), depicted as a hypoechoic area traversing the full thickness of the tendon.

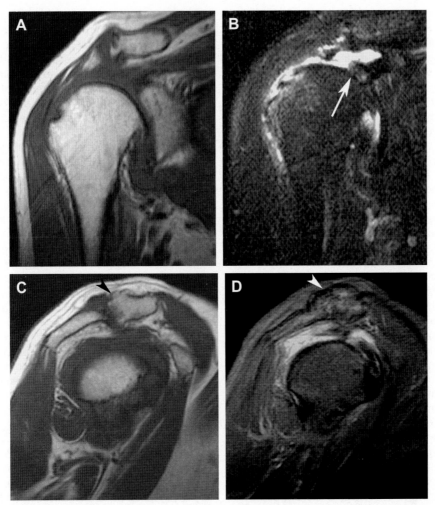

Fig. 12. MR imaging of supraspinatus tear. Coronal (*A*) T1-weighted and (*B*) fat-saturated T2-weighted MR images show a massive supraspinatus tendon tear, with retraction of the stump (*arrow*). Sagittal (*C*) T1-weighted and (*D*) fat-saturated T2-weighted MR images show degenerate and hypertrophic acromioclavicular joint (*arrowhead*), which is very likely to be the predisposing factor for the tendon tear.

tears can be identified with up to 100% sensitivity and specificity.[36]

Degeneration of the Spine

Disk degeneration is part of the normal ageing process and with biomechanical loading over time, there is a decrease in the proteoglycan concentration and number of chondrocytes,[37] leading to alterations in disk structure. As degeneration progresses from the nucleus pulposus to the peripheral annulus, cracks and fissures form, predisposing the central disk material toward herniation through the annulus. Depending on the location of the disk herniation, the pathologic signs and symptoms can range from myelopathy or neurogenic claudication associated with central canal stenosis, to radiculopathy associated with lateral herniations. Disk bulges are symmetric extensions of the disk beyond the margins of the vertebral end plate. The disk is considered herniated only if nuclear material is expelled through a discrete annular defect. It is classified as a disk protrusion if the fragment herniates through the annulus beyond the posterior margin of the vertebral end plate. If the fragment is expelled further and the fragment is in continuity with the central disk (often by a pedicle), then it is classified as a disk extrusion. A sequestered disk fragment is one that has migrated remotely and has no direct contact with the disk.[38]

With worsening degeneration, alterations in the biomechanics of the vertebral body and facet joints occur, with loss in disk height. The body's response to these structural changes may result in osteophyte formation at the facet joints and adjacent to the vertebral end plates. As the disk space collapses, the neural foramen can narrow and impinge on nerve roots, resulting clinically in radicular symptoms. The facets may hypertrophy, causing ligamentum flavum buckling in response to degenerative changes, narrowing the spinal canal. Spondylolithesis can occur eventually. Central compression of neural elements can lead to myelopathy in the cervical spine and neurogenic claudication in the lumbar spine. The central cord syndrome is characterized by disproportionately greater motor impairment in upper compared with lower extremities, bladder dysfunction, and variable degree of sensory loss below the level of injury. It most often occurs after hyperextension injury in an individual with long-standing cervical spondylosis. Injury may result from both posterior pinching of the cord by the buckled ligamentum flavum or from anterior compression by osteophytes. This syndrome is generally associated with a favorable prognosis.

Degenerative changes are particularly common in the mid-lower cervical and the lower lumbar spinal segments. Disk space narrowing, osteophytes, facet joint changes, and spondylolithesis are easily demonstrated on radiographs. Oblique views are useful in showing the encroachment of the neural foramina by posterior osteophytes. CT is useful if any further delineation of bony changes is required. MR imaging is highly effective in demonstrating changes of disk degeneration, canal stenosis, and nerve impingement. Disk degeneration results in decreased signal intensity of the nucleus pulposus on T2-weighted images. Annular tears appear as focal areas of T2-hyperintensity. The morphology of disk herniation and its relation to the nerve roots and adjacent structures are well demonstrated on MR imaging. Narrowing of the central canal, lateral recesses, and neural foramina can also be assessed (**Fig. 13**). Other changes that may contribute to nerve impingment or canal stenosis, such as thickening of the hypointense ligamentum flavum and the T2-hyperintense synovial cyst, can also be detected on MR imaging.

Provocative diskography is the only diagnostic test that provides both anatomic and functional information about a suspected abnormal disk, and is usually performed on the lumbar spine. The most useful and important aspect of diskography is the provocation of diskogenic pain by injection of contrast agent into the nucleus pulposus of the intervertebral disk. Disk morphology, including annular tears and disk herniations, can also be assessed radiographically or on CT, or both. Provocative diskography is considered when other noninvasive imaging modalities have failed to explain the patient's pain or have failed to localize the symptomatic disk levels for surgical planning.[39] Although the complication rate of diskography is low (<1%),[40] it should be performed only as a complementary test, and after careful patient selection.

Diffuse Idiopathic Skeletal Hyperostosis

Diffuse idiopathic skeletal hyperostosis (DISH) (also known as "hyperostostic spondylosis," Forestier disease) is a multifocal entity characterized by a tendency toward ossification of ligaments, particularly the paraspinal ligaments. DISH is usually asymptomatic. The condition occurs more commonly in men (65%), and most often in

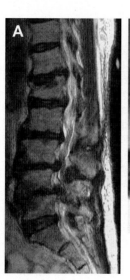
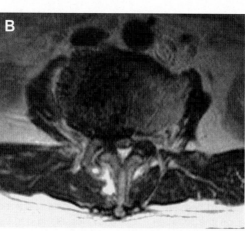

Fig. 13. Lumbar spondylosis. (*A*) Sagittal T2-weighted MR image of the lumbar spine shows multiple levels of disk degeneration with osteophytes, posterior disk protrusions, and mild L4-L5 degenerative spondylolithesis. (*B*) Axial T1-weighted MR image of L4-L5 disk space shows marked narrowing of the central canal and bilateral facet hypertrophy.

persons aged 50 to 75 years. Its estimated frequency in the elderly is 5% to 15%.[41] Although DISH occurs more commonly in Europeans and North Americans, the associated ossification of the posterior longitudinal ligament occurs more frequently in the Japanese population.[42] DISH diagnostic criteria include the following:[41]

1. Flowing calcifications and ossifications along the anterolateral aspect of at least four contiguous vertebral bodies, with or without osteophytes
2. Preservation of disk height in the involved areas and an absence of excessive disk disease
3. Absence of bony ankylosis of facet joints and absence of sacroiliac erosion, sclerosis, or bony fusion, although narrowing and sclerosis of facet joints are acceptable

Unlike ankylosing spondylitis, DISH does not involve the sacroiliac joint. DISH is also distinct from marginal osteophytes that form in response to degenerative disk disease. Lower thoracic spine involvement is typical of DISH, but the lumbar and cervical spine also can be affected. The left side of the spine is typically spared or less involved, which may be attributable to the pulsating aorta. Any extraspinal ligamentous hyperostosis is most frequently seen in the pelvis, calcaneum, ulna, olecranon, and patella. The diagnosis is made on radiographs (**Fig. 14**). When better anatomic definition is required, CT with multiplanar reconstruction is useful. MR imaging is usually not indicated for diagnosis, but is valuable for determining any mass effect on the thecal sac and the presence of cord compression, especially when there is associated ossification of the posterior longitudinal ligament.

INFLAMMATORY, AUTOIMMUNE, AND METABOLIC ARTHROPATHY
Rheumatoid Arthritis

The primary manifestation of rheumatoid arthritis (RA) is a symmetric inflammatory polyarthritis, and can affect any of the synovial joints. RA is relevant to geriatrics for several reasons: (1) as a chronic condition, a large portion of patients survive into old age and late complications are common; (2) although typically presenting initially in a younger age group, initial presentation at old age can occur; (3) diagnosis and management can be difficult because of frequent pre-existing joint symptomatology in old age; and (4) RA may present differently in older adult patients, compared with younger patients.[43,44] Although the hallmark of RA is its symmetry, an exception occurs in a hemiplegic patient, where the paralyzed

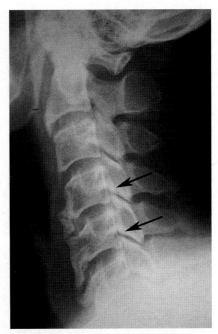

Fig. 14. DISH with ossification of the posterior longitudinal ligament. Lateral radiograph shows features of early DISH, seen as vertically oriented ossification of the anterior longitudinal ligament, more prominent in the lower cervical vertebra. Note that the intervertebral disk spaces are preserved and the facet joints are normal. There is an associated ossification of the posterior longitudinal ligament (*arrows*) located posterior to C4 and C5 vertebral bodies.

side is often spared. Compared with the younger patients, the older patient is more likely to have

1. More equal gender distribution
2. Acute onset
3. Frequent large joint involvement, particularly the shoulders, hips, and wrists, with sparing of the hands (mimicking polymyalgia rheumatica)
4. More systemic features
5. Higher erythrocyte sedimentation rate elevations
6. Lower frequency of rheumatoid factor

On radiography, RA is characterized by a diffuse, usually multicompartmental, symmetric joint space narrowing associated with marginal or central erosions, periarticular osteoporosis, and periarticular soft tissue swelling. Subchondral sclerosis is minimal or absent, and typically there is also a lack of osteophyte formation. Osteophyte formation, however, often occurs and probably represents the overlap of osteoarthritis and RA that occurs in many patients, particularly in the elderly. Large joints, such as the knee, hip, shoulder, and elbow, may be involved (**Fig. 15**). In advanced stages, axial

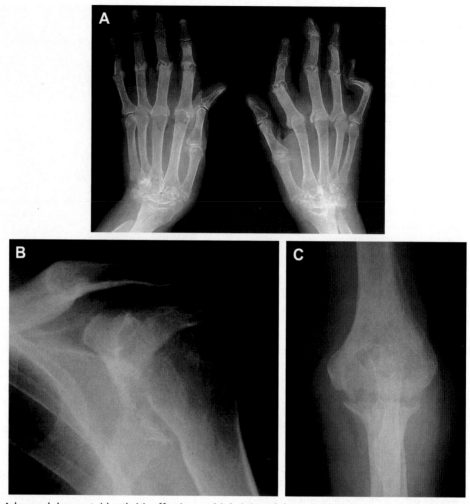

Fig. 15. Advanced rheumatoid arthritis affecting multiple joints. (*A*) Frontal hand radiograph shows bilateral and symmetric involvement of all the finger and wrist joints. There are extensive severe erosions, with dislocations and subluxations of some of the metacarpophalangeal joints bilaterally. The carpal bones are destroyed and fused. Both distal ends of the radii are eroded, with severe ulnar resorption bilaterally. (*B*) Anteroposterior radiograph of the left shoulder shows humeral head erosions and pseudowidening of the acromioclavicular joint caused by distal clavicular resorption. (*C*) Anteroposterior radiograph of the left elbow shows extensive periarticular erosion with a large distal humeral defect. Similar changes were present in the right shoulder and elbow (not shown).

migration of the hip may result in acetabular protusio. Destructive changes in the shoulder joint and rotator cuff rupture may result in superior migration of the humeral head. Pencil-like resorption of the distal clavicle is also a well-described feature (see **Fig. 15**). Synovial cysts and pseudocysts present as radiolucent defects usually seen close to the joints (see **Fig. 15**). They may or may not communicate with the joint space. Joint effusions are also common in the large joints.

RA typically affects the small joints of the wrists, and the metacarpophalangeal and proximal interphalangeal joints of the hands and feet (see **Fig. 15**). Symmetry is most common in the wrist.[45] Typically, the distal interphalangeal joints in the

hands are spared. The most common locations for marginal erosions are the radial aspects of the second and third metacarpal heads, and the radial and ulnar aspects of the bases of the proximal phalanges. Marginal erosion of the styloid tip is caused by synovial inflammation in the prestyloid recess. Chronic inflammation of the small joints of the hand can lead to characteristic deformities, such as swan neck and boutonnière deformity. Subluxations and dislocations of the fingers are common in advanced stages, with ulnar deviation of the fingers at the metacarpophalangeal joints and radial deviation of the wrist in the radiocarpal articulation being characteristic features. In far-advanced disease, a main-en-lorgnette or "telescoping" appearance of the fingers results from destructive shortening of the fingers associated with metacarpophalangeal dislocations (see **Fig. 15**).

Spinal involvement is common, typically the cervical spine, whereas thoracic and lumbar involvement is rare. Erosions of the odontoid process and apophyseal joints can be seen. Ankylosis of the apophyseal joints, however, is uncommon. Subluxation of the lower cervical vertebrae also occurs, most commonly at C3-C4 level. The most frequent cervical abnormality is laxity of the transverse ligament, which results in subluxation of the atlantoaxial joints and cervical myelopathy. The most common atlantoaxial subluxation is the anterior type, typified by abnormal separation between the anterior arch of the atlas and the odontoid process of the axis. Generally, the interosseous distance between the posterior aspect of the anterior arch of the atlas and the anterior aspect of the odontoid process should not exceed 2.5 mm in adults. Upper spinal cord compression develops when C1-C2 subluxation is greater than 9 mm, and in the presence of atlantoaxial impaction.[46] Vertical subluxation with superior migration of the odontoid process is next most common, and when extensive, can be fatal. It is also known as "cranial settling" or "atlantoaxial impaction" and results from the combined bone and cartilage loss in the atlantoaxial and atlanto-occipital articulations. Posterior and lateral atlantoaxial subluxations are rarer. Cervical myelopathy in the absence of significant subluxation has been reported in patients with long-standing severe disease, and is attributed to ligamentous and granulation tissue forming a constricting ring in the posterior half of the extradural space.[47]

Scleroderma

Scleroderma occurs primarily in late middle age, and is occasionally seen in patients aged 65 years or older, either a new onset or in patients who have grown old with their disease. The characteristic features are thickening and atrophy of the skin of the hands and face. As the disease progress, hand changes progress to sclerodactyly, with limited motion of the interphalangeal joints. Radiographs may show bone loss from the distal phalanges and occasionally calcinosis. Other manifestions include esophageal dysmotility, and progressive fibrosis or vascular changes in the lungs, heart, gastrointestinal tract, and kidneys.

Gout

The frequency of gout increases with age, especially in postmenopausal women, in whom the frequency is equal to that of men at a comparable age. Gout is more common in older individuals because this condition generally appears only after 20 to 30 years of hyperuricemia. Diagnosis is suspected on clinical grounds and is confirmed by demonstration of urate crystals in synovial fluid. Normouricemia does not exclude gout, because only about 80% of patients are hyperuricemic at the time of acute attack. The first metatarsophalangeal joint is the most common site of involvement in gouty arthritis (**Fig. 16**). Other frequently affected sites include the ankle, knee, wrist, and elbow. Less commonly affected areas include the sacroiliac, sternoclavicular, and shoulder joints. In gouty arthritis, characteristic radiographic features include sharply marginated erosions that are initially periarticular and later extend into the joint, with an "overhanging edge" being a frequent identifying feature. Intraosseous defects secondary to intraosseous tophi formation are occasionally seen. An asymmetrical distribution and a striking lack of osteoporosis help to differentiate gout from rheumatoid arthritis. In chronic tophaceous gout, there are urate deposits in and around the joint. A dense mass frequently associated with calcifications, known as a "tophus," is formed. Although randomly and asymmetrically distributed, they are more often seen on the dorsal aspects of the hands or feet.

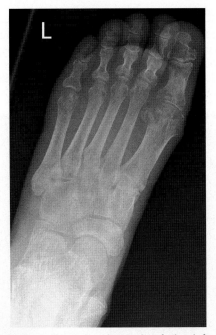

Fig. 16. Gout. Frontal radiograph of the left foot shows large periarticular erosions with "overhanging edges" affecting the first metatarsophalangeal joint.

Calcium Pyrophosphate Arthropathy

In contrast to gout, calcium pyrophosphate arthropathy results from intra-articular deposits of calcium pyrophosphate dehydrate crystals. Patients are usually middle aged and older. It affects men and women fairly equally, in contrast to gout, which has a male predominance. Septic arthritis, gout, and calcium pyrophosphate arthropathy can present in very similar ways, and often cannot reliably be distinguished on clinical grounds. Joint fluid analysis under a polarized light is helpful in differentiating between urate and calcium pyrophosphate dehydrate crystals. Prior history of gout or pseudogout does not rule out the possibility of acute septic arthritis, because septic arthritis is more common in patients with a history of crystal-induced arthritis. The wrist, elbow, shoulder, ankle, and patellofemoral joints are characteristically involved. Radiographically, the condition is characterized by chondrocalcinosis, and arthritic changes are similar to those in osteoarthritis. Chondrocalcinosis refers to calcification of the hyaline (articular) cartilage and fibrocartilage (menisci) (**Fig. 17**). The tendons, ligaments, and joint capsule may also be calcified. It is important to note that chondrocalcinosis is a characteristic but not unique feature of calcium pyrophosphate arthropathy, because it may also be present in other diseases, such as gout, hyperparathyroidism, hemachromatosis, and Wilson's disease.

Hemochromatosis

Hereditary hemochromatosis is a fairly common disease in whites and is a result of iron deposition in hepatocytes, myocardial fibers, and other visceral cells. The classic tetrad of manifestations resulting from hemochromatosis consists of (1) cirrhosis, (2) diabetes mellitus, (3) hyperpigmentation of the skin, and (4) cardiac failure. Clinical consequences also include hepatocellular carcinoma, impotence, and arthritis. Secondary hemochromatosis is related to iron overload (eg, transfusion or dietary intake) and may be associated with alcohol abuse. It is more common in men and generally diagnosed between 40 and 60 years of age. Women tend to have a later onset of disease. Serum iron levels are elevated and biopsy of the liver or synovium may be performed for diagnosis. A total of 50% of patients have a slowly progressing arthritis. The disease starts in the small joints of the hands, and may eventually involve the large joints and cervical-lumbar intervertebral disks. In the hands, the second and third metacarpophalangeal joints are characteristically affected. Hook-like osteophytes of the metacarpal heads are typical. Other small joints, such as the interphalangeal and carpal articulations, may be involved. Chondrocalcinosis, loss of articular space, eburnation, and subchondral cyst formation are also prominent features.

Neuropathic Arthropathy

Neuropathic arthropathy (or Charcot's joint) occurs in a number of diseases that have neurologic sequelae. Neuropathic arthropathy related to diabetes mellitus, syphilis, and leprosy is the most common in the elderly population. Each neuropathy type has a predilection for certain joints. Tabes dorsalis of neurosyphilis affects the dorsal (sensory) roots and hence could affect any joint but has a predilection for the spine and lower limbs. Diabetic neuropathy tends to affect the extremities, notably the toes, midfoot, and ankle, and

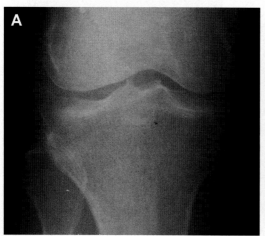
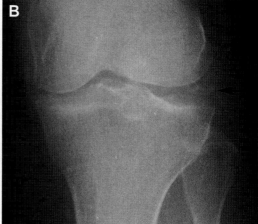

Fig. 17. Bilateral knee chondrocalcinosis. Frontal radiographs of the right (*A*) and left (*B*) knees show calcifications of all the menisci, more prominently involving the lateral menisci (*arrows*) bilaterally.

may cause a neuropathic spine. The interphalangeal joints of the hands and the metatarsophalangeal joints of the feet are commonly affected in patients with leprosy. Gross joint manifestations are characteristic of neuropathic arthropathy. Neuropathic arthropathy can simulate osteoarthritis, however, in the early stages. The usual distinctive characteristics are large joint effusion, joint instability manifested by subluxation or dislocation, marked lysis of adjacent bones often leaving sharply defined margins, bone and calcified debris, preservation of regional mineral content, and excessive sclerosis.

Paget's Disease

Paget's disease is a localized disorder of bone characterized by an increase in osteoclast-mediated bone resorption and accompanied by osteoblast-mediated formation of architecturally inferior new bone. This results in a propensity for fractures and skeletal deformities in advanced cases. The exact etiology is still unknown, although it is believed that there is a viral etiology, and possible agents, such as respiratory syncytial virus and paramyxovirus, have been suggested. Genetic predisposition to the development of Paget's disease also may exist. The prevalence varies considerably in different parts of the world. It is rare in Asians and reaches its greatest incidence in Great Britain, Australia, and New Zealand. It is slightly more common in men than women (3:2). With an average onset between 45 and 55 years of age, the disease has a prolonged course, lasting well into the geriatric age group. Skeletal abnormalities are frequently asymptomatic and may be an incidental finding. Symptoms are often related to complications of the disease, such as deformity, bone pain, fractures, secondary osteoarthritis, neural compression, and sarcomatous change. Paget's disease may be monostotic but is more commonly polyostotic. The following bones, in order of decreasing frequency, are most often affected: pelvis, femur, skull, tibia, lumbar and thoracic vertebrae, clavicle, humerus, and ribs (Fig. 18).

There are three phases of Paget's disease, and these may coexist in the same long or flat bone. In the long bones, the disease typically starts from one articular end (usually proximal) and advances to the other. In the initial osteolytic or hot phase, the terms "advancing wedge," "blade of grass," and "candle flame" have all been commonly used to describe the radiolucent wedge or elongated area representing active bone resorption along the shafts of long bones. In flat bones, such as the ilium or calvarium, there may be

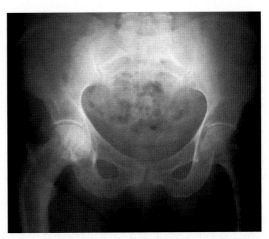

Fig. 18. Polyostotic Paget's disease. Anteroposterior radiograph of the pelvis shows sclerosis of the right proximal femur caused by coarsened thickened trabeculae. There is extensive cortical thickening with medullary encroachment, especially when compared with the normal left femur. Subtler changes are present in the right superior and inferior pubic rami, where there is patchy sclerosis, mild but definite generalized cortical thickening, and loss of corticomedullary differentiation.

a well-demarcated radiolucent area of osteolysis, known as "osteoporosis circumscripta." In the skull, the frontal and occipital bones are most commonly affected and both inner and outer tables are involved. In the intermediate phase or mixed phase, osteolysis is accompanied by new bone formation, which tends to predominate. There is thickening of the cortex and coarse trabeculation of cancellous bone. In the skull, patchy densities give a characteristic "cotton-ball" appearance. Cortical thickening and sclerosis of the iliopectineal and ischiopubic lines can be observed in the pelvis (see Fig. 18). In the spine, coarse trabeculated bone forming around the vertebral body gives a "picture-frame" appearance. The cool or sclerotic phase is marked by a diffusely increased bone density, with bone widening and enlargement. In the long bones, there is marked thickening of the bone cortex and loss of normal differentiation between the cortex and spongiosa (see Fig. 18). In the skull, the diploic space can be obliterated. The vertebral bodies become densely sclerotic, giving an "ivory vertebra" appearance. Several conditions may mimic Paget's disease and vice versa. In the long bones, monostotic disease may mimic monostotic fibrous dysplasia. In the spine, "ivory vertebra" can be mistaken for metastases or lymphoma. Secondary hyperparathyroidism and vertebral hemangioma can also have similar appearance to Paget's disease of the vertebra.

Fracture is the most common complication of Paget's disease. In the osteolytic phase, fractures are more likely to occur. Complete fractures transversing the bone are described as "banana-type" and are characteristic. Insufficiency fractures may occur, characteristically represented by short horizontal radiolucent lines involving the convex cortical surface (**Fig. 19**). Bowing of the long bones may occur, as the normal bone is replaced by architecturally inferior new bone. Secondary osteoarthritis is common, usually affecting the knee and hip joint. Acetabular protusio can also occur in hip involvement. Most neurologic complications are secondary to involvement of the skull and spine. Bone enlargement may narrow the neural foramina in the spine and skull. Softening of the skull can lead to basilar invagination. Fractures of the spinal vertebrae can cause spinal block and cord compression. Secondary sarcomatous change in pagetic bone is the most lethal complication, occurring in approximately 1% of patients with Paget's disease. These sarcomas are aggressive and prognosis is poor. The gender incidence is probably the same as that of the primary disease. Multicentric disease may occur. The pelvis, femur, and humerus are the most common affected sites, and the spine is typically spared. Radiographically, sarcomatous change is indicated by a lytic lesion, often with a wide transition

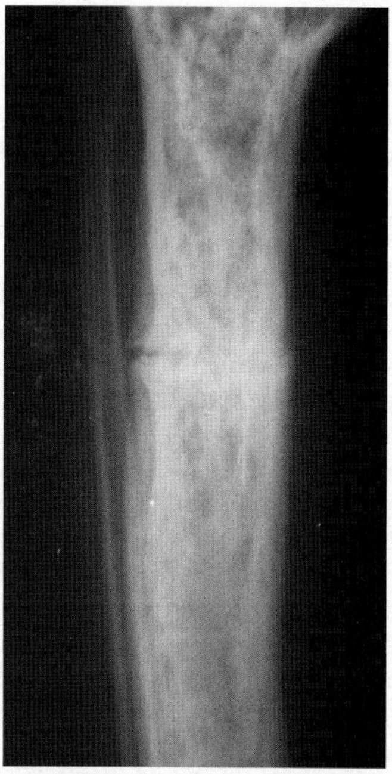

Fig. 19. Paget's disease with fracture. Anteroposterior radiograph of the right tibia shows prominent bone expansion, cortical thickening, areas of sclerosis, and thickened trabeculae. An incremental fracture runs transversely across the proximal tibial shaft.

zone, cortical breakthrough, and a soft tissue mass. Periosteal reaction is uncommon. Osteosarcoma is most frequent, with fibrosarcoma and malignant fibrous histiocytoma accounting for most of the remaining tumors. It is often difficult to differentiate the cell type radiologically, and biopsy is usually required.

Bone scintigraphy is useful in surveying the different sites of involvement in polyostotic disease. Scintigraphy tends to follow the physiologic activity of disease and may also be used to monitor treatment. Characteristically, a marked uptake of radiopharmaceutical in the involved bones is observed. Late-stage involvement may not reveal intense radiopharmaceutical uptake, however, and osteoporosis circumscripta may demonstrate only a peripheral rim of increased uptake. Scintigraphic diagnosis of malignant transformation is not particularly useful, because there may already be high intake by the pagetic bones. MR imaging is occasionally used to exclude disease involvement of the soft tissue or assessment for complications, such as basilar invagination, cord compression, and sarcomatous degeneration.

TUMORS

Bone tumors may present with bone pain, pathologic fractures, disability, or as an incidental finding. The clinical presentation of benign and malignant tumors may be similar. The age of the patient is perhaps the most essential clinical information required in the assessment of a bone tumor. In elderly patients, any newly discovered bone lesion or one developing within a known pre-existing lesion should be assumed to be malignant, until proved otherwise.

Metastases

Metastatic deposits from carcinoma are by far the commonest malignant tumors affecting the skeleton in the elderly, and should always be considered first in the differential diagnosis of any bone lesion. Although often multiple, 9% of carcinoma metastases to bone are solitary.[48] A solitary metastasis is still more common than a primary neoplasm. Metastases involve bone by three main mechanisms: (1) direct extension, (2) retrograde venous flow, and (3) seeding of tumor emboli by the blood circulation. Seeding occurs initially in the red marrow; this process accounts for the predominant distribution of metastatic lesions in the red marrow–containing areas in adults. Metastasis by seeding is also a relatively late occurrence because the lungs trap most tumor emboli. As a metastatic lesion grows in the medullary cavity, the surrounding bone is remodeled by means of either osteoclastic or osteoblastic processes and determines whether a predominant lytic, sclerotic, or mixed pattern is seen on radiographs. The relative degree of resultant bone resorption or deposition is highly variable and depends on the type and location of the tumor. The frequency of carcinoma-caused metastases depends on the prevalence of a particular cancer in a given population. In general, metastasis to the bones is commonest in the following carcinomas: breast, bronchus, prostate, kidney, and thyroid. In North America, overall commonest bone metastases from carcinoma for both genders are breast, prostate, lung, colon, and stomach.

Bone metastases may appear osteolytic, sclerotic, or mixed on radiographs. Lesions usually start in the medullary cavity, spread to destroy the medullary bone, and then involve the cortex. The specific appearance of bone metastases and location is often useful in suggesting the nature of the underlying primary malignancy. Most metastases involve the red marrow–containing axial skeleton (skull, spine, and pelvis) and the proximal segments of long bones. Metastasis distal to the knees or elbows is rare, and 50% of these are from breast or bronchus. Primary tumors arising from the pelvis have a predilection for spread to the lumbosacral spine. Osteolytic metastases are encountered most frequently, especially in breast and lung carcinomas (**Fig. 20**). Metastases from certain primary sites (eg, renal cell or thyroid carcinomas) are almost always osteolytic. Metastatic renal carcinoma has a characteristic expanded, "blown-out" appearance on radiographs. In elderly men, multiple round dense foci or diffuse bone density caused by sclerotic metastases are commonly prostatic in origin (**Fig. 21**). Other malignancies associated with sclerotic metastases include breast carcinoma, colonic carcinoma, melanoma, bladder carcinoma, and soft tissue sarcoma. The finding of sclerotic metastases almost always excludes an untreated renal tumor or hepatocellular carcinoma. A few characteristic features of metastatic lesion may be helpful in distinguishing between single metastasis from primary malignant and benign tumors: (1) metastatic lesion usually shows minimal or lack of adjacent soft tissue involvement; (2) periosteal reaction is uncommon unless the cortex is breached; (3) in the spine, clues to metastatic involvement include pedicular destruction, an associated soft tissue mass, and an angular or irregular deformity of the vertebral end plates.

The response to therapy can be evaluated by using radiographs and by correlating the radiographic changes with bone scintiscan findings and clinical and laboratory data. With healing, an osteolytic metastatic lesion first shows sclerotic rim, which then increases and advances to its

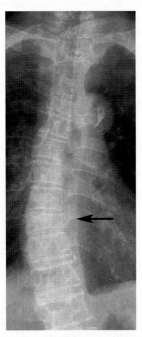

Fig. 20. Osteolytic metastasis. Anteroposterior radiograph of the thoracic spine shows a pathologic compression fracture of T10 vertebra caused by osteolytic metastasis (*arrow*).

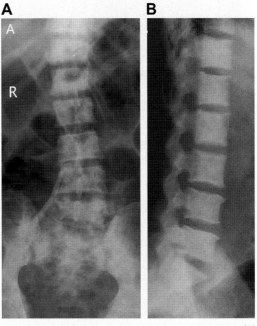

Fig. 21. Osteosclerotic metastases. Anteroposterior (*A*) and lateral (*B*) radiographs of the lumbosacral spine show diffuse sclerosis caused by extensive prostatic metastases. All the vertebrae, sacrum, and pelvis are involved.

center, decreases in size, and eventually resolves. For a mixed osteolytic-sclerotic lesion, a healing response to therapy is demonstrated as uniform lesional sclerosis, whereas increasing osteolysis indicates disease progression. Purely sclerotic lesions are more difficult to assess. Decrease in size or resolution after therapy signifies disease regression, whereas size increase and destruction implies progression. Compared with other imaging techniques, radiography is relatively insensitive in detecting bone metastases, especially subtle lesions. As a general rule, only lesions 2 cm or larger are apparent on radiographs. In addition, metastases to bone become apparent on radiographs only after the loss of more than 50% of the bone mineral content at the site of disease. In an osteoporotic skeleton, even larger lesions may not be revealed on conventional radiographs. Compared with radiographs, CT has superior lesion detection and characterization. It can also demonstrate soft tissue extension, and involvement of neurovascular structures. It is useful for assessment of radiographically negative areas. CT is also useful in guiding needle biopsy of lesions in bones with complex shapes, such as the vertebrae and the ilia (**Fig. 22**). Because considerable cortical destruction is required for visualization of a metastasis by CT, the sensitivity of CT in detecting early malignant bone involvement is relatively low.[49] In addition, skeletal coverage is limited with CT because of its relatively high radiation dose, which makes CT unsuitable as a screening tool.

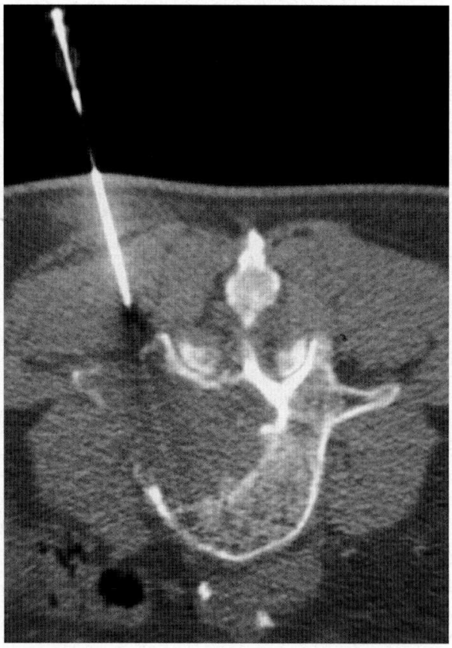

MR imaging has good spatial and contrast resolution. It is an optimal imaging modality for bone marrow assessment. MR imaging can detect an early intramedullary malignant lesion before there is any cortical destruction or reactive processes. On MR imaging, metastatic lesions are typically T1-hypointense and T2-isointense to T2-hyperintense, and usually enhance after administration of intravenous gadolinium–diethylenetriamine pentaacetic acid (**Fig. 23**). MR imaging is superior to CT in detection of malignant marrow infiltration. In addition, MR imaging has a better contrast resolution for visualizing soft tissue and spinal cord lesions, and is superior to CT in differentiating benign and malignant causes of spinal cord compression and vertebral compression fracture. MR imaging is less sensitive than CT for detecting cortical bone destruction, however, because cortical bone appears hypointense on both T1- and T2-weighted sequences. Nevertheless, differentiating benign from malignant compression vertebral fractures with MR imaging may be difficult, particularly if secondary criteria, such as posterior vertebral body bulging, signal intensity changes extending into the pedicle, and paravertebral soft tissue spread, are absent. On diffusion-weighted imaging, malignant fractures have been demonstrated to have a higher signal compared with benign fractures.[50,51] The apparent diffusion coefficients can also be useful in differentiating benign from malignant acute vertebral body compression fractures, with a much larger value in the former. This method is not useful in sclerotic metastases, however, which had a very low apparent diffusion coefficients value, and also fails to distinguish malignant fractures from tuberculous spondylitis.[52] Some authors have shown that MR imaging is more sensitive than ^{99m}Tc bone scintiscans in the detection of bone metastases.[53,54] It has been shown that whole-body MR imaging is a feasible alternative to bone scintiscans in evaluating the entire skeleton for metastatic disease.[55] Whole-body MR imaging with a 32-channel scanner has also been showed to be superior to positron emission tomography–CT in detection of skeletal metastases.[56] Long acquisition time is a concern, however, in whole-body MR imaging.

Tc-99m bone scintigraphy is an effective method of screening the whole body for bone metastases. Areas of increased uptake are seen where metastatic bone deposits induce increased

Fig. 22. CT-guided biopsy of vertebral metastasis. Axial CT image taken with the patient lying prone shows the biopsy needle being directed into an osteolytic lesion that has destroyed the pedicle and ipsilateral vertebral body.

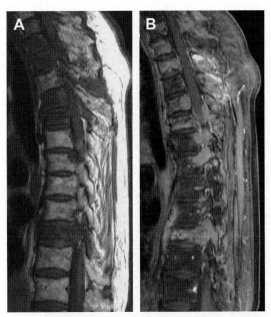

Fig. 23. MR imaging of vertebral metastases. (*A*) Sagittal T1-weighted MR image of the thoracic spine shows replacement of normal hyperintense fatty marrow by hypointense metastases in several vertebrae. (*B*) Corresponding sagittal postcontrast fat-saturated T1-weighted MR image shows enhancement at the metastatic sites. Note extensive posterior element involvement.

osteoblastic activity. The classical pattern of bone metastases consists of multiple randomly distributed focal lesions throughout the skeleton (**Fig. 24**). Other variant patterns that may lead to diagnostic difficulties include a solitary uptake area, superscan (diffuse uptake); cold lesions (minimal or no uptake); and the flare phenomenon. In general, bone scintigraphy is a sensitive but nonspecific technique. 18f-Fluorodeoxyglucose positron emission tomography has the ability to detect early increased glucose metabolism of tumor cells. Because 18f-fluorodeoxyglucose positron emission tomography is limited by its low spatial resolution, complementary CT or MR imaging is usually required for better lesion localization. It is also difficult to assess the presence of bone metastases in the vicinity of physiologic uptake sites. For instance, it is difficult to detect skull metastases because of the high physiologic 18f-fluorodeoxyglucose uptake in the adjacent brain. Single-photon emission CT or positron emission tomography–CT not only overcomes some of these limitations,[57,58] but also offers superior sensitivity and specificity.[59,60]

Myeloma

Myeloma is the commonest primary malignant neoplasm of the bone, originates from the bone marrow, and is a disease of the elderly. A total of 75% of patients are over the age of 50 years, with a peak in those aged over 80 years,[61] and a male predominance of 2:1. Fever, pain, backache, and weakness are common symptoms. Production of abnormal monoclonal immunoglobulins results in Bence Jones proteinuria. The erythrocyte sedimentation rate is raised and serum electrophoresis demonstrates IgG and IgA peaks. Because Bence Jones proteinuria is associated with chronic renal failure, intravenous contrast studies should always be performed with caution. In addition, amyloidosis is a frequent finding in patients with myeloma, and further contributes to renal parenchymal dysfunction. Calculi are often found because of elevated uric acid and calcium levels. The unequivocal diagnosis of myeloma is made when the following three criteria are satisfied: (1) a minimum 10% to 15% of a bone marrow aspirate demonstrates plasma cells, (2) radiographic survey demonstrates lytic lesions, and (3) monoclonal immunoglobulins are present in the urine or blood.

The preferred initial radiographic examination for the staging and diagnosis of myeloma remains the skeletal survey. Patients suspected of having multiple myeloma based on bone marrow aspirate results or hypergammaglobulinemia should undergo a radiographic skeletal survey. Conventionally, this skeletal survey consists of a lateral radiograph of the skull; anteroposterior and lateral

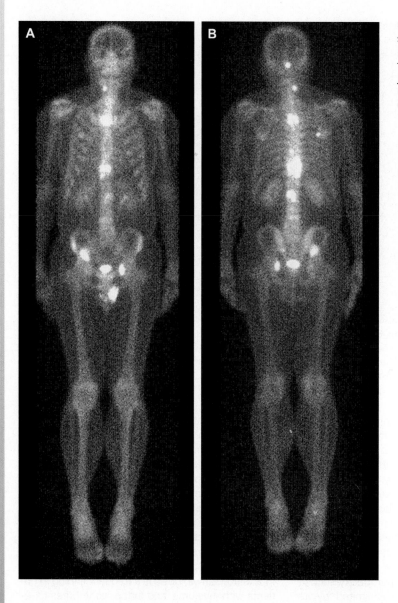

Fig. 24. Scintigraphy of widespread bone metastases. Tc-99m bone scintiscans taken in the anterior (*A*) and posterior (*B*) projections show multiple foci of radiotracer uptake caused by metastases.

radiographs of the spine; and anteroposterior radiographs of the pelvis, ribs, femora, and humeri. There is usually widespread involvement of the skeleton, with the axial skeleton and proximal ends of the limb bones being most commonly involved. It can present rarely as a solitary lesion as a plasmacytoma. The classical appearance of myelomatosis is that of multiple, well-circumscribed, lytic, punched-out, round lesions (**Fig. 25**). Because these lesions are within the medullary compartment, characteristic scalloping of the inner cortical margin can be observed. There is usually no sclerosis or periosteal reaction. Generalized osteopenia is an important presentation in the elderly, because it can be easily dismissed as senile osteoporosis. In the spine, multiple

compression fractures may be present, but it may be seen only as diffuse osteopenia. Myelomatosis should always be suspected in the elderly and appropriate hematologic tests initiated. Sclerotic lesions are rare, making up less than 1% of myeloma, and are known as "sclerosing myelomatosis." Compared with classical myeloma, sclerosing myelomatosis is commonly associated with polyneuropathy. In addition, patients tend to be younger, show fewer marrow plasma cells, and have a better prognosis. A rare variant of sclerosing myeloma is known as "'POEMS" syndrome (polyneuropathy, organomegaly, endocrinopathy, monoclonal gammopathy, and skin changes). The main differential diagnosis of osteolytic multiple myeloma is metastasis. Apart from marrow,

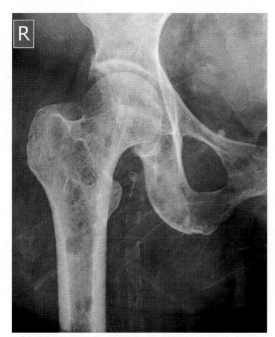

Fig. 25. Multiple myeloma. Anteroposterior radiograph of the right hip shows multiple "punched-out" osteolytic lesions.

blood, and urine tests, some radiologic features are useful in differentiating the two:

1. Destruction of pedicles by metastasis and not myeloma.
2. Destruction of intervertebral disks by myeloma and not metastasis.
3. Soft tissue mass is associated with bony lesion in myeloma and less so in metastasis.
4. Myeloma is common in the mandible, whereas metastasis is rare.
5. Negative bone scinticans are more common in myeloma.

CT depicts well the osseous involvement in myeloma. CT is not required in most patients because the standard skeletal surveys usually show most of the lesions that CT can detect. The single clinical situation in which CT may be of value is in cases in which the patient has bone pain and a negative radiograph.[62] CT can also guide percutaneous biopsies, especially of osseous or extraosseous lesions that are suspected to be plasmacytomas. MR imaging may be useful for evaluating multiple myeloma because of its superior soft tissue resolution. The typical appearance of a myeloma deposit is a round T1-hypointense and T2-hyperintense (relative to muscle) focus. Myeloma lesions tend to enhance with intravenous gadolinium–diethylenetriamine pentaacetic acid administration.

In addition, diffuse areas of replacement of the normal fatty marrow may be seen, resulting in large T1-hypointense regions. Bone scintiscans rely on osteoblastic activity (bone formation) for diagnosis. Myeloma is a disease that results in overactivity of osteoclasts and many lesions show normal or negative radionuclide uptake. Bone scintigraphy underestimates the extent and severity of disease, and is not used routinely.[63]

Lymphoma

Lymphoma is a malignancy of the lymphatic and reticuloendothelial system, which when secondarily involves bone usually indicates extensive or late (stage IV) disease. Histologically, lymphomas may be subdivided into non-Hodgkin or Hodgkin lymphomas. Both subtypes occur in a wide range of ages, but the incidence of non-Hodgkin lymphoma increases with age. Approximately half of all non-Hodgkin lymphomas now occur in individuals greater than or equal to 60 years of age.[64] Hodgkin lymphoma incidence rates, however, are higher in adolescents and young adults. Secondary involvement, however, is common in both Hodgkin and non-Hodgkin lymphoma. Rosenberg and colleagues[65] found osseous involvement in 16% of cases during the entire course of the disease. The most frequent areas of metastatic involvement are the spine, pelvis, and skull. In non-Hodgkin lymphoma, osteolytic metastatic lesions with permeative bone destruction are the most common radiologic findings. Cortical destruction is often associated with involvement of adjacent muscle and soft tissue. In Hodgkin disease, metastatic lesions can be either osteosclerotic, osteolytic, or of a mixed pattern, with sclerotic lesions accounting for up to 45% of all bone lesions.[66] Preservation of the cortex of the vertebral end plate is a feature favoring Hodgkin disease.

Primary lymphoma of bone is rare, accounting for less than 5% of all primary bone tumors,[67] and is usually a non-Hodgkin lymphoma, with Hodgkin disease being rare. It occurs in the second to seventh decades, with a peak occurrence from 45 to 75 years. A slight male predominance is observed. The definition of primary lymphoma of bone continues to be debated. Most authors exclude disseminated or recurrent disease in which the bone is only one of many sites of involvement. To be considered primary lymphoma of bone, the following criteria should be met:[68]

1. Histologic documentation of lymphoma in the bone
2. Solitary bone lesion or multiple skeletal lesions with no prior involvement of lymph nodes or other lymphoid tissue

3. No lymph node involvement or only involvement of regional lymph nodes
4. Soft tissue extension from the bone lesion is acceptable, and the involved soft tissue may be sampled to document malignant lymphoma

In primary lymphoma of the bone, the radiographic features include the following:[67]

1. Lytic lesions with permeative lytic pattern being the most common. Mixed pattern is also encountered, whereas sclerotic lesions are rare.
2. Metadiaphyseal location is the most common. Long bones are more commonly involved than flat bones and most commonly in the femur and tibia. Extension across a joint rarely is seen.
3. Periosteal reaction has been reported in about 60% of cases and may be lamellated (onion-peel appearance). Broken or interrupted periosteal new bone is believed to be a helpful radiographic sign that indicates a poorer prognosis.
4. Soft tissue mass is present in about 50% of cases and is best demonstrated on MR imaging. Presence of a soft tissue mass and cortical breakthrough also indicates an aggressive lesion. An imaging pattern, although not specific but suggestive of primary bone lymphoma, is the presence of soft tissue without large areas of cortical destruction.[67]
5. Sequestrum formation has been reported in 11% to 16% of patients with primary lymphoma of bone, and may help differentiate it from most other diagnostic possibilities.[69]

Primary bone lymphoma can present with near absence of detectable abnormalities on radiographs. Cases with remarkably normal-appearing radiographs may show striking abnormalities on bone scintiscans and MR images. As a result, in patients with symptoms but negative radiographic findings, further assessment with a second, more sensitive modality, such as scintigraphy or MR imaging, is required.[70] Findings in bone scintigraphy are nonspecific, with increased uptake usually noted. Bone scintigraphy is also useful in exclusion of multiple myeloma, because the latter usually shows poor radionuclide uptake. MR imaging signal intensities of primary bone lymphoma are nonspecific, with typically homogeneously T1-isointense to T1-hypointense signal, variable T2 signal intensity, and enhancement after intravenous gadolinium–diethylenetriamine pentaacetic acid.[67,71]

Sarcomas

In the elderly population, most sarcomas are usually secondary to a pre-existing disorder of bone,

such as Paget's disease. Radiation-induced sarcoma may arise from areas of normal bone exposed to radiation or benign conditions treated by radiation, such as fibrous dysplasia or giant cell tumor. Generally, at least 3000 rad is administered within a 4-week period before a sarcoma can develop. The latency period varies from a range 4 to 40 years, with an average of 11 years. Osteosarcoma, malignant fibrous histiocytoma, and fibrosarcoma are the most frequently reported secondary tumors.[72,73]

Chondrosarcoma

Chondrosarcoma is the second most frequent primary malignant tumor of bone, representing approximately 25% of all primary osseous neoplasms. Chondrosarcoma is a malignant tumor of cartilaginous origin, in which the tumor matrix formation is chondroid in nature. Because of the chondroid nature of the tumor, calcifications are a common feature. Chondrosarcomas are classified as central (originating within the intramedullary canal) or peripheral. Juxtacortical lesions may be rarely seen. Lesions are classified as primary when they arise de novo, or as secondary when they occur within a pre-existing lesion, such as an enchondroma or osteochondroma. Tumors are further categorized by grade. Grade 1 represents the least aggressive in terms of histologic features, and grade 3 represents the most aggressive. Most chondrosarcomas are pathologically classified as conventional. Other subgroups (clear cell, mesenchymal, and dedifferentiated) are rare. Conventional and clear cell chondrosarcomas are less aggressive than the mesenchymal and dedifferentiated tumors, which are associated with poor prognosis. Secondary chondrosarcomas are usually of low-grade malignancy, carrying a prognosis that is more favorable than the conventional type.

Most tumors arise in patients older than 40 years and increase with age, peaking in the geriatric age population.[74] Patients with dedifferentiated chondrosarcoma are older than those with conventional lesions, usually between 50 and 70 years old, with an average age of approximately 60 years.[75,76] The risk of chondrosarcoma is increased in people with enchondromatosis syndromes and in those with hereditary multiple exostosis (ie, diaphyseal aclasis). These secondary tumors tend to present earlier than the geriatric population (20–40 years of age).[74] Most conventional chondrosarcomas are slow-growing and often discovered incidentally. If symptomatic, pain is the usual complaint and often long-standing. Chondrosarcomas most commonly involve the pelvic bones, femur, humerus, ribs, scapula, sternum, or spine. In tubular bones, the metaphysis is the most commonly affected in long bones and more commonly proximal. Chondrosarcoma is rare in the hands and feet and, if present, is usually a complication of the enchondromatosis syndrome. Extraskeletal chondrosarcomas are far less common than their intraosseous counterparts. The histologic types of lesions that account for extraskeletal chondrosarcoma are myxoid, mesenchymal, and, very rarely, low grade. Extraskeletal myxoid chondrosarcoma is the most common histologic type, with the mean age at presentation being approximately 50 years. Most lesions arise in the extremities with the thigh being the single most common location. Most lesions are in the deep soft tissue. The more aggressive mesenchymal tumor is uncommon in the geriatric age group. Imaging features are similar to their intraosseous counterparts.

On radiographs, less aggressive chondrosarcoma appears as an osteolytic expanded lesion in the medulla. There may be thickening of the cortex and characteristic endosteal scalloping (**Fig. 26**). Endosteal scalloping greater than two thirds of the normal thickness of the long bone cortex suggests chondrosarcoma rather than the benign enchondroma. Extensive, longitudinal, endosteal scalloping in long bone lesions (greater than two thirds of lesion length) is also more suggestive of conventional chondrosarcoma than enchondroma. Popcornlike, annular, or comma-shaped calcifications are seen and a soft tissue mass may sometimes be present in conventional chondrosarcoma. Aggressive bony destruction and presence of a large soft tissue mass raise suspicion of more aggressive cell types. Aggressive tumors also contain irregular calcifications, and often have large areas showing no calcification at all. On CT, chondroid matrix calcification is easily appreciated (see **Fig. 26**). Endosteal scalloping and cortical destruction are also more easily seen on CT than on radiographs. Low-grade conventional chondrosarcomatous elements typically demonstrate low attenuation, reflecting the high water content of hyaline cartilage. CT performed after intravenous contrast administration demonstrates mild peripheral rim and septal enhancement. Higher-grade lesions may show higher CT attenuation, isodense to that of muscle, and more prominent diffuse or nodular contrast enhancement, caused by increased cellularity and resultant reduced water content. CT can also be used to guide percutaneous biopsy, and it is the modality of choice for investigating possible pulmonary metastatic disease.

MR imaging, by virtue of its high tissue contrast capability, provides the best technique for evaluation of the cartilage cap thickness and the relationship of the lesion to the surrounding tissues. It is the imaging method of choice for patients with suspected malignant transformation, independent of the anatomic site of the lesion.[77] On MR imaging, conventional chondrosarcomas demonstrate the lobular architecture typical of all hyaline cartilage neoplasms. The lobulated nonmineralized chondroid lesions show T1-hypointensity and T2-hyperintensity, again a reflection of the high water content of hyaline cartilage. The lobules are commonly separated by low signal intensity septa. Areas of matrix calcification are shown as signal voids on all sequences, but small amounts may not be identifiable. The presence of soft tissue involvement essentially excludes the possible diagnosis of enchondroma. The presence of septa of low signal intensity on T2-weighted images and septal or ring-and-arc enhancement on T1-weighted images has been reported to represent additional criteria that suggest the diagnosis of a low-grade chondrosarcoma (see **Fig. 26**). These enhancement patterns are discussed controversially in the literature, however, because they may also be seen in benign cartilage-forming tumors. Use of dynamic contrast-enhanced MR imaging and subtraction techniques may be helpful in the differentiation of benign from malignant lesions, with vascularity of the tumor being used as a criterion for differentiation. Unlike conventional chondrosarcoma, myxoid chondrosarcoma frequently contains hemorrhage, which appears as areas of high signal intensity on all MR imaging pulse sequences, particularly in the large associated soft tissue components.[78] In aggressive lesions, high-grade noncartilaginous areas demonstrate variable T2 signal intensity, ranging from low to high (although lower in signal intensity than the conventional chondrosarcomatous component) and there is a more prominent diffuse or nodular contrast enhancement (see **Fig. 26**). This can result in a biphasic pattern, with a clear demarcation seen between the hyperintense low-grade tumor and the comparative hypointense high-grade tumor. Tumor necrosis and large soft tissue mass are also indicators of aggressiveness.[78] On bone scintigraphy, central chondrosarcomas typically show significantly increased uptake of the radioisotope on bone scintiscans, but cannot reliably differentiate between chondrosarcoma and enchondroma. The absence of increased uptake makes malignancy highly unlikely.[79,80]

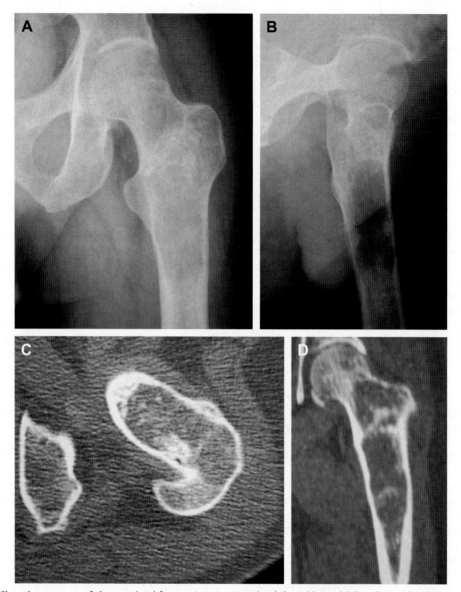

Fig. 26. Chondrosarcoma of the proximal femur. Anteroposterior (*A*) and lateral (*B*) radiographs show an ill-marginated osteolytic lesion in the proximal left femur, with endosteal scalloping and areas of internal calcifications. Axial (*C*) and reformatted (*D*) coronal CT images better show the lesion extent and irregularly calcified matrix. Axial T1-weighted (*E*), fat-saturated T2-weighted (*F*), and postcontrast fat-saturated T1-weighted (*G*) MR images of the femoral neck show a lesion that is largely T1-hypointense; markedly T2-hyperintense; and has peripheral, septal, and nodular enhancement. The histologic diagnosis was dedifferentiated chondrosarcoma.

Chordoma

Chordomas are relatively rare malignant tumors that arise from embryonic remnants of the primitive notochord. Consequently, these tumors occur almost exclusively in the midline of the axial skeleton. Chordomas are considered to be locally invasive, but rarely metastasize.[81,82] Chordomas account for 1% of intracranial tumors and 4% of all primary bone tumors.[83] They are the commonest primary malignant bone tumor in the sacrum. Most chordomas occur in the sacrococcygeal region, with the other common location being the spheno-occipital region. They may occur at any age but usually affect patients between 30 and 60 years of age, and spinal chordomas show a male predominance.[84] The most characteristic appearance of intracranial chordoma is of a centrally located soft tissue mass arising from the

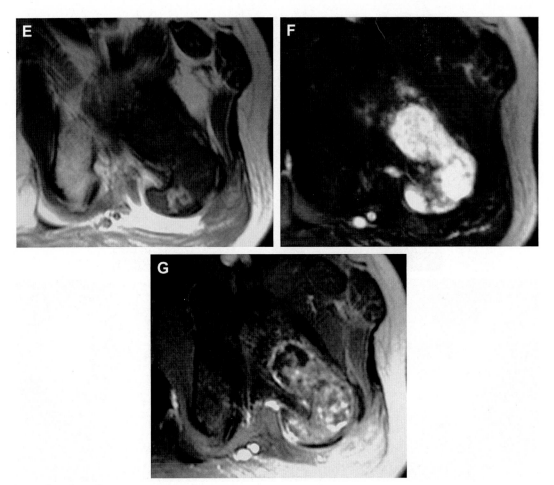

Fig. 26. (*continued*)

clivus, and causing adjacent bone destruction and lateral spread to the petrous apex. A typical appearance of sacral chordomas is the destruction of several sacral vertebrae associated with a soft tissue mass anterior to the sacrum, typically involving the fourth and fifth sacral segments (**Fig. 27**). The size of the presacral mass averages 10 cm, and may displace the rectum and bladder.[85] Regional lymph nodes are usually involved in sacral chordomas.

On radiographs, chordomas appear as a highly destructive lesion with irregular scalloped borders. Bone sclerosis and matrix calcifications are sometimes present on radiographs. On CT, the tumor appears homogeneously isodense to muscle, and enhances heterogeneously. Calcification is common but may be difficult to differentiate from sequestered bone fragments (see **Fig. 27**). Low-density areas may be present and probably represent the myxoid and gelatinous material.[86] On MR imaging, chordomas are T1-hypointense to T1-isointense and prominently T2-hyperintense, with these features likely to reflect the high fluid content of vacuolated cellular components. Small T1-hyperintense foci may sometimes be seen, representing intratumoral hemorrhage or a mucous. Hypointense septations that separate T2-hyperintense lobules are commonly seen, corresponding to the multilobulated gross morphologic features of the tumor. T2-weighted images are also excellent for differentiating tumor from adjacent neural structures. Chordomas have variable enhancement and may have a characteristic honeycomb pattern.[86,87] Occasionally, enhancement may be slight or even absent.

INFECTION

Infection of the bones and joints present in the elderly in a similar fashion as in younger patients. Similar infective organisms affect patients in all age groups, without any particular predilection, although the elderly do have an increased incidence of infection from nosocomial organisms, caused

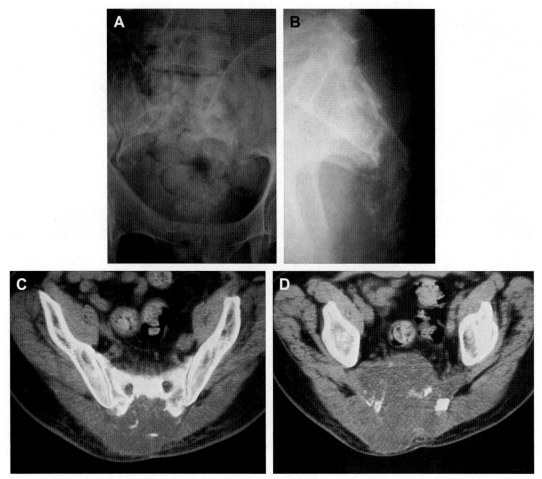

Fig. 27. Sacral chordoma. Anteroposterior (*A*) and lateral (*B*) radiographs show a large expanded osteolytic lesion with amorphous internal calcifications. (*C, D*) Axial CT images of the lower sacrum show a large soft tissue component that extends anteriorly into the presacral space and posteriorly into the gluteal muscles.

by institutionalization and hospitalization. Elderly patients are also more prone to infection, and have poorer outcomes because of comorbidities and ageing.

Osteomyelitis

Osteomyelitis is a common infectious disease among elderly patients. Older adults are predisposed to osteomyelitis, either because of an increased incidence of disorders that predispose to osteomyelitis (eg, diabetes mellitus, peripheral vascular disease, and poor dentition) or because of surgical procedures frequently performed in the elderly population (eg, dental extractions, open heart surgery, and prosthetic joint replacement). Elderly persons frequently fall, which may result in closed or open bone trauma. Acute osteomyelitis may be acquired hematogeneously after closed trauma, and is usually caused by

Staphylococcus aureus. In acute hematogeneous osteomyelitis, the bacteria reach the metaphyseal blood vessels of bone to initiate the infectious process. Subacute osteomyelitis in the elderly population is most commonly caused by vertebral osteomyelitis (**Fig. 28**) or osteomyelitis associated with prosthetic joint replacement. Vertebral osteomyelitis may occur through hematogeneous dissemination from a distant infected source, most commonly *S aureus*. Rarely, vertebral osteomyelitis may occur iatrogenically as a complication of disk space injections or spinal surgery.

Attempts should be made to differentiate pyogenic from tuberculous vertebral osteomyelitis, which is also common among elderly patients. In general, both pyogenic and tuberculous vertebral osteomyelitis destroy adjacent vertebral bodies and involve the disk space. Features that favor a pyogenic etiology of vertebral osteomyelitis include rapid rate of disk space destruction, lower

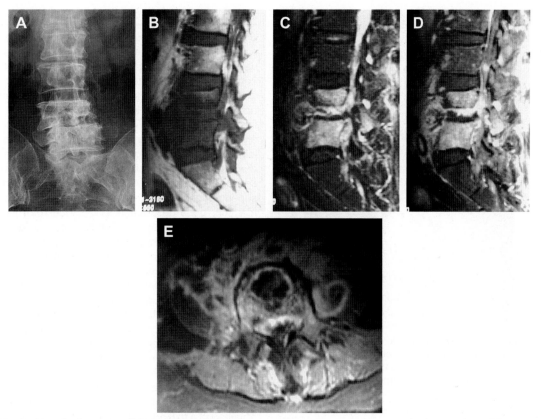

Fig. 28. Vertebral osteomyelitis and diskitis. (*A*) Anteroposterior radiograph shows marked narrowing of the L4-L5 disk space, with mild subluxation, end plate destruction, and L4 and L5 vertebral body sclerosis. Sagittal T1-weighted (*B*), STIR (*C*), and postcontrast fat-saturated T1-weighted (*D*) MR images show destruction of the lower L4 vertebral body with extensive marrow signal changes that are T1-hypointense, T2-hyperintense, and prominently enhancement within L4 and L5 vertebral bodies. The L4-L5 disk is also T2-hypertinese and strongly enhancing. (*E*) Axial postcontrast fat-saturated T1-weighted MR image taken through L4 vertebral body shows extensive soft tissue involvement, with bilateral psoas abscesses.

incidence of abscess formation, less bony changes, and usually limited to a single disk space or adjoining vertebra. In contrast, tuberculous osteomyelitis has a slow and indolent process, a higher incidence of abscess formation, and more bone destruction. Extension into the psoas muscle, forming a "cold" abscess, is also common in tuberculous infection. Typically, but not always, tuberculous osteomyelitis involves more than two contiguous vertebral bodies or disk spaces.

Chronic osteomyelitis is an indolent, slow process with few systemic symptoms and has duration of at least 6 weeks. Chronic osteomyelitis may be associated with performance of certain surgical procedures (eg, sternal osteomyelitis after open heart surgery); occurs secondary to poor dentition or dental extraction (mandibular osteomyelitis); and most commonly may be associated with systemic disorders (eg, peripheral vascular disease and diabetes mellitus). Patients with

diabetes mellitus who have chronic, deep-penetrating foot ulcers or a chronic draining sinus tract of the foot should be considered as having chronic osteomyelitis, until proved otherwise (**Fig. 29**). Elderly patients who are unable to turn themselves over in bed frequently develop pressure sores or decubitus ulcers. Superficial decubitus ulcers (ie, stage 1 or 2) are not associated with osteomyelitis. Decubitus ulcers of the deepest variety (ie, stage 3 or 4) are often complicated by osteomyelitis. Chronic osteomyelitis is usually present when bone is visible in a long-standing deep decubitus ulcer.

Radiographs are usually unhelpful diagnostically in the early phases of acute hematogeneous osteomyelitis. The earliest radiographic signs are usually encountered within 24 to 48 hours, consisting of nonspecific soft tissue edema and loss of fascial planes. A destructive osteolytic lesion may be seen within the first 7 to 10 days of infection. Within 2 to 6 weeks, progressive cortical and medullary

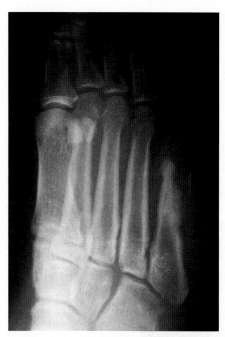

Fig. 29. Chronic osteomyelitis in diabetic foot. Frontal radiograph shows previous amputation of the 5th ray, with sclerosis, irregularity, and deformity of the remnant metatarsal. Small adjacent bony fragments are present.

destruction with periosteal reaction is noted. By 6 to 8 weeks, chronic osteomyelitis is established, and sequestra surrounded by a dense involucrum can be seen. Bone scintigraphy is more useful, yielding positive results within the first 2 or 3 days in acute osteomyelitis. Nuclear medicine studies used in the work-up of osteomyelitis include three-phase Tc-99m bone, gallium 67, and labeled leukocyte scintigraphy. The overall accuracy of bone gallium 67 imaging is about 65% to 80%.[88] Combined leukocyte-marrow imaging has an overall accuracy rate of about 90%.[88] The earliest sign of osteomyelitis at US is nonspecific soft tissue swelling adjacent to the affected bone. Although a diagnosis of osteomyelitis cannot be established on the basis of demonstration of such fluid collections at US, the main role of US lies in the performance of immediate US-guided fluid aspiration to obtain specimens for microbiologic examination.[89] Typical MR imaging findings within the bone marrow include ill-defined, hypointense signal on T1-weighted images, hyperintense signal on T2-weighted, or short tau inversion recovery MR images, in keeping with marrow edema or pus. Enhancement of the affected area is seen,[90] and intravenous contrast administration is also useful in the evaluation of associated soft tissue infection (see **Fig. 28**).[91]

Septic Arthritis

Similar to osteomyelitis, elderly patients are also susceptible to septic arthritis.[92] In addition, advanced age is also a risk factor for poor outcome.[93] Imaging is not the primary means of diagnosing septic arthritis. Joint fluid aspiration and evaluation are the keys to diagnosis. The earliest radiographic findings are soft tissue swelling around the joint and a widened joint space from joint effusion. With progression of the disease, radiographs reveal joint space narrowing as articular cartilage is destroyed. Radiographic findings of superimposed osteomyelitis, such as periosteal reaction, bone destruction, and sequestrum formation, may develop. CT findings are similar to those seen on radiographs. US is limited in the evaluation of septic arthritis. It is a sensitive modality for the detection of joint effusions, but is not reliable in characterizing the effusion or its cause.[94] Scintigraphy, although not very specific, remains the most rapid method for determination of the site and distribution of joint infection. The simplest procedures are three- or four-phase bone scanning using Tc-99m methylenediphosphonate. Early phase (blood flow) and later (blood pool) images show increased activity at the joint and on both sides of the affected area. Delayed images obtained at 4 to 6 hours demonstrate continued increased activity in the bone with associated osteomyelitis.[95]

MR imaging findings in septic joints include synovial thickening and enhancement, perisynovial edema, and joint effusions. Infected and noninfected joint effusions have the same signal intensity characteristics and cannot be reliably distinguished by using MR imaging, although synovial enhancement and the presence of a joint effusion have been reported to have the highest correlation with the clinical diagnosis of a septic joint.[96] Areas of abnormal marrow changes (T1-hypointense and T2-hyperintense) together with intravenous enhancement may represent reactive marrow edema or associated osteomyelitis. Often, it is difficult to differentiate between the two, although diffuse abnormal marrow signal seen on T1-weighted images has the highest association with concomitant osteomyelitis.[96]

SUMMARY

Rising life expectancy and worldwide population ageing is increasing demand on medical resources to meet the needs of the geriatric population. The etiology and outcome of bone diseases in the elderly are very much related to the normal process of ageing and pre-existing comorbidities. Falls are common in the elderly and concurrent osteoporosis results in frequent low-impact fractures. Imaging is important not only in the diagnosis and assessment of fracture, but also the exclusion of any pathologic fracture from underlying malignancy or metastasis, which is also common in the elderly. Unavoidable degeneration of the joints eventually occurs in the elderly and results in pain and disability. Degeneration of the spine can lead to neurologic symptoms and imaging is important in confirming the level and severity of anatomic compromise, enabling accurate presurgical planning. With better treatment, care, and increased life expectancy, patients with chronic inflammatory joint diseases will have to cope with the chronic manifestations and disabilities. Imaging is important in monitoring disease progression, response to treatment, and diagnosing complications.

REFERENCES

1. Day JC. Population projections of the United States by age, sex, race, and Hispanic origin: 1995 to 2050. Washington, DC: US Bureau of the Census; 1996. p. 25–1130.
2. Eliastam M. Elderly patients in the emergency department. Ann Emerg Med 1989;18:1222–9.
3. Graafmans WC, Ooms ME, Hofstee HM, et al. Falls in the elderly: a prospective study of risk factors and risk profiles. Am J Epidemiol 1996;143:1129–36.
4. Nevitt MC, Cummings SR, Hudes ES. Risk factors for injurious falls: a prospective study. J Gerontol 1991; 46:M164–70.
5. Pentecost RL, Murray RA, Brindley HH. Fatigue, insufficiency, and pathologic fractures. JAMA 1964; 187:1001–4.
6. Quek ST, Peh WCG. Radiology of osteoporosis. Semin Musculoskelet Radiol 2002;6:197–206.
7. Harris WH, Heaney RP. Skeletal renewal and metabolic bone disease. N Engl J Med 1969;280:303–11.
8. Mayo-Smith W, Rosenthal DI. Radiographic appearance of osteopenia. Radiol Clin North Am 1991;29: 37–47.
9. Nordell E, Jarnlo GB, Jetsen C, et al. Accidental falls and related fractures in 65–74 year olds: a retrospective study of 332 patients. Acta Orthop Scand 2000; 71:175–9.
10. Gullberg B, Johnell O, Kanis JA. World-wide projections for hip fracture. Osteoporos Int 1997;7:407–13.
11. Oden A, Dawson A, Dere W, et al. Lifetime risk of hip fractures is underestimated. Osteoporos Int 1998;8: 599–603.
12. Barnes R, Brown JT, Garden RS, et al. Subcapital fractures of the femur: a prospective review. J Bone Joint Surg Br 1976;58:2–24.
13. Frihagen F, Nordsletten L, Tariq R, et al. MRI diagnosis of occult hip fractures. Acta Orthop 2005;76: 524–30.
14. Chana R, Noorani A, Ashwood N, et al. The role of MRI in the diagnosis of proximal femoral fractures in the elderly. Injury 2006;37:185–9.
15. Legroux Gerot I, Demondion X, Louville AB, et al. Subchondral fractures of the femoral head: a review of seven cases. Joint Bone Spine 2004;71:131–5.
16. Rafii M, Mitnick H, Klug J, et al. Insufficiency fracture of the femoral head: MR imaging in three patients. AJR Am J Roentgenol 1997;168:159–63.
17. Alost T, Waldrop RD. Profile of geriatric pelvic fractures presenting to the emergency department. Am J Emerg Med 1997;15:576–8.
18. O'Brien DP, Luchette FA, Pereira SJ, et al. Pelvic fracture in the elderly is associated with increased mortality. Surgery 2002;132:710–4.
19. Kiuru MJ, Pihlajamaki HK, Ahovuo JA. Fatigue stress injuries of the pelvic bones and proximal femur: evaluation with MR imaging. Eur Radiol 2003;13:605–11.
20. Balseiro J, Brower AC, Ziessman HA. Scintigraphic diagnosis of sacral fractures. AJR Am J Roentgenol 1987;148:111–3.
21. Davies AM, Evans NS, Struthers GR. Parasymphyseal and associated insufficiency fractures of the pelvis and sacrum. Br J Radiol 1988;61:103–8.
22. Peh WCG, Khong PL, Yin Y, et al. Imaging of pelvic insufficiency fractures. Radiographics 1996;16: 335–48.
23. Grangier C, Garcia J, Howarth NR, et al. Role of MRI in the diagnosis of insufficiency fractures of the sacrum and acetabular roof. Skeletal Radiol 1997;26: 517–24.
24. Peh WCG. Intrafracture fluid: a new diagnostic sign of insufficiency fractures of the sacrum and ilium. Br J Radiol 2000;73:895–8.
25. Peh WCG, Cheng KC, Ho WY, et al. Transient bone marrow oedema: a variant pattern of sacral insufficiency fractures. Australas Radiol 1998;42:102–5.
26. Lyles KW. Management of patients with vertebral compression fractures. Pharmacotherapy 1999;19:21–4.
27. Lee YL, Yip KM. The osteoporotic spine. Clin Orthop Relat Res 1996;(323):91–7.
28. Peh WCG, Gilula LA. Percutaneous vertebroplasty: an update. Semin Ultrasound CT MRI 2005;26: 52–64.
29. Greenspan A, Norman A, Tchang FK. Tooth sign in patellar degenerative disease. J Bone Joint Surg Am 1977;59:483–5.
30. Chakravarty KK, Webley M. Disorders of the shoulder: an often unrecognised cause of disability in elderly people. BMJ 1990;300:848–9.
31. Hattrup SJ. Rotator cuff repair: relevance of patient age. J Shoulder Elbow Surg 1995;4:95–100.
32. Wiener SN, Seitz WH Jr. Sonography of the shoulder in patients with tears of the rotator cuff: accuracy

and value for selecting surgical options. AJR Am J Roentgenol 1993;160:103–7.

33. Burk DL Jr, Karasick D, Kurtz AB, et al. Rotator cuff tears: prospective comparison of MR imaging with arthrography, sonography, and surgery. AJR Am J Roentgenol 1989;153:87–92.

34. Zlatkin MB, Iannotti JP, Roberts MC, et al. Rotator cuff tears: diagnostic performance of MR imaging. Radiology 1989;172:223–9.

35. Tirman PF, Palmer WE, Feller JF. MR arthrography of the shoulder. Magn Reson Imaging Clin N Am 1997; 5:811–39.

36. Palmer WE, Brown JH, Rosenthal DI. Rotator cuff: evaluation with fat-suppressed MR arthrography. Radiology 1993;188:683–7.

37. Biyani A, Andersson GB. Low back pain: pathophysiology and management. J Am Acad Orthop Surg 2004;12:106–15.

38. Jensen MC, Brant-Zawadzki MN, Obuchowski N, et al. Magnetic resonance imaging of the lumbar spine in people without back pain. N Engl J Med 1994;331:69–73.

39. Peh WCG. Provocative discography: current status. Biomed Imaging Interv J 2005;1:e2.

40. Willems PC, Jacobs W, Duinkerke ES, et al. Lumbar discography: should we use prophylactic antibiotics? A study of 435 consecutive discograms and a systematic review of the literature. J Spinal Disord Tech 2004;17:243–7.

41. Cammisa M, De Serio A, Guglielmi G. Diffuse idiopathic skeletal hyperostosis. Eur J Radiol 1998; 27(Suppl 1):S7–11.

42. Resnick D, Guerra J Jr, Robinson CA, et al. Association of diffuse idiopathic skeletal hyperostosis (DISH) and calcification and ossification of the posterior longitudinal ligament. AJR Am J Roentgenol 1978;131:1049–53.

43. Deal CL, Meenan RF, Goldenberg DL, et al. The clinical features of elderly-onset rheumatoid arthritis: a comparison with younger-onset disease of similar duration. Arthritis Rheum 1985;28:987–94.

44. Healey LA. Rheumatoid arthritis in the elderly. Clin Rheum Dis 1986;12:173–9.

45. Halla JT, Fallahi S, Hardin JG. Small joint involvement: a systematic roentgenographic study in rheumatoid arthritis. Ann Rheum Dis 1986;45:327–30.

46. Weissman BN, Aliabadi P, Weinfeld MS, et al. Prognostic features of atlantoaxial subluxation in rheumatoid arthritis patients. Radiology 1982;144:745–51.

47. Kudo H, Iwano K, Yoshizawa H. Cervical cord compression due to extradural granulation tissue in rheumatoid arthritis: a review of five cases. J Bone Joint Surg Br 1984;66:426–30.

48. Johnston AD. Pathology of metastatic tumors in bone. Clin Orthop Relat Res 1970;73:8–32.

49. Muindi J, Coombes RC, Golding S, et al. The role of computed tomography in the detection of bone metastases in breast cancer patients. Br J Radiol 1983;56:233–6.

50. Baur A, Stabler A, Bruning R, et al. Diffusion-weighted MR imaging of bone marrow: differentiation of benign versus pathologic compression fractures. Radiology 1998;207:349–56.

51. Spuentrup E, Buecker A, Adam G, et al. Diffusion-weighted MR imaging for differentiation of benign fracture edema and tumor infiltration of the vertebral body. AJR Am J Roentgenol 2001;176:351–8.

52. Chan JH, Peh WCG, Tsui EY, et al. Acute vertebral body compression fractures: discrimination between benign and malignant causes using apparent diffusion coefficients. Br J Radiol 2002;75:207–14.

53. Algra PR, Bloem JL, Tissing H, et al. Detection of vertebral metastases: comparison between MR imaging and bone scintigraphy. Radiographics 1991; 11:219–32.

54. Aitchison FA, Poon FW, Hadley MD, et al. Vertebral metastases and an equivocal bone scan: value of magnetic resonance imaging. Nucl Med Commun 1992;13:429–31.

55. Steinborn MM, Heuck AF, Tiling R, et al. Whole-body bone marrow MRI in patients with metastatic disease to the skeletal system. J Comput Assist Tomogr 1999;23:123–9.

56. Schmidt GP, Schoenberg SO, Schmid R, et al. Screening for bone metastases: whole-body MRI using a 32-channel system versus dual-modality PET-CT. Eur Radiol 2007;17:939–49.

57. Keidar Z, Israel O, Krausz Y. SPECT/CT in tumor imaging: technical aspects and clinical applications. Semin Nucl Med 2003;33:205–18.

58. Kostakoglu L, Hardoff R, Mirtcheva R, et al. PET-CT fusion imaging in differentiating physiologic from pathologic FDG uptake. Radiographics 2004;24: 1411–31.

59. Even-Sapir E, Metser U, Flusser G, et al. Assessment of malignant skeletal disease: initial experience with 18F-fluoride PET/CT and comparison between 18F-fluoride PET and 18F-fluoride PET/CT. J Nucl Med 2004;45:272–8.

60. Even-Sapir E. Imaging of malignant bone involvement by morphologic, scintigraphic, and hybrid modalities. J Nucl Med 2005;46:1356–67.

61. Singer CR. ABC of clinical haematology: multiple myeloma and related conditions. BMJ 1997;314: 960–3.

62. Schreiman JS, McLeod RA, Kyle RA, et al. Multiple myeloma: evaluation by CT. Radiology 1985;154:483–6.

63. Ludwig H, Kumpan W, Sinzinger H. Radiography and bone scintigraphy in multiple myeloma: a comparative analysis. Br J Radiol 1982;55:173–81.

64. Namboodiri KK, Harris RE. Hematopoietic and lymphoproliferative cancer among male veterans using the Veterans Administration Medical System. Cancer 1991;68:1123–30.

65. Rosenberg SA, Diamond HD, Jaslowitz B, et al. Lymphosarcoma: a review of 1269 cases. Medicine (Baltimore) 1961;40:31–84.

66. Mulligan ME, McRae GA, Murphey MD. Imaging features of primary lymphoma of bone. AJR Am J Roentgenol 1999;173:1691–7.

67. Malloy PC, Fishman EK, Magid D. Lymphoma of bone, muscle, and skin: CT findings. AJR Am J Roentgenol 1992;159:805–9.

68. Coley BL, Higinbotham NL, Groesbeck HP. Primary reticulum-cell sarcoma of bone: summary of 37 cases. Radiology 1950;55:641–58.

69. Mulligan ME, Kransdorf MJ. Sequestra in primary lymphoma of bone: prevalence and radiologic features. AJR Am J Roentgenol 1993;160:1245–8.

70. Krishnan A, Shirkhoda A, Tehranzadeh J, et al. Primary bone lymphoma: radiographic-MR imaging correlation. Radiographics 2003;23:1371–83.

71. White LM, Schweitzer ME, Khalili K, et al. MR imaging of primary lymphoma of bone: variability of T2-weighted signal intensity. AJR Am J Roentgenol 1998;170:1243–7.

72. Smith J. Radiation-induced sarcoma of bone: clinical and radiographic findings in 43 patients irradiated for soft tissue neoplasms. Clin Radiol 1982; 33:205–21.

73. Lorigan JG, Libshitz HI, Peuchot M. Radiation-induced sarcoma of bone: CT findings in 19 cases. AJR Am J Roentgenol 1989;153:791–4.

74. Larsson SE, Lorentzon R. The incidence of malignant primary bone tumours in relation to age, sex and site: a study of osteogenic sarcoma, chondrosarcoma and Ewing's sarcoma diagnosed in Sweden from 1958 to 1968. J Bone Joint Surg Br 1974; 56B:534–40.

75. Frassica FJ, Unni KK, Beabout JW, et al. Dedifferentiated chondrosarcoma: a report of the clinicopathological features and treatment of seventy-eight cases. J Bone Joint Surg Am 1986;68:1197–205.

76. Mercuri M, Picci P, Campanacci L, et al. Dedifferentiated chondrosarcoma. Skeletal Radiol 1995;24: 409–16.

77. Shah ZK, Peh WCG, Wong Y, et al. Sarcomatous transformation in diaphyseal aclasis. Australas Radiol 2007;51:110–9.

78. Murphey MD, Walker EA, Wilson AJ, et al. From the archives of the AFIP. Imaging of primary chondrosarcoma: radiologic-pathologic correlation. Radiographics 2003;23:1245–78.

79. Hudson TM, Chew FS, Manaster BJ. Radionuclide bone scanning of medullary chondrosarcoma. AJR Am J Roentgenol 1982;139:1071–6.

80. Murphey MD, Flemming DJ, Boyea SR, et al. Enchondroma versus chondrosarcoma in the appendicular skeleton: differentiating features. Radiographics 1998;18:1213–37.

81. McMaster ML, Goldstein AM, Bromley CM, et al. Chordoma: incidence and survival patterns in the United States, 1973–1995. Cancer Causes Control 2001;12:1–11.

82. Soo MY. Chordoma: review of clinicoradiological features and factors affecting survival. Australas Radiol 2001;45:427–34.

83. Dahlin DC, Maccarty CS. Chordoma. Cancer 1952; 5:1170–8.

84. Meyer JE, Lepke RA, Lindfors KK, et al. Chordomas: their CT appearance in the cervical, thoracic and lumbar spine. Radiology 1984;153:693–6.

85. Peh WCG, Koh WL, Kwek JW, et al. Imaging of painful solitary lesions of the sacrum. Australas Radiol 2007;51:507–15.

86. Erdem E, Angtuaco EC, Van Hemert R, et al. Comprehensive review of intracranial chordoma. Radiographics 2003;23:995–1009.

87. Wetzel LH, Levine E. Pictorial essay. MR imaging of sacral and presacral lesions. AJR Am J Roentgenol 1990;154:771–5.

88. Palestro CJ, Torres MA. Radionuclide imaging in orthopedic infections. Semin Nucl Med 1997;27: 334–45.

89. Bureau NJ, Chhem RK, Cardinal E. Musculoskeletal infections: US manifestations. Radiographics 1999; 19:1585–92.

90. Morrison WB, Schweitzer ME, Bock GW, et al. Diagnosis of osteomyelitis: utility of fat-suppressed contrast-enhanced MR imaging. Radiology 1993;189: 251–7.

91. Marcus CD, Ladam-Marcus VJ, Leone J, et al. MR imaging of osteomyelitis and neuropathic osteoarthropathy in the feet of diabetics. Radiographics 1996; 16:1337–48.

92. Kaandorp CJ, Van Schaardenburg D, Krijnen P, et al. Risk factors for septic arthritis in patients with joint disease: a prospective study. Arthritis Rheum 1995;38:1819–25.

93. Gavet F, Tournadre A, Soubrier M, et al. Septic arthritis in patients aged 80 and older: a comparison with younger adults. J Am Geriatr Soc 2005;53: 1210–3.

94. van Holsbeeck M, Introcaso JH. Musculoskeletal ultrasonography. Radiol Clin North Am 1992;30: 907–25.

95. Greenspan A, Tehranzadeh J. Imaging of infectious arthritis. Radiol Clin North Am 2001;39:267–76.

96. Karchevsky M, Schweitzer ME, Morrison WB, et al. MRI findings of septic arthritis and associated osteomyelitis in adults. AJR Am J Roentgenol 2004;182: 119–22.

Imaging of Metabolic Bone Diseases

Giuseppe Guglielmi, MD[a,b],*, Silvana Muscarella, MD[a,b],
Antonio Leone, MD[c],
Wilfred C.G. Peh, MBBS, MHSM, MD, FRCPE, FRCPG, FRCR[d]

KEYWORDS

- Aging • Osteoporosis • Radiographs
- DXA (dual X-ray absorptiometry)
- QCT (quantitative computed tomography)
- MR (magnetic resonance) • QUS (quantitative ultrasound)

As people age, they are more likely to encounter disease and disability requiring medical and social interventions. Involutional osteoporosis is the most important metabolic bone disease in geriatric patients. It has unfortunate negative consequences involving social and physical issues in the aging population.[1] Vertebral compression fractures, as a complication of the disease, often produce acute and chronic pain, and represent underappreciated cause of morbidity and mortality in the elderly.[2–4] In addition to physical limitations, vertebral compression fractures may produce a psychosocial and emotional burden on an aging person who already faces losses of independent function.

Moreover, because the age group of those older than 65 years is the fastest growing segment of the population, the incidence of this age-specific fracture is likely to increase.

BASIC CONSIDERATIONS
Definition

Osteoporosis is a disorder characterized by qualitatively normal, but quantitatively deficient, bone with consequent increased bone fragility and susceptibility to fractures.

Involutional osteoporosis is classified as a type I or postmenopausal osteoporosis and a type II or senile osteoporosis.[5,6] Postmenopausal osteoporosis is believed to represent that process occurring in a subset of postmenopausal women, typically between ages 50 and 65. There is accelerated trabecular bone resorption related to estrogen deficiency, and the fracture pattern in this group of women involves primarily the spine and wrist. In senile osteoporosis, there is proportionate loss of cortical and trabecular bone. Characteristic fractures of senile osteoporosis include fractures of the hip, proximal humerus, tibia, and pelvis in elderly women and men. Even though the importance of estrogen deficiency for postmenopausal osteoporosis has been established, the distinction between the two types of osteoporosis sometimes may be arbitrary, and the assignment of fracture sites to the different types of osteoporosis is uncertain. Besides this kind of osteoporosis, known as generalized osteoporosis, there is a regional osteoporosis, affecting only a part of the skeleton, usually the appendicular skeleton, such as osteoporosis resulting from immobilization or disuse, reflex sympathetic syndrome, or transient osteoporosis of large joint.

Epidemiology

Involutional osteoporosis is the most common metabolic disease in elderly. The problem is

[a] Department of Radiology, University of Foggia, Viale L. Pinto 1, 71100 Foggia, Italy
[b] Department of Radiology, Scientific Institute "Casa Sollievo della Sofferenza" Hospital, Viale Cappuccini, 1 - 71013 San Giovanni Rotondo, Italy
[c] Department of Radiology, Catholic University, Largo A. Gemelli 8, 00168 Rome, Italy
[d] Department of Diagnostic Radiology, Alexandra Hospital, 378 Alexandra Road, 159964 Singapore, Republic of Singapore
* Corresponding author. Department of Radiology, University of Foggia, Viale L. Pinto 1, 71100 Foggia, Italy.
E-mail address: g.guglielmi@unifg.it (G. Guglielmi).

Radiol Clin N Am 46 (2008) 735–754
doi:10.1016/j.rcl.2008.04.010

considerable given that internists spend three quarters of their time with patients aged 65 years or older.

Although osteoporosis has long been considered a disease of women, in the earliest reports of the epidemiology of osteoporosis it was apparent that the classical age-related increase in fractures seen in women also is evident in men.

Women diagnosed with a compression fracture of the vertebra have a 15% higher mortality rate than those who do not experience fractures.[7] Although less common in older men, compression fractures are a major health concern in this group.[8–10] Some studies demonstrate that the incidence of all fractures is higher in men than in women early in life, probably as a result of serious trauma.[11,12] At approximately age 40 to 50 there is reversal of this trend for fractures in general and, in particular and more commonly in women, those of the pelvis, humerus, forearm, and femur. The incidence of fractures resulting from minimal to moderate trauma (in particular hip and spine), however, also increases rapidly with aging in men and reflects an increasing prevalence of skeletal fragility.[13]

Few studies have assessed the prevalence and incidence of vertebral fractures in nonwhite ethnic groups.[14] Among Americans, the incidence of hip fractures is considerably lower in blacks than in whites.[15,16] A higher bone mineral density (BMD) is observed consistently in blacks compared with whites.[17,18] This difference could be partly due to serum 1,25-(OH)$_2$D, significantly higher in blacks than in whites, and to a higher bone turnover in blacks than in whites.[19] Moreover, urinary calcium excretion consistently is lower in blacks than in whites.[19–22]

Etiology and Risk Factors

Nutritional and lifestyle influences (lack of adequate dietary calcium and vitamin D or excessive alcohol or tobacco use) may compound the imbalance in bone remodelling[23,24] and largely contribute to age-related bone loss[6] in men and women. Vitamin D deficiency, in particular, is common in older individuals as a result of limited exposure to sunlight and a low dietary intake in vitamin D and calcium.[25,26]

With advancing age, conversion of 25(OH)D$_3$ to 1,25(OH)$_2$D$_3$ decreases, resulting in a reduction in intestinal calcium absorption,[27,28] which adds to the effects of the often low dietary calcium intake.[29] The calcium and vitamin D deficiency stimulates the production of parathyroid hormone (PTH), which accelerates bone turnover,[30] thereby causing bone loss. Alternatively, the formation of vitamin D$_3$ in the skin is much less efficient in the elderly than in younger people. As a consequence, secondary hyperparathyroidism is proposed as

the principal mechanism whereby vitamin D deficiency could contribute to the pathogenesis of hip fractures, which are a major source of morbidity and mortality in the elderly.[31,32]

Other causes of secondary hyperparathyroidism in the elderly are represented mainly by decrease in renal function, loss of estrogen, and, in men, changes in gonadal function.

Renal function decreases slowly with aging. This is associated with a gradual increase of serum PTH with age.[33,34] Multiple regression analysis in studies of elderly patients who have hip fracture show renal function in association with serum 25(OH)D as determinants of serum PTH.[35–37]

In postmenopausal women it is well established that estrogen deficiency is a major determinant of the accelerated bone loss; on average, women lose between one third and one half of their bone within up of 10 years after menopause.[38] Although the rate of bone loss slows after that point, low estrogen levels continue to contribute to diminution of bone mass later in life. In postmenopausal women, interactions between estrogen status and serum PTH are reported. The rise in serum PTH with aging does not occur in women receiving estrogen replacement therapy.[39]

In men, aging also is associated with changes in gonadal function, in particular in the hypothalamic-pituitary-gonadal axis, that result in notable declines in total and free testosterone levels.[40,41] Although serum testosterone levels vary remarkably between individuals, it is generally accepted that androgen levels decline with aging. Androgens are important regulators of bone metabolism. This is best illustrated by the fact that osteoporosis is a main feature of overt hypogonism.[42–44]

Besides these, other risks factors, such as presence of dementia, susceptibility to falling, history of fractures in adulthood, history of fractures in a first-degree relative, frailty, impaired eyesight, insufficient physical activity, and low body weight, can contribute in part to the development of involutional osteoporosis and its complications.

Physiopathology

Age-related osteopenia may result from inversely related changes in the pool size of hematopoietic osteoclast precursor cells and osteogenic stromal cells; reduced production of osteoprotegerin would additionally promote the formation of osteoclasts. Many investigators have demonstrated an age-related decline in trabecular bone volume in men and women.[45–47] In both genders a negative effect of aging on cortical bone mass also is demonstrated at distinct sites of the axial and the appendicular skeleton.[48]

Bone loss results from any imbalance of bone turnover when the rate of bone resorption exceeds that of bone formation. Moreover, individual bone loss is determined by two factors: (1) the peak bone mass (the amount of bone mass achieved at skeletal maturity) and (2) the subsequent rate of bone loss. Considering the pathogenesis of osteoporosis, it should be taken into account that, in addition to interindividual variations, there is an important gender-related difference in peak bone mass achieved during adolescence. In women, bone mass increases during childhood and adolescence, and peak bone mass is achieved by the early to late 20s, so that on average young women have a significantly lower peak bone mass than young men, in whom bone mass is achieved later.

Complications

Vertebral compression fractures are recognized as the hallmark of osteoporosis.

Generally, some trauma occurs with each compression fracture. In cases of severe osteoporosis, however, the cause of trauma may be simple, such as stepping out of a bathtub or vigorous sneezing, or the trauma may result from the load caused by muscle contraction.[49] Up to 30% of compression fractures occur while patients are in bed.[50] Vertebral fractures typically occur at the thoracolumbar junction (T12-L1) and the midthoracic area (T7-T8).[51]

The applied force usually causes the anterior part of the vertebral body to crush, forming an anterior wedge fracture. As the collapsed anterior vertebrae fuse together, the spine bends forward, causing a kyphotic deformity and a significant loss of height. Because the majority of damage is limited to the anterior vertebral column, the fracture is usually stable and rarely associated with neurologic compromise.[52] Progressive loss of stature results in shortening of paraspinal musculature requiring prolonged active contraction for maintenance of posture, resulting in pain from muscle fatigue. The rib cage presses down on the pelvis, reducing thoracic and abdominal space. In severe cases, this results in impaired pulmonary function, a protuberant abdomen, and—because of compressed abdominal organs—early satiety and weight loss.[53]

Besides the spine, other common sites of involvement are the neck and intertrochanteric region of the femur, distal radius, and tibia. The proximal femur is the most important site of osteoporotic fracture. The incidence of hip fracture rises exponentially in men with aging, as it does in women. Unfortunately, the number of hip fractures is projected to increase dramatically as the elderly population expands.[54] The occurrence of a distal forearm fracture[55] or a tibial fracture[56] in men indicates a considerably increased risk for subsequent hip fracture, presumably as a result of low bone mass or increased risk for falling.

DIAGNOSTIC IMAGING OF OSTEOPOROSIS

Diagnostic imaging of osteoporosis has two principle aims: (1) to identify the presence of osteoporosis and (2) to quantify bone mass by using semiquantitative (conventional radiography) or quantitative methods (densitometric techniques).

Conventional Radiography

The radiologic appearances of osteoporosis are essentially the same, irrespective of the cause. Despite the advent of newer and highly accurate and precise quantitative techniques, such as dual x-ray absorptiometry (DXA) and quantitative CT (QCT), osteoporosis still is most commonly and probably best diagnosed on conventional radiographs that are widely available and remain useful, alone and in conjunction with other imaging techniques (such as bone scintigraphy and MR imaging), for the detection of complications of osteopenia (eg, fractures), for the differential diagnosis of osteopenia, or for follow-up examinations in specific clinical settings (progression of soft tissue calcifications or signs of secondary hyperparathyroidism and osteomalacia in renal osteodystrophy).

Conventional radiography, however, is relatively insensitive in detecting early disease, as a substantial amount (approximately 30%) of bone loss must occur before it can be detected radiographically;[57] also, variability in technical factors, such as radiographic exposure factors, film development, and soft tissue thickness of patients, could make a diagnosis difficult.

The main radiographic features of generalized osteoporosis are (1) increased radiolucency and (2) cortical thinning.

Increased radiolucency
Increased radiolucency is a common feature in osteoporosis and is the result of resorption and thinning of the trabeculae, some of which may be lost. As a consequence, the term, *osteopenia* (poverty of bone), is used as a generic designation for radiographic signs of decreased bone density (**Fig. 1**).

The trabecular bone responds faster to metabolic changes than does cortical bone.[58] Trabecular bone changes are most prominent in the axial skeleton and in the ends of the long and trabecular bones of the appendicular skeleton

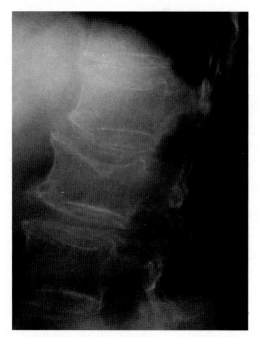

Fig. 1. Lateral radiograph of the dorsolumbar junction showing increased radiolucency and radiodense end plates. There is loss of the secondary trabeculae with relative prominence of the primary vertical trabeculae. Multiple vertebral fractures associate.

(juxta-articular) (eg, proximal femur and distal radius). These are sites with a relatively great proportion of trabecular bone. Loss of trabecular bone (in cases of low rates of loss, as in senile osteoporosis) occurs in a predictable pattern. The process initially selectively affects secondary trabeculae. As a result, the primary trabeculae may develop relative prominence, as they are affected only at a later state. For example, early changes of osteopenia in the lumbar spine include a rarefaction of the horizontal (secondary) trabeculae accompanied by a relative accentuation of the vertical (primary) trabeculae (see **Fig. 1**). This may lead to an appearance of vertical striation, which may simulate hemangioma. Similarly, in the femur, there is accentuation of the principal compressive and tensile trabeculae, with increased prominence of the sparsely trabeculated area between them, known as Ward's area (an area on radiographs of the proximal femur enclosed by the principle and secondary compressive and the tensile group).[59]

Cortical thinning

Cortical thinning is the result of osseous resorption in the cortex. The structural changes seen in cortical bone represent bone resorption at different sites (eg, the inner and outer surface of the cortex

or within the cortex in the haversian and Volkmann canals). These three sites (endosteal, intracortical, and periosteal) may react differently to distinct metabolic stimuli.

Cortical bone remodelling typically occurs in the endosteal envelope, resulting in a scalloping of the inner margin of the cortex. With increasing age, there is a widening of the marrow canal as a result of imbalance of endosteal bone formation and resorption that leads to a trabeculization of the inner surface of the cortex. Endosteal scalloping resulting from resorption of the inner bone surface is the least specific radiographic finding of osteoporosis and it can be seen in high bone turnover states, such as postmenopausal osteoporosis (and also hyperparathyroidism, osteomalacia, renal osteodystrophy, and acute osteoporoses from disuse or the reflex sympathetic dystrophy syndrome). Nevertheless, the interpretation of subtle changes in this layer may be difficult.

With intracortical resorption, prominent longitudinal striations within the cortex, also known as cortical tunneling, are observed. Intracortical tunneling is slightly more specific as a hallmark of rapid bone turnover, so that it usually is not apparent in disease states with low bone turnover, such as senile osteoporosis.

Finally, subperiosteal resorption also may be seen. It is associated with an irregular definition of the outer bone surface. It most specific finding in diseases with a high bone turnover. It also rarely may be present, however, in other diseases.

Axial Skeleton

One of the first methods introduced to classify radiolucency in the axial skeleton was the Saville index.[60] According to this method, it was possible to distinguish four grades of radiographic appearance of the vertebra: 0, normal bone density; 1, minimal loss of density and end plates begin to stand out giving a stenciled effect; 2, vertical striation is more obvious and end plates are thinner; 3, more severe loss of bone density than grade 2 and end plates becoming less visible; 4, ghost-like vertebral bodies, density is no greater that soft tissue, and no trabecular pattern is visible (**Fig. 2**). This index, however, has never gained widespread acceptance as it is prone to great subjectivity and experience of the reader.

As a result of loss of adjacent trabecular bone, the thinning of the cortex usually remains sharp and clear in osteoporosis, thus giving rise to a well-demarcated outline of the vertebral body (usually described as picture framing or empty box).

Vertebral fractures often complicate osteoporosis and even though osteopenia per se may not be

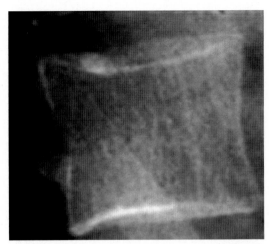

Fig. 2. Radiograph of a single vertebra displaying characteristic features of osteoporosis, including an overall increased radiolucency and verticalization of the trabeculae (Saville index II).

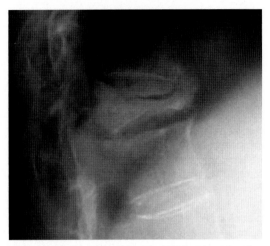

Fig. 3. Lateral radiograph of dorsal spine showing a severe wedge fracture with vacuum phenomenon. There is generalized osteoporosis.

diagnosed reliably from spinal radiographs, spinal radiography continues to be of substantial aid in diagnosing and following-up vertebral fractures and as a complement for the several quantitative morphometric methods for measurements of vertebral heights introduced to reduce the subjectivity of a radiologist's reading.[61,62]

Compression fractures can occur anywhere from the occiput to the sacrum, although they usually occur at the lumbodorsal junction, namely T8-T12, L1, and L4.[50] It is important to image the entire spine, in a lateral and anteroposterior projection, because 20% to 30% of vertebral compression fractures are multiple. The presence and number of vertebral fractures correlate well with the degree of osteoporosis: the greater the degree of osteoporosis, the greater the number of fractures present. Careful scrutiny of the bone beneath the vertebral end plate is helpful in differentiating deformities that result from fractures. Despite limitations, the degree of deformity is used most commonly to define vertebral fractures. Fractures generally are described as wedge when the anterior height is reduced in relation to posterior height; as end plate when the midheight is reduced in relation to posterior height; and as crush when all heights of a vertebra are reduced in relation to the dimensions of adjacent vertebrae. Because the posterior height of the thoracic vertebrae normally is 1 to 3 mm more than the anterior height, a loss of height greater than 4 mm is considered a true vertebral fracture deformity (**Figs. 3** and **4**).[63,64] This criterion also is used for lumbar vertebrae, although differences between anterior and posterior heights are less in lumbar vertebrae than in vertebrae in the thoracic spine.

The shape of vertebrae and their dimensions not only should be defined according to their posterior border but also should be compared with those of adjacent vertebrae. Altered appearance is suspicious and could be the result of fracture of the whole end plate with height loss of the complete vertebral body.[65]

Another method for fracture definition commonly used was described by Genant and colleagues[66]: a vertebral deformity in T4-L4 of

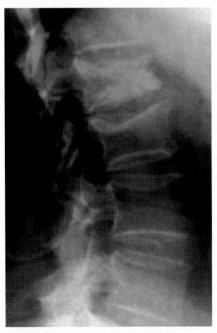

Fig. 4. Involutional osteoporosis of the dorsolumbar spine showing wedge fracture and end plate fracture.

more than 20% of loss in height with a reduction in area of more than 10% to 20% is defined as a fracture. Using this fracture threshold, a semiquantitative score to grade the severity of vertebral fractures as visually determined from radiographs also was described by Genant and colleagues.[66] In this score, four grades are differentiated: grade 0, no fracture; grade 1, mild fracture (reduction in vertebral height of 20%–25% compared with adjacent normal vertebrae); grade 2, moderate fracture (reduction in height 25%–40%); grade 3, severe fracture (reduction in height of more that 40%). From this semiquantitative assessment, a spinal fracture index can be calculated as the sum of all grades assigned to the vertebrae divided by the number of the vertebrae evaluated. Involvement of multiple vertebral bodies leads to kyphosis of the thoracic spine, a clinically obvious deformity known as dowager's hump.

In contrast to fractures of long bones, osteoporotic vertebral fractures rarely are associated with a demonstrable break in the cortex or accompanied by significant callus formation. Isolated fractures above T7 level are rare in osteoporosis and should alert clinicians to a cause other than osteoporosis.[67]

Appendicular Skeleton

The axial skeleton is not the only site where characteristic changes of osteopenia and osteoporosis can be depicted radiographically. Changes in the trabecular and cortical bone also can be seen in the appendicular skeleton. They are first apparent at the ends of long and tubular bones due to the predominance of cancellous bone in these regions. The main sites where these changes are evident are hand, proximal femur, and calcaneus.

Radiologic imaging of the hand is a fundamental step in evaluating grade and type of osteoporosis, thanks to anatomic peculiarities of this anatomic region that allow a detailed evaluation through high-resolution systems (eg, industrial films).

Metacarpal bones (usually II, III, and IV) are investigated. Spongious and cortical compartments are evaluated separately. The corticomedullar index, based on the evaluation of the cortical thickness at metacarpal bone II, represents a good semiquantitative measure for grading osteoporosis at this site.[68]

For evaluation of proximal femur, Singh and colleagues[69] in 1972 proposed a femoral index for the diagnosis of osteoporosis, based on the assumption that the trabeculae in the proximal femur disappear in a predictable sequence depending on their origin thickness. The investigators considered that the thickness and spacing

of trabeculae in the various trajectorial groups (principal compressive, secondary compressive, greater trochanter, principal tensile, and secondary tensile group) depend on the intensity of stresses normally carried by these trabeculae, and with advancing bone loss, trabeculae that are thinner become invisible first on the radiograph. Singh and coworkers introduced a classification ranging from grade VI (normal, all trabeculae groups visible) to grade I (markedly reduction in even the principal compressive trabeculae) according to the degree of bone loss. Singh and colleagues[69] added a grade VII to their scale for individuals who have dense bone, as the Ward's triangle contained trabeculae that were as dense as the other surrounding trabeculae (**Fig. 5**).

Finally, the calcaneus is an optimal site for the morphologic evaluation of trabecular pattern because it allows, through a semiquantitative index, measuring the grade of osteopenia related to resorption of trabecular groups. It is known as Jhamaria index and is performed on radiographic films of calcaneus in a lateral projection.[70]

Dual Energy X-Ray Absorptiometry

As discussed previously, judging bone density on a radiograph can be imprecise. Although whether or not a patient suffers a fracture depends on

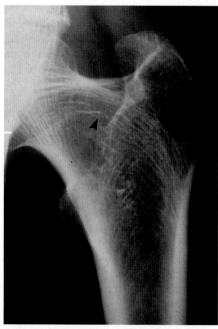

Fig. 5. Singh femoral index: the radiograph of the proximal femur demonstrates principal tensile trabeculae group (*arrowhead*); the other trabeculae (principal compressive group) are less evident.

several factors (propensity to fall and the nature of, and response to, a fall), approximately 60% to 70% of bone strength and what determines whether or not a fracture occurs are related to BMD.

These factors indicate the importance of having accurate and reproducible methods available to quantitate the BMD of the skeleton to

1. Diagnose osteoporosis early
2. Predict fracture risk
3. Determine therapeutic intervention
4. Monitor response to therapy and changes with time (the diagnostic and management role of bone densitometry)[71]

DXA was introduced in 1987[72] and, to date, represents the most widely used technique for diagnosis of osteoporosis in the clinical practice. The World Health Organization (WHO) has defined the threshold levels for the diagnosis of osteopenia and osteoporosis using DXA technique. As a consequence, DXA measures currently are the gold standard for clinical diagnosis of osteoporosis by bone densitometry.

A DXA machine consists of a mobile source of radiographs, a patient couch, a detection system on which fall radiations emerged from the bones under examination. The x-ray source is under the couch and moves together with the detection system, which is located opposite to it over the body of the patient. The main characteristic of DXA lies in that it uses an x-ray beam composed of two different photon energies (constant and pulsed). The energy used is selected to compensate the different attenuation coefficients of mineralized bone and soft tissues of the skeletal site analyzed. Practically, the intensity of high-energy photons and that of low-energy photons are analyzed separately after they have passed through bones and soft tissues. Using a particular computing algorithm, the attenuations of soft tissues are subtracted, obtaining the attenuation values of bone. The attenuation of the skeleton is related to its BMD by comparing the values obtained with standard values determined on phantoms of known density (higher attenuation–higher density). The original DXA scanners used a pencil x-ray beam and a single detector and scanned in a rectilinear fashion across the anatomic site examined. Technical developments in DXA in recent years include fan-beam x-ray sources and a bank of detectors. Fan-beam machines use wider beams that permit more rapid scanning (approximately 3–5 minutes per site; times are similar for whole-body scans), improved image quality, and spatial resolution of 0.5 to 0.7 mm. Newer machines have the capacity to perform

lateral scanning. This is permitted by a C-arm structure on which the x-ray tube is mounted that can be rotated along 90°. Lateral scanning increases measurement accuracy, avoiding the superimposition of vertebral posterior elements, marginal osteophytes, and vascular calcifications that may artificially increase bone density in the posteroanterior (PA) measurement of the lumbar spine. DXA examination is a monoplanar bone density. The measurements provided by DXA are bone mineral content in grams and projected area of the measured site in square centimeters. By dividing the bone mineral content by the area, BMD is given as g/cm^2. So, evaluation and the densitometric findings (BMD) are expressed as a planar density. BMD results are provided as SD by means of T-score and Z-score. T-score describes the difference between the BMD of the patient under examination and the BMD of a standard young adult population (20–30 years) and refers to the peak of bone mass; the Z-score shows a patient's results as the difference from the mean of age and gender-matched controls. Z-score is important particularly for patients aged 75 or more. The WHO has defined osteopenia T-score values as between −1 and −2.5 SD, osteoporosis T-score values equal to or lower than −2.5 SD, and severe osteoporosis T-score values lower than −2.5 SD associated with radiologic evidence of one or more fractures.[73] DXA results are reported as numeric values of T-score and Z-score and by a graphic curve normalized for gender and age. This definition is applied to DXA measurements made in the lumbar spine, the proximal femur, and the forearm. The definition does not apply to other techniques (eg, QCT) or other anatomic sites (eg, calcaneus).[74–76]

Axial dual x-ray absorptiometry

Axial DXA can be applied to sites of the skeleton where osteoporotic fractures occur, such as the lumbar spine (L1-L4) and proximal femur (total hip, femoral neck, trochanter, and Ward's area) (Fig. 6). As the DXA image is a two-compartment (2C) image of 2-D objects (ie, an areal, rather than a true volumetric density), the depth of the bones cannot be taken into account with a single PA projection. This results in one of the limitations of DXA, as the measurement is size dependent. Because whether or not a patient develops a fracture depends on factors in addition to BMD (if the patient falls, the nature of the fall, and the patient's response to the fall), it is impossible for BMD techniques to completely discriminate between those who have and who do not have fractures. The lower the BMD, however, the more at risk the patient is for suffering a fracture.[77] Although the

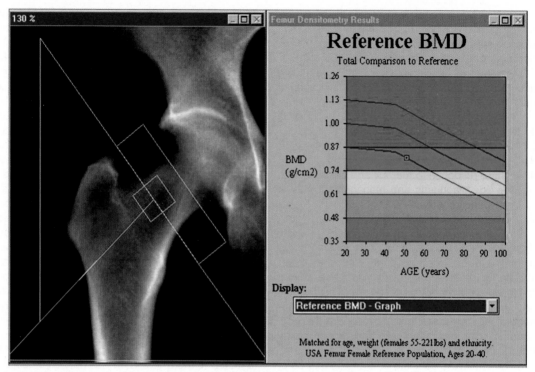

Fig. 6. DXA of the proximal femur showing ROIs analyzed: femoral neck (*oblong box*), Ward's area (*box*), and trochanter. Patient's age and BMD for the total femur plotted with respect to the reference range also are reported.

ionizing radiation from these DXA scanners is low, ionizing radiation regulations apply to their installation and operation. Dedicated and highly motivated technical staff who have appropriate training can ensure high quality of positioning of patients and good precision of results.

Different manufacturers use different edge detection algorithms and analyze different regions of interest (ROIs) for analysis in the hip. For this reason, results from different scanners are not interchangeable. In longitudinal studies, it is vital to use the same scanner and software program.

Peripheral Dual X-Ray Absorptiometry

An increasing number of small, portable DXA scanners are becoming available for application to peripheral sites (distal radius and the calcaneus). For monitoring changes in BMD, the forearm site, predominantly cortical bone, is not a sensitive site; the calcaneus, 95% trabecular bone, offers more potential for this purpose. BMD measurements in these sites are as predictive of fractures in all sites as the more conventional measurements in axial sites. The forearm measurements are particularly predictive of wrist fractures and are performed in particular conditions, such as hyperparathyroidism or when evaluation of other sites is impossible; the calcaneus

measurements are particularly predictive of spine fractures, even in the elderly, in whom spinal DXA is confounded by degenerative disease.[77–79] As discussed previously, although the WHO criterion for the diagnosis of osteoporosis (T-score less than −2.5) is applicable to the forearm, it is not to the calcaneus. T-scores between −1.0 and −1.5 for BMD in the calcaneus are suggested as more appropriate in this site, but the definitive threshold for diagnosis is still to be determined.[80]

Quantitative CT

QCT is different from DXA because it provides separate estimates of trabecular and cortical bone BMD as a true volumetric mineral density in mg/cm^3. It can be performed at axial sites and peripheral sites.

Axial quantitative CT

Axial CT provides a measure of trabecular bone in consecutive vertebrae of the spine (usually two to four vertebrae out of T12 to L4) using commercial CT scanners and a bone mineral reference standard to calibrate each scan. Beginning from an initial localized image and using a low-dose technique with the gantry angled parallel to the vertebral end plate, single 8 to 10 mm–thick sections are obtained through the midplane of each of these vertebrae. A ROI is positioned manually in the anterior portion of trabecular bone of the vertebral body for analysis.[81–83] Software automatically locates the vertebral body, maps its outer edges, and uses anatomic landmarks, such as spinous process and spinal canal, and calculates size and location of the ROIs. Hounsfield units, also known as CT numbers, are used to measure the CT density of the selected area of interest within a slice through a vertebral body. Then, comparing the CT number of the trabecular bone to that of the compartments of the calibration standard, it is possible to achieve a conversion to bone mineral equivalent values expressed in milligrams of calcium hydroxyapatite per cubic centimeter. Usually a calibration phantom made of different concentrations of calcium hydroxyapatite in water-equivalent plastic is used. The calculated densities for the vertebrae are averaged and compared with those of a normal population.[84] Normative data are gender and race specific (Fig. 7).[85]

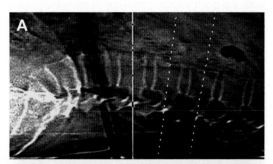

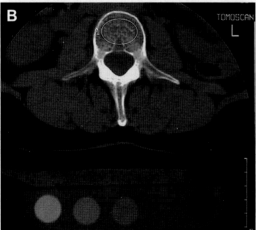

Fig. 7. Scout view (A) and axial slice (B) trough lumbar vertebral bodies. Scout view shows location of slices through vertebral lumbar bodies. The elliptic ROI measuring purely trabecular bone of the vertebral body is shown in the axial slice along with the QCT calibration phantom used to convert Hounsfield units to mg/cm³ of calcium hydroxyapatite.

Densities are given per vertebral body and a mean value for all vertebral bodies measured. Absolute normal bone density values are race dependent, as black men and women have higher bone density values then white men and women. As with all bone densitometry techniques, the results of the measurements usually are given in the form of absolute values and as Z-scores and T-scores.

QCT has an excellent ability to predict vertebral fractures and to serially measure bone loss, generally with better sensitivity than projectional methods, such as DXA, because it selectively assesses the metabolically active and structurally trabecular bone in the center of the vertebral body.

Through the selective trabecular measurement, QCT also is sensitive in measuring changes in a short follow-up period. Nevertheless, myelofibrosis and marrow changes in hematopoietic disorders can affect the measurements.

Some studies have examined BMD decrements between normal subjects and those who have vertebral fractures. These studies showed that the decrement as measured by spinal QCT is significantly higher than that observed by PA-DXA and that QCT usually allows superior vertebral fracture discrimination. Moreover, QCT shows a comparatively good sensitivity for measurement of age-related bone loss after menopause, because the metabolic rate in the vertebral trabecular bone is substantially greater than that of the surrounding cortical bone.

The main theoretic advantages of QCT over DXA are the exclusion from the measurement of structures that do not contribute to spine mechanical resistance, yet contribute to DXA BMD values, and the possibility to selectively measure trabecular tissue, considered the main determinant of compressive strength in the vertebrae.[86]

Although the use of standard QCT has been based on 2C characterization of vertebral trabecular bone, three-compartment, or volumetric QCT, is a new technique that allows improving spinal measurements and extending QCT assessments to the proximal femur.[87] Volumetric QCT devices encompass the entire object of interest with stacked slices, or spiral CT scans, and can use anatomic landmarks to automatically generate relevant projections. Volumetric QCT can not only determine BMD of the entire bone or subregion, such as vertebral body or femoral neck, but also provide separate analysis of the trabecular or cortical components.

Peripheral quantitative CT

Besides its cited advantages with respect to DXA technique, spinal QCT has several disadvantages that have limited its widespread application: high radiation dose, poor precision that limits its applicability to longitudinal assessments, high costs for QCT scanners, high degree of operator dependence, space requirements, and limited access to the scanners. Moreover, axial QCT is used only for the assessment of spine volumetric BMD because the complexity of the hip architecture has precluded the development of reliable methods for densitometric assessment in this clinically important region.

To obviate the limitations of DXA and axial QCT, a peripheral QCT (pQCT) device has been developed. It not only allows separate assessments of cortical and trabecular bone but also provides also direct information on bone geometry at several appendicular sites. From the analysis of cross-sectional images provided by pQCT, information on mass and distribution of bone material can be integrated into indexes of bone stability in response to bending and torsional loads, which are the most important biomechanical measures of susceptibility fracture and may improve accuracy in the prediction of fractures (**Fig. 8**).[88,89]

Morphometry

Vertebral fractures are the most common of osteoporotic fractures. A diagnosis of vertebral fracture is a frequently used endpoint in clinical trials and epidemiologic studies investigating the effectiveness of different therapeutic regimes on osteoporosis.[90,91] As discussed previously, vertebral fractures are classified as anterior wedging, biconcavity, and crushing resulting from the loss of anterior, middle, and posterior heights of vertebral bodies. On conventional radiographs,

osteoporotic vertebral fractures often appear as mild vertebral deformities, atraumatic and asymptomatic, so that the visual radiologic approach may lead to disagreement about whether or not a vertebra is fractured.[92] In an effort to reduce the high subjectivity and poor reproducibility of qualitative readings, more than a decade ago morphometric methods based on vertebral height measurements to definite vertebral fractures were introduced.[93] Quantitative vertebral morphometry involves making measurements of vertebral body heights. The measurements may be made on conventional spinal radiographs (morphometric x-ray radiography) or on absorptiometric images (morphometric x-ray absorptiometry [MXA]) (**Fig. 9**).

MRX was introduced in 1960 by Barnett and Nordin.[94] Before performing the measurement of vertebral heights, a reader has to identify the vertebral levels. The vertebral bodies should be marked so that they can be identified more easily in other reading sessions or when compared with follow-up radiographs. On lateral radiographs with six-point digitization—the most widely used technique—the four corner points of each vertebral body from T4 to L5 (or L4, because of the highly variable shape of L5) and additional points in the middle of the upper and lower end plates are marked. The manual point placement is done, according to Hurxthal[63], by excluding the uncinate process at the posterosuperior border of the thoracic vertebrae from vertebral height measurement, Schmorl's nodes, and osteophytes.

Some investigators[95–98] have assessed the vertebral dimensions from digital images of spine radiographs captured by means of a videocamera or scanner. Postprocessing of the digital images

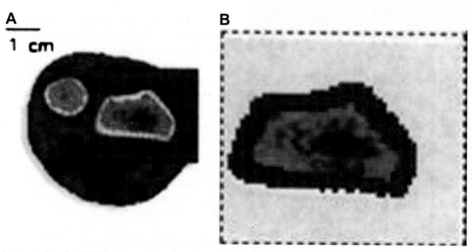

Fig. 8. Cross-sectional pQCT images easily separate the cortical and trabecular region at distal forearm (*A*) and radius (*B*).

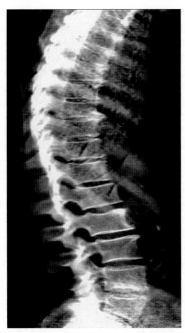

Fig. 9. MXA scan image of dorsolumbar spine.

can highlight the end plate and the four corners of vertebral bodies allowing points to be placed more precisely. After the radiographs are digitized, an operator manually selects the four corners of the vertebra. The software automatically determines the midpoints between the anterior and posterior corner points of the upper and lower end plates and calculates the posterior, middle, and anterior heights (Hp, Hm, and Ha, respectively) of each vertebra and specific indices derived from height measurements for defining vertebral deformities.

MXA currently is the most widespread digital technique for assessing vertebral height. Some systems perform a PA projection of the thoracic and lumbar spine before lateral scans are acquired; this PA image is useful for visualizing spinal anatomy to determine the centerline of the spine; the lateral scan covers the distance from L4 to T4. After a lateral scan, the program automatically identifies vertebral levels and indicates the centers of the vertebrae. The six-point placement for the determination of the vertebral heights is semiautomated. The operator uses a mouse-pointing device to specify the 13 locations of the anterior inferior corner of the vertebrae L4 to T4. Then, the MXA software computes the positions of the remaining five vertebral points for each vertebral body. A vertebral body is fractured if any of three height ratios—anterior to posterior height (Ha/Hp for wedge), middle to posterior height (Hm/Hp for biconcavity), and posterior to posterior height of adjacent vertebra (ratio Hp for

crush)—is reduced by more than 15% compared with the normal ratio for level.

After the analysis is finished, a final report is displayed. It gives information on the measured vertebral body height and their ratios and includes an assessment of a patient's fracture status based on normative data and different models for fracture assessment using quantitative morphometry.

The quantitative morphometry is unable to distinguish osteoporotic vertebral fractures by vertebral deformities due to other factors, such as degenerative spine and disc disease. Although visual interpretation of radiographs is subjective, an expert eye can distinguish between true fractures and vertebral anomalies better than quantitative morphometry can.

Quantitative Ultrasound

Quantitative ultrasound (QUS) is used to measure quantitative parameters and assess tissue properties. QUS offer advantages of small size, quick and simple measurements, no need for ionizing radiation, and low cost compared with axial DXA or QCT devices. These advantages explain the motivation for using QUS for the assessment of osteoporosis, assuming that performance is comparable. Ultrasound waves are affected not only by the amount of material but also by its elasticity and structure. As a consequence, QUS might be able to yield additional information about bone fragility so that, at present, QUS devices mostly are used for the prediction of osteoporotic fracture risk. Because of these characteristics, QUS has continued to be of interest in the past 2 decades.

Because of the strong attenuation of high-frequency ultrasound in bone, especially trabecular bone, the frequency range typically is limited to 0.1 to 2 MHz. The interactions of bone and ultrasound wave are analyzed, and from this analysis, quantitative parameters are derived that are associated with properties of the skeletal site (such as a density, structure, or strength).

Commercial bone QUS has used transit time velocity measurement (the time for the arrival of ultrasound signal at the receiving transducer), with different definition: bone velocity, heel velocity, and speed of sound. For attenuation, more uniformity is present among commercial devices; attenuation typically is characterized by broadband ultrasound attenuation (BUA), the slope at which attenuation increases with frequencies, generally between 0.2 MHz and 0.6 MHz.

Velocity and BUA provide quantitative information on ultrasound interaction with the medium. Theory suggests that BUA is determined by bone density and bone microarchitecture, whereas speed of sound is influenced by the elasticity of bone and bone density. Recently it has been demonstrated, in human calcaneal specimens, that QUS reflects BMD especially and, to a lesser extent, bone microarchitecture.[99] The calcaneus is the most studied skeletal site for QUS assessment for several reasons: it has a high percentage of trabecular bone (95%), which has a turnover higher than cortical bone, allowing early evidence of metabolic changes; it is easily accessible; and the mediolateral surfaces are fairly flat and parallel, thus reducing repositioning error.

In cadaver studies, calcaneal ultrasound correlates with femoral and vertebral strength, but the predictive ability is less than, not independent of, BMD measurements.[100,101] In contrast to these results, however, Lochmuller and colleagues[102] found that calcaneal QUS correlates with failure load of the proximal femur similarly to femoral neck BMD. In conclusion, qualitative evidence for the influence of structure on ultrasound exists, but there are no conclusive data demonstrating that ultrasound provides useful information on specific structural parameter at clinical sites.

Other skeletal sites explored are metaphysis of the phalanx, radius, and tibia.

The phalanx is a long bone consisting of a trabecular component and a cortical component. This site is strongly predictive of the condition of the bone tissue throughout the skeletal system and predictive of osteoporotic-type, vertebral, hip, and forearm fractures. The phalanx is measured by QUS at metaphyseal level, where trabecular bone (at approximately 40%) and cortical bone are present. The metaphysis of the phalanx, moreover, is characterized by a high bone turnover, and thus is a site extremely sensitive to changes regarding the skeleton, whether or not natural (growth and aging), the result of metabolic disease (hyperparathyroidism), or drug induced (treatment with glucocorticoids).[103–107]

In tibia and radius, propagation occurs mainly along the external surface of the bone, providing indications mostly on the cortical bone tissue. Investigations at tibia and radius are sensitive to phenomena of endosteal reabsorption.[108]

QUS results can be expressed in absolute values or as T-scores and Z-scores thanks to well established and validated normative reference curves, allowing bone loss to be followed with time.[99,109–113]

Currently there is a lack of diagnostic criteria that would make QUS suitable for the diagnosis of osteoporosis. It has been demonstrated that the WHO criteria cannot simply be used with QUS. Different QUS approaches may show very different age-related declines. Consequently, the number of subjects who fall below a T-score of -2.5 threshold varies and different percentages of subjects are identified as osteoporotic, which is inconsistent with the notion of a constant percentage of subjects who have osteoporosis. In addition, the limitation in measuring peripheral bones further restricts the use of QUS for diagnostic purposes. Correlations with the bone density of the main fractures sites in the spine and femur are modest and do not allow a judgment about their bone mass status. Because the decline in bone density is gradual, no fixed threshold can exist above which a person has a healthy skeleton and below which he or she is osteoporotic. For this reason, bone density and QUS results always have to be seen in context of clinical risk factors and patient anamnesis. QUS may be helpful, but it cannot be used as a stand-alone tool for diagnosis of osteoporosis. Estimation of risk fracture is the main field of application for QUS.[114] Many prospective studies show that fractured patients have lower calcaneal ultrasound values than normal patients and that QUS parameters are consistently predictive of osteoporotic fractures.[115–118]

MR Imaging

A more recent development in the assessment of trabecular bone structure is the use of MR imaging, which makes it possible to obtain noninvasive bone biopsies at multiple anatomic sites. Cortical and trabecular bone have a low water content and short T2 and are not detectable using routine MR imaging methods. The marrow surrounding the trabecular bone network, however, if imaged at high resolution, reveals the trabecular network. Using such images, several different image processing and image analysis algorithms have been developed. The goal of all of these is to quantify the trabecular bone structure in 2-D or 3-D.[119] Several calibration and validation studies (in vitro and in vivo)[120–124] have been undertaken in which MR imaging–derived measures of structure are compared with measures derived from other modalities, such as histology, micro-CT, or BMD and with biomechanics.[125] With recent advances in phased-array coils and higher-strength magnets, the potential of MR imaging of bone structure is increasing. The skeletal sites imaged most commonly are the radius and calcaneus (**Fig. 10**). Studies currently underway are exploring the possibility of obtaining microarchitectural features of trabecular bone to understand whether or not bone turnover and microarchitecture are related, clarifying the underlying relationship between turnover, BMD, and architecture.[119]

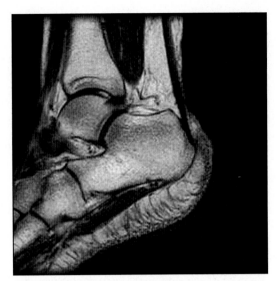

Fig. 10. In vivo high-resolution MR image of calcaneus depicting trabecular bone structure.

Other Imaging Techniques

Other techniques have been proposed to study trabecular microstructure. Ito and colleagues[125] studied performance of multidetector CT as a new technique to study in vivo trabecular bone structure of human vertebrae and concluded that microstructure parameters obtained by MDC, together with volumetric BMD, provide better diagnostic performance for assessing fracture risk than DXA measurement.

In the past decade, MR imaging–based studies have documented physiologic differences in aging bone. Dynamic contrast material–enhanced MR imaging studies across different age groups have revealed that vertebral marrow perfusion is reduced in older subjects.[126–128] Hydrogen 1 MR imaging spectroscopy–based studies have revealed an age-dependent linear increase in vertebral marrow fat content.[129,130] Griffith and colleagues[131] observed that reduction in vertebral marrow perfusion in older male subjects is related to bone density. Subjects who had osteoporosis had significantly reduced vertebral marrow perfusion compared with perfusion in subjects who had osteopenia, and subjects who had osteopenia had significantly reduced vertebral marrow perfusion compared with that in subjects who had normal bone density. Moreover, vertebral marrow fat content is related to bone density. Subjects who had osteoporosis or osteopenia had a significantly increased marrow fat content compared with the fat content in subjects who had normal bone density. Decreasing marrow perfusion and increasing marrow fat content accompany

a reduction in bone density. It is conceivable that within the borders of the vertebral body, an increasing amount of fat simply could compress the intraosseous veins, diminishing blood flow. Also, a clear interplay between lipids, arteriosclerosis, and bone density increasingly is recognized. Accumulation of oxidized lipids in the arterial wall induces arterial wall calcification (as a feature of atherosclerosis), whereas accumulation of the same oxidized lipids within bone can inhibit osteoblastic and promote osteoclastic differentiation.[132,133] In conclusion, compared with bone perfusion in men who have normal bone density, bone perfusion is reduced in men who have osteopenia and further reduced in men who have osteoporosis. In contrast, vertebral marrow fat content is increased in men who have osteopenia or osteoporosis.

DIFFERENTIAL DIAGNOSIS

Apart from senile and postmenopausal states there are various conditions that may be accompanied by generalized osteoporosis.

Hyperparathyroidism may result from autonomous hypersecretion by a parathyroid adenoma or diffuse hyperplasia of the parathyroid glands (primary hyperparathyroidism). Subperiosteal bone resorption is the most characteristic radiographic feature of hyperparathyroidism[134] with consequent multiple erosions at the radial site of medium phalanges (usually II and III), sacroiliac joints, and pubic symphysis. Often an endosteal, subchondral, or trabecular involvement is observed. It is especially prominent in the hand, wrist, and foot. Other skeletal sites of involvement are long bones, such as humerus, femur, and tibia, with thinning of compact and cortex and consequent endosteal resorption and intracortical linear strations. Brown tumors often may occur; they present as focal osteolitic areas with swelling of bone most localized at ribs and long bones of hand and foot.

Hypercortisolism probably is the most common cause of medication-induced generalized osteoporosis, whereas the endogenous form, Cushing's disease, is rare.[135,136] Decreased bone formation and increased bone resorption are observed in hypercortisolism. The typical radiographic appearance of steroid-induced osteoporosis comprises generalized osteoporosis, at predominantly trabecular sites, with decreased bone density and fractures of the axial and appendicular skeleton. A characteristic finding in steroid-induced osteoporosis is marginal condensation of the vertebral bodies resulting from exuberant callus formation. Sometimes, osteonecrosis of the femoral head, tendon rupture, and joint infections associate.

Moreover, there are several differential diagnoses that have to be considered in elderly patients who have vertebral deformities. The most important differential diagnosis is malignant disease (eg, multiple myeloma or metastatic bone disease). In addition, vertebra deformity is found in metabolic bone diseases (such as osteomalacia, renal osteodystrophy, and primary hyperparathyroidism), degenerative disease, Scheuermann's diseases, Paget's disease, hemangioma, infections, and dysplastic changes.

Fractures that are located above the T7 level, that present with a soft tissue mass osseous destruction, and that are in the posterior part of the vertebral body in conventional radiographs most likely have a malignant etiology. A concave posterior border of the vertebra more likely is a sign of benign osteoporotic fracture, in particular if there is some retropulsion of bone parts into the spinal canal, whereas a convex posterior border suggests malignant disease. CT and MR imaging are helpful in differentiating osteoporotic and malignant fractures. Characteristic MR imaging findings in malignant disease include the depiction of multiple lesions or soft tissue masses, with or without encasing epidural masses and destructive changes (Fig. 11). The fluid sign can be an additional sign or recent fracture in osteoporosis and rarely occurs in metastatic fractures.[137] Gadolinium-enhanced MR can allow a better evaluation of metastatic fractures. MR is useful particularly in visualizing marrow pathology: in multiple myeloma, for example, diffuse demineralization may be shown on radiographs, which may not be differentiated from osteoporosis, whereas diffuse bone marrow pathology usually is well visualized with standard MR imaging. CT may provide better information on matrix changes and demonstrate the border of a lesion better, which is important in the differentiation between benign and malignant disease and may provide a specific tumor diagnosis (Fig. 12). CT also depicts vacuum phenomenon more sensitively, which is a sign of benign disease.[138] Characteristic morphologic changes associated with factures include so-called H vertebrae in sickle cell anemia, Gaucher's disease (also sometimes found in thalassemia and congenital hereditary spherocitosis), and Schmorl's nodes found in Scheuermann's disease. H vertebrae show a characteristic step-like depression of the superior and inferior vertebral margins, which is attributed to disturbance in growth at the chondro-osseous junction resulting from vascular occlusion by abnormal red blood cells in hemoglobinopathic disorders. Schmorl's nodes are focal end plate depressions caused by invagination of disc material into the subchondral vertebral body owing to congenital weakness of subchondral bone and superimposed trauma. Vertebral fractures resulting from osteomalacia in adulthood resemble those found in

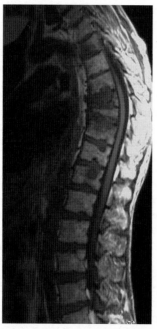

Fig. 11. Sagittal T1-weighted sequence demonstrating a diffuse pathologic bone marrow signal in the spine and several vertebral pathologic fractures consistent with bone marrow infiltration.

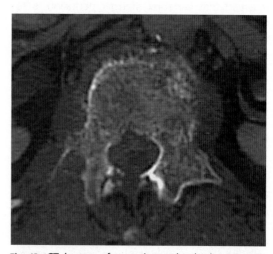

Fig. 12. CT image of a patient who had metastatic disease showing fracture and osteolysis of vertebral body.

osteoporosis but are the result of bone softening and consequent biconcave deformity of the end plates (codfish vertebrae)[139] rather than the microfractures that occur in the brittle bone of the end plates of osteoporosis. Usually osseous deformities at other sites of the skeleton (eg, protrusion acetbul, pseudofractures [Looser's zones] in the pelvis, and bone deformities) are more helpful in differentiating osteoporosis from osteomalacia.[140] In renal osteodystrophy, bone changes are complex and caused by osteomalacia, osteoporosis, and secondary hyperparathyroidism.[141] Vertebral deformities found in this disease typically have a so-called rugger jersey appearance, consisting of bands of subchondral sclerosis beneath the end plates of the vertebrae and more lucent areas in-between. In Paget's disease, the vertebrae may have a coarse, dense, trabecular structure with a more dense periphery on lateral spine radiographs (window pane).[142] The vertebrae are reduced in height but increased in cross-sectional diameter, owing to structural weakness and softening of the bone. In hemangioma, deformity and fracture are rare. Focal, thickened trabeculae may be best shown with CT.

Infection causes erosion of bilateral end plates and loss of disc height and usually has typical imaging features, which differentiates it from osteoporotic fractures. MR imaging criteria with good to excellent sensitivity include the presence of paraspinal or epidural inflammation, disc enhancement, hyperintensity, or fluid-equivalent disc signal intensity on T2-weghted MR images and erosion or destruction of at least one vertebral end plate.[143]

Another important differential diagnosis in osteoporotic vertebral fractures is post-traumatic deformity after compression fractures. If the available clinical history is inadequate then the radiographic appearance may be useful: in post-traumatic deformities, usually the diameter of the vertebrae is enlarged and there are substantial secondary, degenerative changes with osteophytes formation. MR imaging may be useful to determine if there are local pathologic changes in a fractured vertebra and to look for evidence of marrow edema, a sign that a fracture is recent.[144] Generally, the signal abnormality encountered in acute osteoporotic fractures tends to occur adjacent to the fracture site in a band-like configuration. There usually is preservation of some normal marrow signal, especially in the posterior elements and pedicles. The involved vertebral body often shows homogeneous enhancement with gadolinium DTPA, with an absence of an epidural or paravertebral soft tissue mass.

SUMMARY

Osteoporosis is a serious public health problem. The incidence of osteoporotic fractures increases with age. As life expectancy increases, social costs associated with osteoporotic fractures will multiply exponentially. The early diagnosis of osteoporosis thanks to evermore precise devices becomes, therefore, fundamental to preventing complications of disease and unnecessary suffering.

REFERENCES

1. Applegate WB, Blass JP, Williams TF. Instruments for functional assessment of older patients. N Engl J Med 1990;322(17):1207–14.
2. Nevitt MC, Ettinger B, Black DM, et al. The association of radiographically detected vertebral fractures with back pain and function: a prospective study. Ann Intern Med 1998;128(10):793–800.
3. Melton LJ III, Lane A, Cooper C, et al. Prevalence and incidence of vertebral deformities. Osteoporos Int 1993;3(3):113–9.
4. Cummings SR, Black DM, Rubin SM. Lifetime risks of hip, Colle's, or vertebral fracture and coronary heart disease among white postmenopausal women. Arch Intern Med 1989;149(11):2445–8.
5. Albright F. Osteoporosis. Ann Intern Med 1947;27: 861–82.
6. Riggs BL, Melton LJ III. Evidence for two distinct syndromes of involutional osteoporosis. Am J Med 1983;75(6):889–901.
7. Cooper C, Atkinson EJ, Jacobsen SJ, et al. Population-based study of survival after osteoporotic fractures. Am J Epidemiol 1993;137(9):1001–5.
8. Kenny A, Taxel P. Osteoporosis in older men. Clin Cornerstone 2000;2(6):45–51.
9. Resch A, Schneider B, Bernecker P, et al. Risk of vertebral fractures in men: relationship to mineral density of the vertebral body. Am J Roentgenol 1995;164(6):1447–50.
10. Scane AC, Sutcliffe AM, Francis RM. The sequelae of vertebral crush fractures in men. Osteoporos Int 1994;4(2):89–92.
11. Bacon WE, Smith GS, Baker SP. Geographic variation in the occurrence of hip fractures among elderly white US population. Am J Public Health 1989;79(11):1156–8.
12. Melton LJ III, Cummings SR. Heterogeneity of fractures: implications for epidemiology. Bone Miner 1987;2(4):321–31.
13. Orwoll ES, Klein RF. Osteoporosis in men. Endocr Rev 1995;16(1):87–116.
14. Genant HK, Jergas M, Palermo L, et al. Comparison of semiquantitative visual and quantitative morphometric assessment of prevalent and

incident vertebral fractures in osteoporosis. The Study of Osteoporotic Fractures Research Group. J Bone Miner Res 1996;11(7):984–96.

15. Farmer ME, White LR, Brody JA, et al. Race and sex differences in hip fracture incidence. Am J Public Health 1984;74(12):1374–80.

16. Kellie SE, Brody JA. Sex-specific and race-specific hip fracture rates. Am J Public Health 1980;80(3): 326–8.

17. Liel Y, Edwards J, Shary J, et al. The effects of race and body habitus on bone mineral density of the radius, hip and spine in premenopausal women. J Clin Endocrinol Metab 1988;66(6):1247–50.

18. Luckey MM, Meier DE, Mandeli JP, et al. Radial and vertebral bone density in white and black women: evidence for racial differences in premenopausal bone homeostasis. J Clin Endocrinol Metab 1989; 69(4):762–70.

19. Bell NH, Greene A, Epstein S, et al. Evidence for alteration of the vitamin D-endocrine system in blacks. J Clin Invest 1985;76(2):470–3.

20. Bell NH, Yergey AL, Vieira NE, et al. Demonstration of a difference in urinary calcium, not calcium absorption, in black and white adolescents. J Bone Miner Res 1993;8(9):1111–5.

21. Dawson-Hughes B, Harris SS, Finneran S, et al. Calcium absorption responses to calcitriol in black and white premenopausal women. J Clin Endocrinol Metab 1995;80(10):3068–72.

22. Meier DE, Luckey MM, Wallenstein S, et al. Calcium, vitamin D, and parathyroid hormone status in young white and black women: association with racial differences in bone mass. J Clin Endocrinol Metab 1991;72(3):703–10.

23. Hodgson SF, Watts NB, Bilezikian JP, et al. American Association of Clinical Endocrinologists 2001 medical guidelines for clinical practice for the prevention and management of postmenopausal osteoporosis. Endocr Pract 2001;7(4):293–312.

24. Walker-Bone K, Dennison E, Cooper C. Epidemiology of osteoporosis. Rheum Dis Clin North Am 2001;27(1):1–18.

25. Corless D, Gupta SP, Sattar DA, et al. Vitamin D status of residents of an old people's home and long-stay patient. Gerontology 1979;25(6):350–5.

26. McKenna MJ, Freaney R, Meade A, et al. Hypovitaminosis D and elevated serum alkaline phosphatase in elderly Irish people. Am J Clin Nutr 1985; 41(1):101–9.

27. Bullamore JR, Wilkinson R, Gallagher JC, et al. Effect of age on calcium absorption. Lancet 1970; 12(2):535–7.

28. Ireland P, Fordtran IS. Effect on dietary calcium and age on jejunal calcium absorption in humans studied by intestinal perfusion. J Clin Invest 1973;52(1): 2672–81.

29. Fardellone P, Brazier M, Kamel S, et al. Biochemical effects of calcium supplementation in postmenopausal women: influence of dietary calcium intake. Am J Clin Nutr 1998;67(6):1273–8.

30. Brazier M, Kamel S, Maamer M, et al. Markers of bone remodeling in the elderly subject: effects of vitamin D insufficiency and its correction. J Bone Miner Res 1995;10(11):1753–61.

31. Heaney RP, Gallagher JC, Johnston CC, et al. Calcium nutrition and bone health in the elderly. Am J Clin Nutr 1982;36(5S):986–1013.

32. Spencer H, Kramer L, Osis D. Do proteins and phosphorus cause calcium loss? J Nutr 1988; 118(6):657–60.

33. Wiske PS, Epstein S, Bell NH, et al. Increases in immunoreactive parathyroid hormone with age. N Engl J Med 1979;300(25):1419–21.

34. Marcus R, Madvig P, Young G. Age-related changes in parathyroid hormone and parathyroid hormone action in normal humans. J Clin Endocrinol Metab 1984;58(2):223–30.

35. Bruce DG, St John A, Nicklason F, et al. Secondary hyperparathyroidism in patients from Western Australia with hip fracture: relationship to type of hip fracture, renal function, and vitamin D deficiency. J Am Geriatr Soc 1999;47(3):354–9.

36. Stein MS, Scherer SC, Walton SL, et al. Risk factors for secondary hyperparathyroidism in a nursing home population. Clin Endocrinol 1996;44(4): 375–83.

37. Freaney R, McBrinn Y, McKenna MJ. Secondary hyperparathyroidism in elderly people: combined effect of renal insufficiency and vitamin D deficiency. Am J Clin Nutr 1993;58(2):187–91.

38. LeBoff MS, Glowwacki J. Sex steroids, bone and aging. In: Rosen CJ, Glowacki J, Bilezikian JP, editors. The aging skeleton. San Diego (CA): Academic; 1999. p. 159–74.

39. Khosla S, Atkinson EJ, Melton LJ III, et al. Effects of age and estrogen status on serum parathyroid hormone levels and biochemical markers of bone turnover in women: a population-based study. J Clin Endocrinol Metab 1997;82(5):1522–7.

40. Vermeulen A. Clinical review 24: androgens in the aging male. J Clin Endocrinol Metab 1991;73(2): 221–4.

41. Vermeulen A, Kaufman JM. Role of the hypothalamo-pituitary function in the hypoandrogenism of healthy aging. J Clin Endocrinol Metab 1992; 75(3):704–6.

42. Finkelstein JS, Klibanski A, Neer RM, et al. Osteoporosis in men with idiopathic hypogonadotropic hypogonadism. Ann Intern Med 1987;106(3): 354–61.

43. Stepan JJ, Lachmann M, Zverina J, et al. Castrated men exhibit bone loss: effect of calcitonin treatment

on biochemical indices of bone remodeling. J Clin Endocrinol Metab 1989;69(3):523–7.

44. Orwoll ES, Klein RF. Osteoporosis in men: epidemiology, pathophysiology and clinical characterization. In: Marcus R, Feldman D, Kelsey J, editors. Osteoporosis. San Diego (CA): Academic; 1996. p. 745–84.

45. Vedi S, Compston JE, Webb A, et al. Histomorphometric analysis of bone biopsies from the iliac crest of normal British subjects. Metab Bone Dis Relat Res 1982;4(4):231–6.

46. Ballanti P, Bonucci E, Della Rocca C, et al. Bone histomorphometric reference values in 88 normal Italian subjects. Bone Miner 1990;11(2):187–97.

47. Clarke BL, Ebeling PR, Jones JD, et al. Changes in quantitative bone histomorphometry in aging healthy men. J Clin Endocrinol Metab 1996;81(6): 2264–70.

48. Brockstedt H, Kassem M, Eriksen EF, et al. Age- and sex-related changes in iliac cortical bone mass and remodeling. Bone 1993;14(4):681–91.

49. Silverman SL. The clinical consequences of vertebral compression fracture. Bone 1992;13(2S):27–31.

50. Patel U, Skingle S, Campbell GA, et al. Clinical profile of acute vertebral compression fractures in osteoporosis. Br J Rheumatol 1991;30(6):418–21.

51. Cooper C, Atkinson EJ, O'Fallon WM, et al. Incidence of clinically diagnosed vertebral fractures: a population-based study in Rochester, Minnesota, 1985–1989. J Bone Miner Res 1992;7(2):221–7.

52. Rockwood CA Jr, Green DP. Rockwood and Green's fractures in adults, vol. 2. 4th edition. Philadelphia: Lippincott-Raven; 1996. p. 1544–45.

53. Cooper C, O'Neill T, Silman A. The epidemiology of vertebral fractures. European Vertebral Osteoporosis Study Group. Bone 1993;14(1S):89–97.

54. Schneider EL, Guralnik JM. The aging of America. Impact on health care costs. JAMA 1990;263(17): 2335–40.

55. Mallmin H, Ljunghall S, Persson I, et al. Fracture of the distal forearm as a forecaster of subsequent hip fracture: a population-based cohort study with 24 years follow-up. Calcif Tissue Int 1993;52(4): 269–72.

56. Karlsson MH, Hasserius R, Obrant J. Individuals who sustain nonosteoporotic fractures continue to also sustain fragility fractures. Calcif Tissue Int 1993;53(4):229–31.

57. Harris WH, Heaney RP. Skeletal renewal and metabolic bone disease. N Engl J Med 1969;280(6): 303–11.

58. Frost HM. Cybernetic aspects of bone modeling and remodeling, with special reference to osteoporosis and whole-bone strength. Am J Hum Biol 2001;13(2):235–48.

59. Singh M, Nagrath AR, Maini PS. Changes in trabecular pattern of the upper end of the femur as an index of osteoporosis. J Bone Joint Surg Am 1970;52(3):457–67.

60. Saville PD. The syndrome of spinal osteoporosis. Clin Endocrinol Metab. 1973;2(2):177–85.

61. Black DM, Palermo L, Nevitt MC, et al. Comparison of methods for defining prevalent vertebral deformities: the study of osteoporotic fractures. J Bone Miner Res 1995;10(6):890–902.

62. Grampp S, Genant HK, Mathur A, et al. Comparisons of noninvasive bone mineral measurements in assessing age-related loss, fracture discrimination, and diagnostic classification. J Bone Miner Res 1997;12(5):697–711.

63. Hurxthal LM. Measurement of anterior vertebral compressions and biconcave vertebrae. Am J Roentgenol Radium Ther Nucl Med 1968;103(3): 635–44.

64. Lunt M, Ismail AA, Felsenberg D, et al. Defining incident vertebral deformities in population studies: a comparison of morphometric criteria. Osteoporos Int 2002;13(10):809–15.

65. Link TM, Guglielmi G, van Kuijk C, et al. Radiologic assessment of osteoporotic vertebral fractures: diagnostic and prognostic implications. Eur Radiol 2005;15(8):1521–32.

66. Genant HK, Wu CY, van Kuijk C, et al. Vertebral fracture assessment using a semiquantitative technique. J Bone Miner Res 1993;8(9):1137–48.

67. Quek ST, Peh WC. Radiology of osteoporosis. Semin Musculoskelet Radiol 2002;6(3):197–206.

68. Link TM, Rummeny EJ, Lenzen H, et al. Artificial bone erosions: detection with magnification radiography versus conventional high resolution radiography. Radiology 1994;192(3):861–4.

69. Singh M, Riggs BL, Beabout JW, et al. Femoral trabecular-pattern index for evaluation of spinal osteoporosis. Ann Intern Med 1972;77(1):63–7.

70. Jhamaria NL, Lal KB, Udawat M, et al. The trabecular pattern of calcaneum as an index of osteoporosis. J Bone Joint Surg Br 1983;65(2):195–8.

71. Adams JE. Dual-energy X-Ray absorptiometry. In: Grampp S, editor. Radiology of osteoporosis. Berlin-Heidelberg: Springer-Verlag; 2003. p. 87–100.

72. Stein JA, Waltman MA, Lazewatsdy JL, et al. Dual energy X-ray bone densitometer incorporating an internal reference system. Radiology 1987;165: 313–8.

73. World Health Organization. Assessment of osteoporotic fracture risk and its role in screening for postmenopausal osteoporosis. WHO technical report series, no. 843. Geneva (Switzerland): World Health Organization; 1994. p. 5.

74. Grampp S, Jergas M, Gluer CC, et al. Radiologic diagnosis of osteoporosis. Current methods and perspectives. Radiol Clin North Am 1993;31(5): 1133–45.

75. Faulkner KG, Gluer CC, Majumdar S, et al. Noninvasive measurements of bone mass, structure, and strength: currents methods and experimental techniques. Am J Roentgenol 1991;157(6):1229–37.

76. Miller PD, Bonnick SL, Rosen CJ. Consensus of an international panel on the clinical utility of bone mass measurements in the detection of low bone mass in the adult population. Calcif Tissue Int 1996;58(4):207–14.

77. Marshall D, Johnell O, Wedel H. Meta-analysis of how well measures of bone mineral density predict occurrence of osteoporotic fractures. Br Med J 1996;312(7041):1254–9.

78. Cheng S, Suominen H, Sakari-Rantala R, et al. Calcaneal bone mineral density predicts fracture occurrence: a five-year follow-up study in elderly people. J Bone Miner Res 1997;12(7):1075–82.

79. Miller PD, Siris ES, Barrett-Connor E, et al. Prediction of fracture risk in postmenopausal white women with peripheral bone densitometry: evidence from the National Osteoporosis Risk Assessment. J Bone Miner Res 2002;17(12):2222–30.

80. Pacheco EM, Harrison EJ, Ward KA, et al. Detection of osteoporosis by dual X-ray absorptiometry (DXA) of the calcaneus: is the WHO criterion applicable? Calcif Tissue Int 2002;70(6):475–82.

81. Van der Linden JC, Homminga J, verhaar JA, et al. Mechanical consequences of bone loss in cancellous bone. J Bone Miner Res 2001;16(3):457–65.

82. Guo XE, Kim CH. Mechanical consequence of trabecular bone loss and and its treatment: a three-dimensional model simulation. Bone 2002;30(2):404–11.

83. Villani P, Brondino-Riquier R, Bouvenot G. Fragilité des données acquises de la science. L'example du fluor dans l'osteoporose. Presse Med 1998;27(8):361–2.

84. Wilkin TJ. Changing perceptions in osteoporosis. Br Med J 1999;318(7187):862–4.

85. Yu W, Qin M, van Kuijk C, et al. Normal changes in spinal bone mineral density in a Chinese population: assessment by quantitative computed tomography and dual-energy X-ray absorptiometry. Osteoporos Int 1999;9(2):179–87.

86. Guglielmi G, Muscarella S. Axial CT in the diagnosis of osteoporosis. Clin Cases Miner Bone Metabol 2005;2(2):110–2.

87. Guglielmi G, Floriani I, Torri V, et al. Effect of spinal degenerative changes on volumetric bone mineral density of the central skeleton as measured by quantitative computed tomography. Acta Radiol 2005;46(3):269–75.

88. Guglielmi G, van Kuijk C, Li J, et al. Influence of anthropometric parameters and bone size on bone mineral density using volumetric quantitative computed tomography and dual X-ray absorptiometry at the hip. Acta Radiol. 2006;47(6):574–80.

89. Currey JD. Bone strength: what are we trying to measure? Calcif Tissue Int 2001;68(4):205–10.

90. Liberman UA, Weiss SR, Broll J, et al. Effect of oral alendronate on bone mineral density and the incidence of fractures in postmenopausal osteoporosis. N Engl J Med 1995;333:1437–43.

91. Nevitt MC, Ross PD, Palermo L, et al. Association of prevalent vertebral fractures, bone density, and alendronate treatment with incident vertebral fractures: effect of number and spinal location of fractures. The Fracture Intervention Trial Research Group. Bone 1999;25(5):613–9.

92. Hedlund LR, Gallagher JC. Vertebral morphometry in diagnosis of spinal fractures. Bone Miner 1988;5(1):59–67.

93. Guglielmi G, Diacinti D. Vertebral morphometry. In: Grampp S, editor. Radiology of osteoporosis. Berlin-Heidelberg: Springer-Verlag; 2003. p. 101–10.

94. Barnett E, Nordin BE. The radiological diagnosis of osteoporosis: a new approach. Clin Radiol 1960;11:166–74.

95. Jergas M, Felsenberg D. Assessment of vertebral fracture. In: Genant HK, Guglielmi G, Jergas M, editors. Bone densitometry and osteoporosis. Berlin-Heidelberg: Springer-Verlag; 1998. p. 235–46.

96. Nicholson PH, Haddaway MJ, Davie MW, et al. A computerized technique for vertebral morphometry. Physiol Meas 1993;14(2):195–204.

97. Rosol MS, Cohen GL, Halpern EF, et al. Vertebral morphometry derived from digital images. Am J Roentgenol 1996;167(6):1545–9.

98. Diacinti D, Acca M, Tomei E. Metodica di radiologia digitale per la valutazione dell'osteoporosi vertebrale. Radiol Med 1996;91(1–2):13–7.

99. Cortet B, Boutry N, Dubois P, et al. Does quantitative ultrasound of bone reflect more bone mineral density than bone microarchitecture? Calcif Tissue Int 2004;74(1):60–7.

100. Nicholson PH, Lowet G, Cheng XG, et al. Assessment of the strength of the proximal femur in vitro: relationship with ultrasonic measurements of the calcaneus. Bone 1997;20(3):219–24.

101. Cheng XG, Nicholson PH, Boonen S, et al. Prediction of vertebral strength in vitro by spinal bone densitometry and calcaneal ultrasound. J Bone Miner Res 1997;12(10):1721–8.

102. Lochmuller EM, Zeller JB, Kaiser D, et al. Correlation of femoral and lumbar DXA and calcaneal ultrasound, measured in situ with intact soft tissues, with the in vitro failure loads of the proximal femur. Osteoporos Int 1998;8(6):591–8.

103. Guglielmi G, Cammisa M, De Serio A, et al. Phalangeal US velocity discriminates between normal and vertebrally fractured subjects. Eur Radiol 1999;9(8):1632–7.

104. Guglielmi G, Njeh CF, de Terlizzi F, et al. Phalangeal quantitative ultrasound, phalangeal morphometric variables, and vertebral fracture discrimination. Calcif Tissue Int 2003;72(4):469–77.

105. Guglielmi G, de Terlizzi F, Aucella F. Quantitative bone ultrasonography: state of the art and perspectives. G Ital Nefrol 2004;21(4):343–54.

106. Guglielmi G, de Terlizzi F, Torrente I, et al. Quantitative ultrasound of the hand phalanges in a cohort of monozygotic twins: influence of genetic and environmental factors. Skeletal Radiol 2005;34(11): 727–35.

107. Guglielmi G, de Terlizzi F, Aucella F, et al. Quantitative ultrasound technique at the phalanges in discriminating between uremic and osteoporotic patients. Eur J Radiol 2006;60(1):108–14.

108. Barkmann R, Kantorovich E, Singal C, et al. A new method for quantitative ultrasound measurements at multiple skeletal sites: first results of precision and fracture discrimination. J Clin Densitom 2000; 3(1):1–7.

109. Cepollaro C, Gonnelli S, Pondrelli C, et al. The combined use of ultrasound and densitometry in the prediction of vertebral fracture. Br J Radiol 1997; 70(835):691–6.

110. Thompson P, Taylor J, Fisher A, et al. Quantitative heel ultrasound in 3180 women between 45 and 75 years of age: compliance, normal ranges and relationship to fracture history. Osteoporos Int 1998;8(3):211–4.

111. Pluijm SM, Graafmans WC, Bouter LM, et al. Ultrasound measurements for the prediction of osteoporotic fractures in elderly people. Osteoporos Int 1999;9(6):550–6.

112. Hartl F, Tyndall A, Kraenzlin M, et al. Discriminatory ability of quantitative ultrasound parameters and bone mineral density in a population-based sample of postmenopausal women with vertebral fractures: results of the basel osteoporosis study. J Bone Miner Res 2002;17(2):321–30.

113. Ekman A, Michaelsson K, Petren-Mallmin M, et al. Dual X-ray absorptiometry of hip, heel ultrasound, and densitometry of fingers can discriminate male patients with hip fracture from control subjects: a comparison of four different methods. J Clin Densitom 2002;5(1):79–85.

114. Barkmann R, Gluer CC. Quantitative ultrasound. In: Grampp S, editor. Radiology of osteoporosis. Berlin-Heidelberg: Springer-Verlag; 2003. p. 131–41.

115. Heaney RP, Avioli LV, Chesnut CH III, et al. Ultrasound velocity, through bone predicts incident vertebral deformity. J Bone Miner Res 1995;10(3):341–5.

116. Bauer DC, Gluer CC, Cauley JA, et al. Broadband ultrasound attenuation predicts fractures strongly and indipendently of densitometry in older women. A prospective study. Study of Osteoporotic Fractures Research group. Arch Intern Med 1997; 157(6):629–34.

117. Hans D, Dargent-Molina P, Schott AM, et al. Ultrasonographic heel measurements to predict hip fracture in elderly women: the EPIDOS prospective study. Lancet 1996;348(9026):511–4.

118. Porter RW, Miller CG, Grainger D, et al. Prediction of hip fracture in elderly women: a prospective study. Br Med J 1990;301(6753):638–41.

119. Shefelbine SJ, Majumdar S. Imaging bone structure and osteoporosis using MRI. Clin Cases Miner Bone Metabol 2005;2(2):119–26.

120. Guglielmi G, Selby K, Blunt BA, et al. Magnetic resonance imaging of the calcaneus: preliminary assessment of trabecular bone-dependent regional variations in marrow relaxation time compared with dual X-ray absorptiometry. Acad Radiol 1996;3(4):336–43.

121. Link TM, Majumdar S, Augat P, et al. In vivo high resolution MRI of the calcaneus: differences in trabecular structure in osteoporotic patients. J Bone Miner Res 1998;13(7):1175–82.

122. Herlidou S, Grebe R, Grados F, et al. Influence of age and osteoporosis on calcaneus trabecular bone structure: a preliminary in vivo MRI study by quantitative texture analysis. Magn Reson Imaging 2004;22(2):237–43.

123. Fanucci E, Manenti G, Masala S, et al. Multiparameter characterisation of vertebral osteoporosis with 3-T MR. Radiol Med 2007;112(2):208–23.

124. Majumdar S. Magnetic resonance imaging for osteoporosis. Skeletal Radiol 2008;37(2):95–7.

125. Ito M, Ikeda K, Nishiguchi M, et al. Multi-detector row CT imaging of vertebral microstructure for evaluation of fracture risk. J Bone Miner Res 2005; 20(10):1828–36.

126. Chen WT, Shih TT, Chen RC, et al. Vertebral bone marrow perfusion evaluated with dynamic contrast-enhanced MR imaging: significance of aging and sex. Radiology 2001;220(1):213–8.

127. Montazel JL, Divine M, Lepage E, et al. Normal spinal bone marrow in adults: dynamic gadolinium-enhanced MR imaging. Radiology 2003; 229(3):703–9.

128. Baur A, Stabler A, Bartl R, et al. MRI gadolinium enhancement of bone marrow: age-related changes in normals and in diffuse neoplastic infiltration. Skeletal Radiol 1997;26(7):414–8.

129. Schellinger D, Lin CS, Hatipoglu HG, et al. Potential value of vertebral proton MR spectroscopy in determining bone weakness. AJNR Am J Neuroradiol 2001;22(8):1620–7.

130. Kugel H, Jung C, Schulte O, et al. Age- and sex-specific differences in the 1H-spectrum of vertebral bone marrow. J Magn Reson Imaging 2001;13(2): 263–8.

131. Griffith JF, Yeung DK, Antonio GE, et al. Vertebral bone mineral density, marrow perfusion, and fat content in healthy men and men with osteoporosis: dynamic contrast-enhanced MR imaging and MR spectroscopy. Radiology 2005;236(3): 945–51.

132. Parhami F. Possible role of oxidized lipids in osteoporosis: could hyperlipidemia be a risk factor? Prostaglandins Leukot Essent Fatty Acids 2003; 68(6):373–8.

133. McFarlane SI, Muniyappa R, Shin JJ, et al. Osteoporosis and cardiovascular disease: brittle bones and boned arteries, is there a link? Endocrine 2004;23(1):1–10.

134. Camp JD, Oscher HC. The osseous changes in hyperparathyroidism associated with parathyroid tumor: a roentgenologic study. Radiology 1931; 17:63.

135. Adachi JD, Bensen WG, Hodsman AB. Corticosteroid-induced osteoporosis. Semin Arthritis Rheum 1993;22(6):375–84.

136. Brandli DW, Golde G, Greenwald M, et al. Glucocorticoid-induced osteoporosis: a cross-sectional study. Steroids 1991;56(10):518–23.

137. Boehm HF, Link TM. Bone imaging: traditional techniques and their interpretation. Curr Osteoporos Rep 2004;2(2):41–6.

138. Laredo JD, Lakhdari K, Bellaiche L, et al. Acute vertebral collapse: CT findings in benign and malignant nontraumatic cases. Radiology 1995; 194(1):41–8.

139. Resnick DL. Fish vertebrae. Arthritis Rheum 1982; 25(9):1073–7.

140. Adams J. Radiology of rickets and osteomalacia. In: Feldman D, Glorieux FH, Pike JW, editors. Vitamin D. San Diego (CA): Elsevier Academic Press; 1997. p. 967–94.

141. Adams JE. Dialysis bone disease. Semin Dial 2002;15(4):277–89.

142. Whitehouse RW. Paget's disease of bone. Semin Musculoskelet Radiol 2002;6(4):313–22.

143. Ledermann HP, Schweitzer ME, Morrison WB, et al. MR imaging findings in spinal infections: rules or myths? Radiology 2003;228(2):506–14.

144. Guglielmi G, Andreula C, Muto M, et al. Percutaneous vertebroplasty: indications, contraindications, technique, and complications. Acta Radiol 2005; 46(3):256–68.

Gastrointestinal Disorders in Elderly Patients

A. Reginelli, MD[a], M.G. Pezzullo, MD[a], M. Scaglione, MD[b],
M. Scialpi, MD[c], L. Brunese, MD[d], R. Grassi, MD[a],*

KEYWORDS
- Gastrointestinal • Elderly • Swallowing • Pelvic floor
- Acute abdomen

Gastrointestinal (GI) diseases are common in older patients, and the clinical presentation, complications, and treatment may be different from those in younger patients. With the marked increase in population aged 65 years and over, the study and care of GI disorders should be a high priority for both clinicians and researchers. Both the usual course of aging and the accumulation of multiple disease states can lead to impairments in GI function. Older individuals' propensity to use multiple medications, combined with years of acquired lifestyle choices, can disrupt the integrity and functioning of the GI system. Most problems encountered occur at the proximal and distal ends of the GI tract.[1,2] Constipation is the most common GI complaint in of one quarter of elderly men and one third of elderly women.[3]

Acute abdomen in elderly patients poses a difficult challenge for emergency physicians. Elderly patients have a diminished sensorium, allowing pathology to advance to a very dangerous state before developing symptoms. In the presence of serious intra-abdominal pathology, elderly patients are more likely to present with vague symptoms and to have nonspecific findings on examination. Mesenteric ischemia and small bowel obstruction (SBO) must be included in the initial differential diagnosis of abdominal pain, because an early diagnosis minimizes the risk of an unfortunate outcome.[4]

SWALLOWING DISORDERS

Swallowing is an essential biologic function, and any alteration can have severe consequences, such as malnutrition, dehydration, aspiration pneumonia, or airway obstruction. Swallowing disorders have a variety of causes: neurologic disease; neoplasia of the oral cavity, the pharynx and/or the larynx; connective tissue disease; trauma; infection; or iatrogenic illness.

Because dysphagia covers a wide range of symptoms, from a vague or subtle sensation of abnormal swallowing in an ambulatory, alert patient to an apparent inability to swallow at all in a severely handicapped, bedridden patient, a complete evaluation of the swallowing mechanism should be performed.[5–7]

Oral and pharyngeal phase dysfunctions often are caused by central nervous system disorders of pyramidal and extrapyramidal pathways and peripheral nervous system motor impairment. Neurogenic dysphagia may result from cortical (generally bilateral) lesions of the pyramidal tracts, movement disorders (eg, Parkinson's disease), cerebellar disorders, brain stem lesions, lesion of the cranial nerves or their neuromuscular junctions, or lesions of the oral, pharyngeal, or esophageal striated muscles.[8–10] The number of swallowing-impaired persons is substantial, particularly among the

[a] Section of Radiology, Department "Magrassi-Lanzara," Second University of Naples, Piazza Miraglia 2, 80131, Naples, Italy
[b] Department of Radiology, Clinica Pineta Grande, Via Domitiana Km. 30, 81030, Castelvolturno (CE), Italy
[c] Section of Diagnostic and Interventional Radiology, Surgery and Odontostomatology Science, University of Perugia, via Brunamonti 51, 06100, Perugia, Italy
[d] Department of Radiology, Health Science, University of Molise, via De Sanctis, 86100, Campobasso, Italy
* Corresponding author.
E-mail address: roberto.grassi@unina2.it (R. Grassi).

Radiol Clin N Am 46 (2008) 755–771
doi:10.1016/j.rcl.2008.04.013

elderly. It is believed that 30% to 40% of nursing home residents have some form of swallowing impairment. These individuals are particularly prone to episodes of choking during swallowing, a sign that the swallowing mechanism is abnormal.[11–13]

Some of these patients develop compensatory mechanisms of the swallowing process, either voluntary (modifications of the diet and/or of the mechanism of swallowing) or involuntary.

Especially in the elderly, the reduced sensitivity of the oral cavity, pharynx, and/or larynx, together with swallowing mechanism alterations, can allow aspiration or penetration of food into the trachea and bronchi that often is not perceived by the patient but that can lead to respiratory alterations, as laryngospasm, asthma, and airway inflammation.[14]

There are six physiologic stages in swallowing:[15,16]

Stage I. Preparation for swallowing: The bolus is maintained within the mouth by the close apposition of the soft palate to the posterior aspect of the tongue.

Stage II. Initial stage of swallowing: Elevation of the soft palate that is apposed to the posterior pharynx wall that moves anteriorly (Passavant's cushion). The anterior and downward movement of the tongue contributes to create a receiving space of the bolus in the oropharynx with initial filling of the glossoepiglottic valleculae.

Stage III. The bolus in the oropharynx: The epiglottis tilts downward and posteriorly to prevent laryngeal injection. The superior and medium constrictor muscles of the pharynx create a posterior contraction wave (stripping wave) that pushes the bolus into the hypopharynx. The larynx is closed and elevates during swallowing. Free up-and-down motion of larynx is an important factor preventing laryngeal injection. This elevation may be recognized by upward and anterior movement of the hyoid bone toward the mandible during deglutition.

Stage IV. The bolus in the hypopharynx: The hyoid bone and the larynx reach the maximum position. Closure of the larynx results in loss of air from the laryngeal ventricule and produces a "conus" appearance with a straight inferior border of the larynx. The peristaltic wave of the constrictors pushes the bolus into the hypopharynx while the cricopharyngeal muscles are opened.

Stage V. Bolus in the hypopharynx, in the pharyngo-esophageal segment and cervical esophagus: The laryngeal vestibule remains closed from the inward fold movement of the epiglottis.

Stage VI. Reopening of the pharynx and larynx: All the structures return to their initial state with the complete opening of the nasopharynx and the laryngeal vestibule and the reopening of the larynx.

Radiologic contrast examination is essential to evaluate physiologic swallowing dynamics and to detect pathologic impairments. Imaging features allow an accurate study of the tongue, palate, pharynx, and larynx, providing useful information for identifying the cause of the swallowing difficulty and for planning management.

Various nonradiologic techniques, including videoendoscopy, manometry, and electromyography, are used in the dynamic evaluation of swallowing disorders. The videofluorographic examination allows patients who have normal swallowing to be differentiated from patients who have swallowing alterations that require a specific rehabilitation program. Only through the dynamic examination of swallowing is it possible to confirm or exclude the presence of food aspiration or penetration into the airways; this information influences the type of nutrition (oral or nonoral) the patient should receive. Simultaneous examination using videofluoroscopy concurrent with solid-state manometry—videomanometry—provides qualitative, and quantitative information by combining movement analysis with pressure recordings.[17]

Imaging Technique

Videofluoroscopic study is performed with a remote-controlled radiographic apparatus connected to a personal computer workstation that allows analysis of static images and dynamic sequences and the possibility of postprocessing elaborations.

The most recent technique is digital videofluoroscopy with real-time acquisition of a minimum of 12 images/s and a 320 × 240 pixel matrix.

In uncooperative patients (eg, elderly patients who have neurologic disease), the examination could be performed using lateral acquisitions with the patient seated rather than standing.[18]

The technique protocol includes

Precontrastographic phase (plain film)
- A preliminary soft-tissue lateral and frontal view of the neck that displays pharynx and larynx contours and provides information about the surrounding structures, such as

cervical vertebrae, and possible pathologic conditions

Precontrastographic dynamic phase
- Patient erect, frontal projection: examination of the motility of the larynx and vocal chords with a first series of acquisitions during phonation (the patient pronounces the vocal "eee")
- Patient erect, lateral projection: examination of the motility of the soft palate (right-angle lifting of the palate with apposition against Passavant's cushion) with a second series of acquisitions during phonation (the patient says the word "candy") (**Fig. 1**)

Contrastographic dynamic phase
- Patient erect, lateral projection: examination of the oropharynx with acquisition during the swallowing of a high-density barium bolus
- Patient erect, frontal projection: examination of the oropharynx with acquisition during the swallowing of a high-density barium bolus

Small boluses (15–20 mL) of high-density (250% weight/volume) barium are used for the study of the oral and pharyngeal stages of swallowing. For patients suffering from dysphagia to liquids, the study also includes acquisitions during swallowing of small boluses (15–20 mL) of semi-fluid barium (barium sulfate, 60% weight/volume).

The dynamic examinations and/or the individual frames can be examined on the same console.

Pathologic Findings

Deglutition is a complex process that involves many muscular structures and multiple innervations. Swallowing alterations often are a result of several impairments, so they can appear as a complex syndrome with multiple findings rather than as a single, isolated dysfunction.[19]

Moreover, apart from pathologic alteration of deglutition caused by neuromuscular disorders, this physiologic function can be impaired by natural aging processes, leading to a typical pathophysiologic configuration termed "presbyphagia."[20] Characteristic features of presbyphagia, such as weakness of pharyngeal ligaments, lower position of the hyoid bone, quadrangular shape of the valleculae, and expansion of the pharyngeal cavity, should not be considered abnormal findings but rather as paraphysiologic aspects of an aged deglutition system.

The purposes of the dynamic radiologic study of the pharynx are

1. To define the normal anatomy of oropharyngeal region
2. To identify swallowing abnormalities (in the oral and pharyngeal phases)
3. To detect the mechanism responsible for the alteration
4. To determine the circumstances under which the patient can swallow safely

Oropharyngeal incontinence
Drooling of saliva seems to be the consequence of a dysfunction in the coordination of the

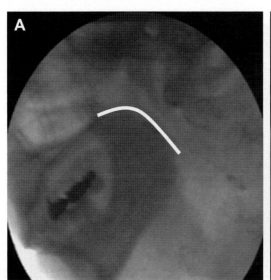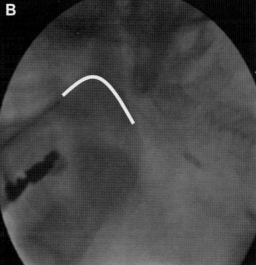

Fig. 1. Examination of the motility of the soft palate. (*A*) At rest the soft palate is in normal position (*white line*). (*B*) Acquisition during phonation (with the patient pronouncing the word "candy") shows right-angle lifting of the palate with apposition against Passavant's cushion (*white line*).

swallowing mechanism, resulting in excess pooling of saliva in the anterior portion of the oral cavity and the unintentional loss of saliva from the mouth.

Incompetence of the seal between the tongue and the palate results in premature leakage of the barium into the oropharynx before initiation of swallowing, with the potential for aspiration into the open, unprotect larynx (**Fig. 2**). Tongue deficiency resulting from atrophy, weakness, or lack of coordination may be compensated by the downward displacement of the palate with the palate "kinking" to appose the tongue.[21,22]

Pharyngeal retention
Normal subjects occasionally retain small amounts of food in the pharyngeal recesses (the glossoepiglottic valleculae and pyriform sinuses) after swallowing. Excessive retention of food in the pharynx after swallowing may be caused by obstruction of the foodway or by weakness or lack of coordination of the pharynx (**Fig. 3**).

Pharyngeal weakness may be caused by a reduction in driving force of the tongue or by weakness of the pharyngeal constrictor muscle resulting from nerve or muscle diseases. Residual bolus spreads throughout pharynx after swallowing and enters the airway as the patient inhales.

Epiglottic dysfunction
Radiologic examination may reveal dysfunction of the epiglottis that can assume a variety of features. A totally immobile epiglottis may lead to altered swallowing. An epiglottis that attains an obliquity

and does not tilt down properly but remains in a transverse position during deglutition, as seen in the anteroposterior projection (**Fig. 4**), may lead to misdirected swallowing.[23]

Penetration
Laryngeal penetration is the entry of swallowed material into the larynx during swallowing, stopping at vocal cord level. It is important to distinguish laryngeal penetration from aspiration (**Fig. 5**).

Aspiration
Aspiration is the entry of liquid or food through the larynx above the vocal cord level. Approximately 40% of patients who are aspirating are not identified during clinical evaluation. On dynamic radiologic study (**Fig. 6**), these patients often are found to have barium aspiration in the airway without coughing (silent aspiration).[24,25] Fifty-eight percent of patients suffering from dysphagia after a stroke present aspiration of contrast bolus during the videofluoroscopic examination despite the absence of clinical symptoms.[26,27] The odds ratio of developing pneumonia is 7.6 times greater for patients who aspirate than for those who do not. The odds ratio of death is 9.2 times greater for patients who aspirate thick liquids or food of more solid consistency than for those who do not aspirate or who aspirate only thin liquids.[28]

The risk of illness caused by aspiration depends on the amount and the nature of material aspirated and on the depth of aspiration, factors that can be demonstrated by dynamic radiologic study.

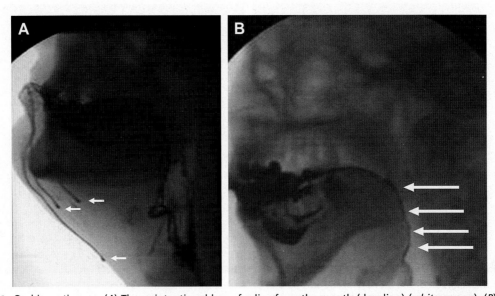

Fig. 2. Oral incontinence. (*A*) The unintentional loss of saliva from the mouth (drooling) (*white arrows*). (*B*) The incompetence of the seal between the tongue and the palate results in premature leakage (*white arrows*).

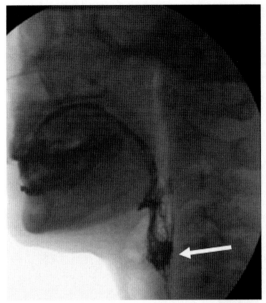

Fig. 3. Excessive retention of barium in the pharynx (*arrow*) after swallowing caused by weakness of the pharyngeal constrictor muscle.

Laryngeal injection through the vocal cords into the trachea may occur during swallowing, before swallowing, or after swallowing. Timing of the injection has important therapeutic implications.

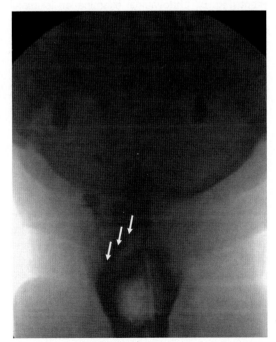

Fig. 4. The epiglottis attains an oblique position and does not tilt down properly but remains in a transverse position during deglutition (*white arrows*).

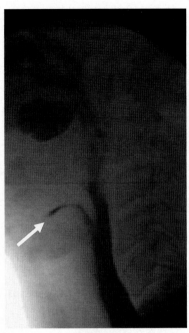

Fig. 5. Laryngeal penetration. Entry of swallowed material into the larynx during swallowing, stopping at the level of the vocal cord (*white arrow*).

During radiologic examination, various therapeutic modifications of head position, laryngeal elevation, bolus size, and swallow/respiration/cough sequencing can be tried, based on the analysis of why and when aspiration occurs.[29,30]

Cricopharyngeal dysfunction

Functional disturbance of the cricopharyngeal muscle makes it incapable of relaxing during swallowing. Such dysfunction often is referred to as "cricopharyngeal achalasia," but this term seems inappropriate, because the muscle does relax in these patients, although the relaxation may be delayed or incomplete. "Cricopharyngeal dysfunction" seems to be a more adequate designation. The classical finding on a dynamic radiologic study is the presence of the horizontal bar (often called the "cricopharyngeal bar") at the level of the C5-C6 vertebral body. This bar makes a posterior indentation in the barium column that persists throughout the swallow.[31]

PELVIC FLOOR PATHOLOGIES

In recent years, diagnostic imaging has renewed interest in the study of morphofunctional disorders characterizing pelvic floor pathologies.

Because of the multiplicity of these disorders and the variety of symptoms (which are not related easily to individual diseases and which present in various associations of symptoms), the clinical

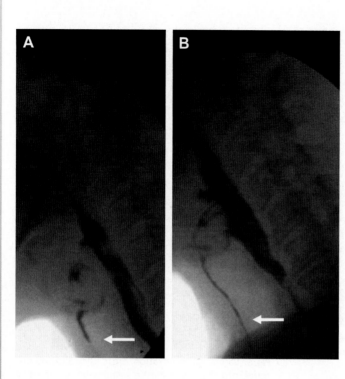

Fig. 6. Aspiration. Entry of swallowed material through the larynx (*A*) (*white arrow*) over vocal cord level (*B*) (*white arrow*).

examination, although necessary as a first approach to the problem, often is insufficient to define the nature of the disorder. Furthermore, it is common for a dynamic radiologic examination of endopelvic structures to reveal multicompartmental dysfunction in patients whose initial clinical observation was oriented to a single-compartment disorder.[32] The classical segregation of the pelvic floor into three compartments—anterior, middle, and posterior—is largely artificial, because the pelvic floor structures are closely interrelated; patients who have abnormalities in one compartment often have disorders in others.[33]

Imaging Techniques

Ultrasound

Ultrasound examination of pelvic floor can be performed by using transabdominal techniques (transperineal imaging) or by using endorectal and/or endovaginal approaches (endocavitary imaging). Endoanal ultrasound of the anal sphincters, achieved by using a mechanically rotated endoprobe, obtains a 360° axial view of the anal canal. In the proximal portion of the anal canal this procedure visualizes the puborectalis muscle as a hyperechoic arch-shaped structure opened anteriorly (**Fig. 7**A). In the middle level of the canal the external sphincter is seen as a complete hyperechoic ring, and the internal sphincter is seen as a thicker hypoechoic structure (**Fig. 7**B). The distal portion of the canal is defined by the subcutaneous

external sphincter that lies below the termination of the internal sphincter (**Fig. 7**C).

This examination allows the radiologist to detect structural abnormalities that may support functional defects of posterior pelvic floor compartment (**Fig. 8**). Endovaginal examination is useful in studying the female sphincter, and it is especially helpful in postoperative assessment and in evaluating an enterocele. It is expected that further information regarding the usefulness of the ultrasound transperineal approach[34] with dynamic acquisition in the contraction and straining phases and of the new three-dimensional processing imaging (**Fig. 9**) will be forthcoming.

Cine colpo-cystodefecography

The radiologic technique of cine colpo-cystodefecography involves dynamic imaging of rectal voiding,[35,36] associated with a cystographic examination[37] and opacification of vaginal canal, to visualize simultaneously the bladder, urethra, vagina, rectal ampulla, and anal canal at rest and during evacuation (**Fig. 10**).

The patient is seated on a portable lavatory seat on the step of the fluoroscopy table, and a lateral pelvic radiograph is taken at rest and during the contraction, straining, and defecatory phases.

At rest, the position of the bladder base with urethra, rectum, anal canal, and vaginal vault are determined by the basal tone of the pelvic floor muscles. In the contraction phase, the strength

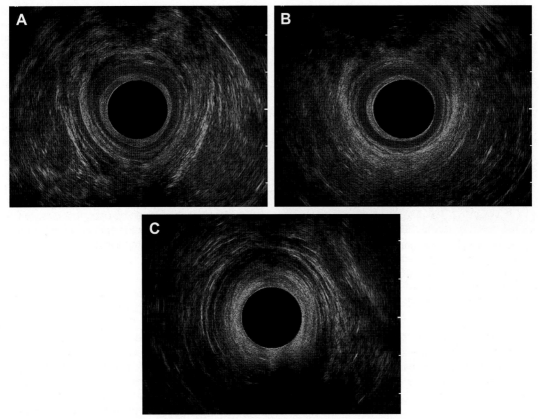

Fig. 7. Endoanal ultrasound. (*A*) At the proximal level the puborectalis muscle is visible as a U-shaped hyperechoic sling. (*B*) At the middle level the internal anal sphincter is visible as a hypoechoic dominant inner ring. Medially to the internal sphincter is the hyperechoic thin ring of the mucosa-submucosa complex. (*C*) At the distal level the subcutaneous external sphincter is visible as a hyperechoic round structure that lies below the termination of the internal sphincter.

of voluntary pelvic floor musculature can be evaluated; if the contraction is valid, the vescicourethral angle and anorectal angle decrease significantly. In the straining phase, the impact on the pelvic viscera of the pelvic muscle relaxation can be demonstrated to assess pelvic floor descent. During evacuation it is possible to observe bladder excursion and the loss of the puborectal impression with the anorectal angle becoming more obtuse; it also is possible to identify any alterations of rectum profile and any change in the relationship between the anterior rectal wall and the posterior portion of vagina.

Dynamic MR imaging

MR imaging has been applied to pelvic floor dynamics to evaluate the complex anatomy and topography of pelvic structures and simultaneously to assess their variations during physiologic dynamic acts.[38] This examination shows the excursion of bladder, rectum, uterus, and vagina, and it analyses the efficacy of puborectalis

muscle contraction and the pelvic floor descent during evacuation (**Fig. 11**).

The rectal ampulla, the bladder, and, in women, the vagina must be opacified: the bladder must be full; the rectum is filled with ultrasonographic gel (250 mL) mixed with gadolinium-diethylenetriamine pentaacetic acid (3 mL); and the vaginal walls are opacified with the same mixture.

The authors perform the examination on a permanent, open-configuration, low-field-strength magnet with a phased array coil, so the patient is free to assume the gynecologic position, which is more comfortable than the supine position for carrying out the whole defecatory act. The protocol consists of T2-weighted sequences in the axial, coronal, and sagittal planes and, for dynamic study, T2-breath-hold sequence (slice, 10 mm; TR, 6.6; TE, 3.3; acquisition time, 01.37; field of view, 380 mm) in the sagittal plane. The MR images so obtained then are assembled in cineview in postprocessing.

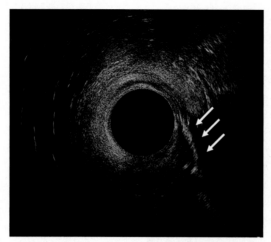

Fig. 8. Endoanal ultrasound. A superficial fistula within the tract that lies medial to the internal sphincter and does not cross any part of it. Note that identification of the fistulous tract is enhanced by hydrogen peroxide injection (*arrows*).

Dynamic MR imaging has better accuracy in detecting and characterizing pelvic organ prolapse but has lower sensitivity than cine colpocystodefecography in detecting parietal and mucosal alterations.

Pathologic Findings

Rectal prolapse

Rectal prolapse is an intussusception that may be external or internal, and it may be limited to mucosa or may involve the full thickness of the rectal wall. An intussusception that remains within the rectum is termed "intrarectal." An intussusception becomes intra-anal if its apex passes into the anal canal and remains there during straining. If the entire thickness of the rectal wall is extruded through the anal canal, the condition is named "complete external rectal prolapse." A prolapse also may be confined to the anterior rectal wall; in that case it is termed an "anterior mucosal prolapse."

Evacuation proctography remains the examination of choice for studying intussusception and mucosal prolapse, because it documents the entire process of intussusception, the segment involved, its location, and any amount of contrast medium not expelled. It also visualizes mucosal prolapse, defines its extent into the anal canal, and reveals any involvement of small intestinal loops. MR imaging provides a level of detail otherwise unobtainable. It can be used to assess pelvic floor mobility with precision and the involvement of anterior and middle compartments.

Rectocele

Rectocele is a protrusion of the anterior rectal wall during evacuation (**Fig. 12**); most rectoceles are not apparent at rest. Rectocele is common in women, because the rectovaginal septum is relatively weak, as is the pelvic floor support, secondary to aging, obesity, pregnancy, and vaginal delivery. A protrusion of the rectum also may be posterior, known as a "posterior rectocele"[39,40] or, more correctly, as "posterior perineal hernia."

Both anterior and posterior rectoceles are well detected with defecography.[41] This imaging modality also evaluates the residual amount of barium at the end of the evacuatory act. MR defecography is the best way to assess rectal ampulla and pelvic floor descent, and it is able to determine if the descent involves only the posterior compartment or if it extends to the anterior and middle compartment structures. Currently, surgical repair of rectocele usually is performed using the double-stapled transanal rectal resection technique.[42]

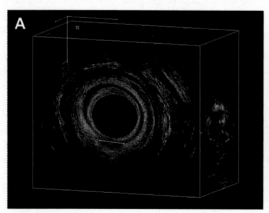
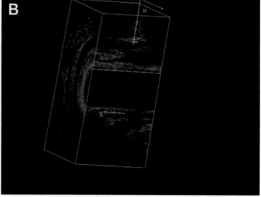

Fig. 9. Image from a three-dimensional data set. Chronic intersphinteric abscess (1) presenting as an area of intermediate reflectivity (*A*) in the frontal view and (*B*) its deep extension in the lateral view.

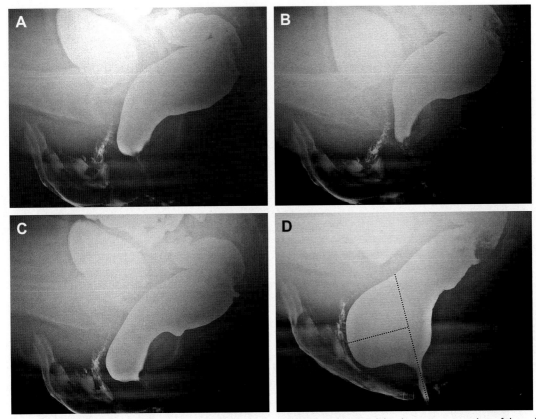

Fig. 10. Radiologic examination. Lateral view of the pelvis (*A*) at rest and during (*B*) voluntary contraction of the pelvic floor muscles ("squeezing"), (*C*) straining, and (*D*) defecation. The depth of a rectocele is measured from its anterior aspect (*horizontal dotted line*) to the vertical from the anterior wall of the anal canal (*vertical dotted line*).

Enterocele, elitrocele, edrocele, (anterior rectal wall hernia) sigmoidocele, and omentocele

Enterocele is a descent of the small bowel, peritoneal fat, or sigmoid colon into the rectogenital space above the superior portion of the vaginal dome. If these structures enter the vaginal fornix posteriorly, there is an elitrocele (posterior vaginal hernia); if they enter the rectum anteriorly, there is an edrocele. An enterocele associated with uterine prolapse is termed a "traction enterocele," whereas an enterocele in a patient who has been hysterectomized is termed a "pulsion enterocele."

Enterocele is easily documented with traditional evacuation proctography, but it is necessary to opacify small bowel loops with barium contrast (four-contrast defecography). Dynamic MR imaging has the advantage of visualizing intestinal descent without the need to opacify bowel loops, and it better assesses pelvic floor excursion and the real dimensions of the hernial orifice (**Fig. 13**). Furthermore, it easily detects omentocele, which is peritoneal fat herniation, and sigmoidocele, which is a descent of sigmoid colon.

Lateral perineal hernias

Perineal hernia is a very rare clinical finding. It occurs when the hernial sac passes through the perineal wall. This pathology is related to a defect in the anatomic structures forming the pelvic diaphragm. The pelvic diaphragm is made up of the levator ani muscle, the coccygeus muscle, the sphincter externus muscle, and the ani and perineal fascia.

Perineal hernias are identified easily with traditional defecography, but it is necessary to integrate the study with anterior/posterior projections. Dynamic MR imaging allows a panoramic view of the whole perineal region, and multiplanar acquisitions can outline the hernial route precisely.

ACUTE ABDOMEN

Elderly patients who have acute abdomen are much less likely to have the classic presentation of this syndrome. Some differences in presentation of the acute abdomen are caused by age-associated physiologic changes. An aged immune system has a decreased ability to react to

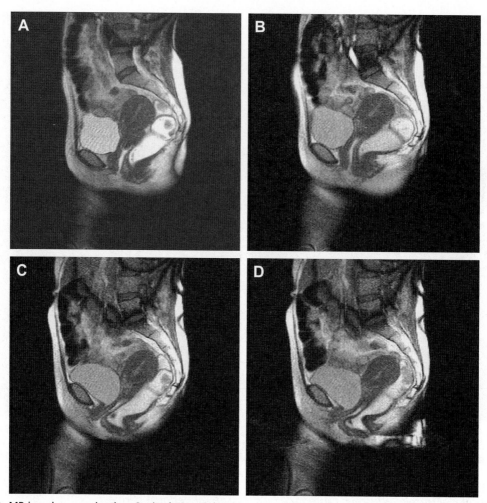

Fig. 11. MR imaging examination. Sagittal T2-weighted images of the pelvis with rectal and vaginal contrast. (*A*) At rest the position of the pelvic viscera is normal. (*B*) In the contraction phase, the efficacy of puborectalis muscle contraction and the excursion of bladder, rectum, uterus, and vagina can be evaluated. (*C*) Position of the pelvic viscera during straining. (*D*) As the patient defecates, there is further descent of the bladder, vaginal angulation, and an anterior rectocele.

common insults, so elderly patients are less likely to have fever or leukocytosis. Their pain often is much less severe than would be expected for a particular disease, because decreased neural sensitivity causes reduced sensation of pain and leads to a delay in the presentation of an acute abdomen. Often, elderly patients who have serious pathology are misdiagnosed initially as having benign conditions such as gastroenteritis or constipation.[3] Moreover, elderly patient often have underlying pathologies, such as chronic cardiovascular and pulmonary disease, diabetes, malignancies, diverticula, abdominal aortic aneurism, peptic ulcer disease, and biliary tract disease. They usually take multiple medications, and they often are unable to explain their symptoms clearly because of an impaired sensorium.

Although SBO and mesenteric ischemia are well-known and common conditions, the diagnosis and the choice of the correct treatment still pose challenges for those working in emergency clinical settings. Clinicians must take into account atypical presentations and the many clinical differentials. Once they have established the diagnosis, they need to decide whether, how, and when to intervene.[43]

Mesenteric Ischemia

Mesenteric ischemia leading to bowel infarction is a relatively common catastrophic occurrence in the elderly. In this condition the diagnosis may be difficult, but time is of the essence for survival, because the prognosis is poor, and the treatment

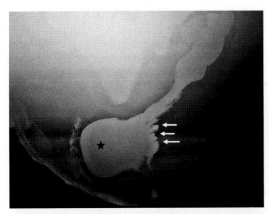

Fig. 12. Barium trapping in rectocele. The postdefecation image shows considerable trapping of barium within a large rectocele (*black star*) and mucosal internal prolapse (*arrows*).

is almost inconsequential if performed too late.[44,45] Acute mesenteric ischemia is a true surgical emergency. Risk factors for acute mesenteric ischemia in patients of advanced age include atherosclerosis, arrhythmias, hypovolemia, congestive heart failure, recent myocardial infarction, valvular disease, deep venous thrombosis, intra-abdominal malignancy, and the use of medications with vasoconstrictive effect on the splanchnic vascular district, such as digitalis, beta-blockers, somatostatin, and vasoactive amines. The diagnosis of acute mesenteric ischemia may be overlooked because of the vague nature of the patient's symptoms.[46–48] Patients may present with recurrent episodes of postprandial abdominal pain (intestinal angina), but often the clinical presentation consists of vomiting or diarrhea with occasional blood in the stool and localized or generalized abdominal pain of either acute or subacute onset. The characteristic of this disease is that symptoms typically are out of proportion to findings.

Acute mesenteric ischemia is a syndrome in which inadequate blood flow through the mesenteric circulation causes ischemia and eventual gangrene of the bowel wall. The etiology could be arterial or venous; the arterial disease can be subdivided into nonocclusive and occlusive ischemia.[49,50]

Occlusion of the superior mesenteric artery may be caused by embolism or thrombosis. Emboli may occlude the proximal portion or one of the distal branches of the superior mesenteric artery, whereas thrombosis more frequently involves the origin of superior mesenteric artery, where wall aortic atheromatous apposition may cause partial obstruction of the orifice. When the superior mesenteric artery is obstructed at the origin by an embolus, most of the small intestine and the right colon are subject to ischemia.[51]

Nonocclusive mesenteric ischemia, most frequent in the elderly, results from decreased arterial perfusion that is not related to the presence of endovascular obstruction but rather is caused by an insufficient cardiac output from congestive heart failure, from myocardial infarction, or from a decreased blood pressure with a low-flow state caused by hypovolemia or shock.[52]

Occlusion of the superior mesenteric vein may be caused by thrombosis at the origin or in its distal branches. It can be primary, or it can be observed in cirrhotic patients who have portal hypertension or in patients who have coagulation disorders. Occlusion of he superior mesenteric vein leads to intramural hemorrhage from impaired venous drainage of the bowel wall.

Chronic mesenteric ischemia may be the precursor of any of these conditions. When the arterial lumen is narrowed secondary to atherosclerosis, an increased metabolic demand (eg, in digestion) exceeds the possible blood supply and can result in severe abdominal pain and possibly infarction.[53]

The superior mesenteric vessels are involved more frequently than the inferior mesenteric vessels, but blockage of the latter often is silent because of better collateral circulation. Damage to the affected bowel portion may range from reversible ischemia to transmural infarction with necrosis and perforation.[54]

Imaging Techniques

Diagnostic imaging plays the main role in detecting the degree and severity of intestinal ischemia and in assessing for evidence of infarction.[55]

Plain abdominal films

Findings on plain films of the abdomen often are normal in the presence of acute mesenteric ischemia. Positive findings usually are late and nonspecific. Plain films, however, are warranted to exclude identifiable causes of abdominal pain such as perforation with free intraperitoneal air. In the earliest phase of ischemia, plain films show a gasless abdomen from spastic ileus. There may be a mild gaseous dilatation of the loops with total loss of tone. In a more advanced phase, small bowel walls may appear thickened, with a "thumbprinting" appearance, sparse and subtle valvulae conniventes, and evidence of air-fluid levels. In the necrotic phase, there is evidence of intestinal and portal pneumatosis.[56]

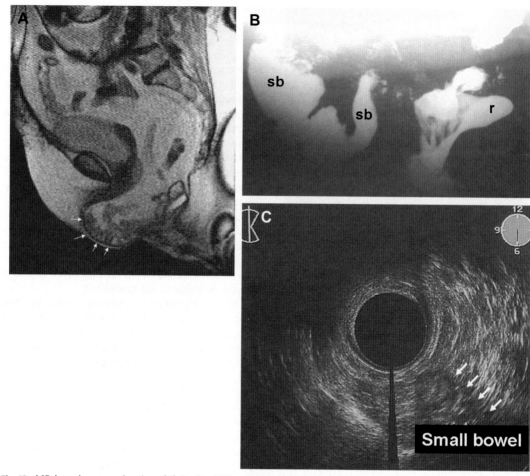

Fig. 13. MR imaging examination. (*A*) Sagittal T2-weighted images of the pelvis with rectal contrast during defecation. There is widening of the rectovaginal space with descending of small bowel loops (*white arrows*); the rectum lies low in the pelvis because of perineal descent. (*B*) The same case studied with the radiologic technique shows small bowel loops (sb) and rectum (r). The intussuscepting rectal wall is invaginating into the anal canal. (*C*) Axial two-dimensional endosonographic image of the anal canal with evidence of small bowel loops (*arrows*).

Ultrasonography

Ultrasound is considered a second-line study for mesenteric ischemia. This technique may be of interest in the follow-up of patients who have an acute abdomen of indeterminate origin or to monitor a pathologic condition that does not require immediate surgery, especially in emergency departments that have a consistent amount of patient admittance with a low prevalence of significant pathologies. The examination may show a thrombus or absent flow in the involved arteries or veins. It cannot detect clots beyond the proximal main vessels, and it cannot be used to distinguish ischemia from hypoperfusion.[57] It often is less useful in the presence of dilated, fluid-filled bowel loops. Possible findings that may be seen in advanced phases include bowel wall thickening with hypoechogenicity of the layers caused by edema, evidence of extraluminal fluid, and decreased peristalsis.

Multidetector CT

Multidetector CT is the study of choice to make a diagnosis of mesenteric ischemia and to exclude other causes of abdominal pain.[58,59] The examination is performed from the diaphragmatic dome to the pubic symphysis with intravenous contrast enhancement injection (120–150 mL volume; 2.5–3 mL/s flow). In acute abdomen of indeterminate cause, a delay of 60 seconds from the start of injection usually is observed. When the clinical suspicion is for intestinal infarction, a biphasic study (arterial and venous phases) may be performed. Multidetector CT allows multiplanar reformatting that may be helpful to study the mesenteric vascular pattern, especially for the terminal branches. The examination is performed without endoluminal opacification by orally or rectally administered contrast medium.

CT findings that must be evaluated to assess a suspected intestinal ischemia are wall thickening, contrast enhancement, caliber of intestinal loops, presence of air-fluid levels, mesenteric arterial and venous vessel viabilities, streaking of mesentery, solid organ infarction, and mural and/ or portal/mesenteric pneumatosis. These findings can be correlated with various phases of intestinal changes from ischemia and infarction.[60]

At an earlier phase of arterial mesenteric ischemia, findings may be normal, with normal or thinned ("paper-thin") bowel wall thickness and normal enhancement, so the diagnosis depends

entirely on the direct visualization of endovascular occlusion. For this reason, an early diagnosis of nonocclusive ischemia is extremely difficult to make, because it would be based only on small bowel appearance. Diagnosis of ischemia with a venous etiology is easier, because an early thickening of intestinal wall caused by intramural hemorrhage and submucosal edema, with the typical alternating layers of different density (the "target sign"), may be observed. This stage of impaired flow may be reversible, but if the vascular injury persists, and no reperfusion therapy is performed, the process evolves to intestinal infarction. Parietal enhancement is a significant sign for assessing bowel segment vitality, because necrotic tissue enhances poorly. Diminished enhancement

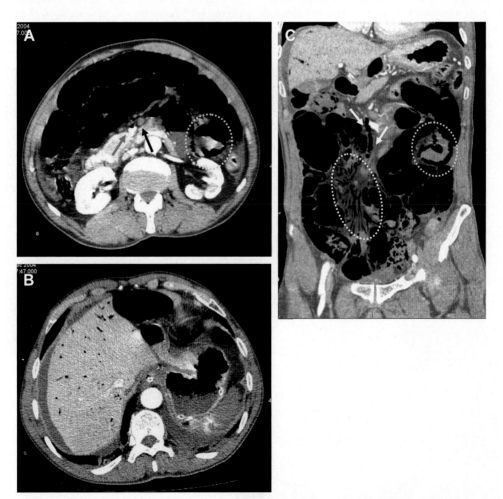

Fig. 14. Late stage of small bowel infarction caused by thrombosis of the superior mesenteric artery. (*A*) Axial multidetector CT demonstrates "paper-thin" small bowel wall distended only by gas, pneumatosis of a small bowel loop at the left flank (*yellow circle*), gas in the superior mesenteric vein (*red arrow*), and occlusion of the superior mesenteric artery (*black arrow*). (*B*) Axial multidetector CT shows portal pneumatosis, splenic infarction, and free fluid in the peritoneal spaces. (*C*) Coronal reformation demonstrates pneumatosis of the mesenteric root (*white circle*) and an ileal loop (*yellow circle*) and gas in the superior mesenteric vein (*arrows*). Signs of portal pneumatosis and free fluid are visible also.

means that the bowel segment is no longer recoverable and must be resected.

In the latest phases of mesenteric ischemia (**Fig. 14**), CT findings show peritoneal fluid, intramural and portal-mesenteric pneumatosis, and, in case of venous etiology, mesenteric engorgement.

Serial CT angiograms can be used to monitor patients treated nonsurgically with anticoagulation therapy.

ACUTE SMALL BOWEL OBSTRUCTION

An SBO is one of the most common causes of admission in emergency departments. The leading cause of SBO in developed countries is postoperative adhesions (60%), followed by malignancy, Crohn's disease, and hernias. Based on surgical and imaging findings, SBOs can be classified as simple, unbalanced, or complicated.[61]

Simple obstruction is characterized by a "bowel picture," and has the most favorable patient prognosis and outcome. In these patients nonoperative management is the first-line clinical approach. Unbalanced SBOs involve both the bowel loops and the peritoneal cavity when there is initial impairment in fluid reabsorption and microvascular wall changes caused by increased luminal tension. This increased tension leads to abnormal permeability and fluid in the adjacent loop spaces and in the peritoneal cavity. In complicated SBOs there is vascular involvement of the "bowel-mesentery" complex with possible ischemic injury.[62] This condition is quite rare, can be partial or complete, and is a real surgical emergency. If not properly diagnosed and treated, complicated SBOs may lead to bowel ischemia and further morbidity and mortality.[63] Because as many as 40% of patients have strangulated obstructions, differentiating the characteristics and causes of obstruction is

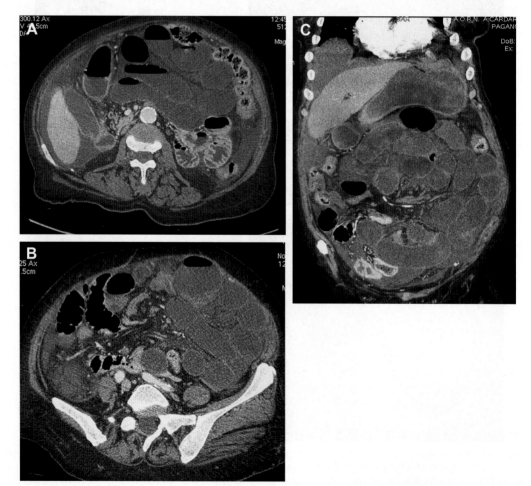

Fig. 15. Complicated small bowel obstruction caused by strangulation. (*A, B*) Two contiguous axial multidetector CT scans show fluid-filled small bowel loops with vascular changes (decreased enhancement) and free fluid at the peritoneal cavity. Note abnormal location of the dilated loops. (*C*) Multiplanar reconstruction on coronal plane gives optimal depiction of these findings.

critical to proper patient treatment. From a clinical viewpoint, differentiating simple, unbalanced, and complicated SBO is not always straightforward, especially in critically ill elderly patients. In the management of SBOs, it is often said, "Never let the sun rise or set on small bowel obstruction," because they sometimes are fatal if treatment is delayed. Furthermore, in the emergency setting, other important emergencies (such as small bowel infarcts or acute pancreatitis) initially may mimic the signs and symptoms of SBOs.[64] Thus, in this context, plain film and CT studies are extremely useful tools in the emergency room. The radiologist's task is to provide accurate details concerning the pathophysiologic aspects of the complex "bowel-mesentery" status, thus supporting the appropriate management decision process.

Imaging Techniques

Plain film and ultrasonography

Plain film radiographs remain the first-line radiologic measure for patients in whom acute SBO is suspected. Plain radiographs are more accurate diagnostically in cases of simple obstruction. Combining plain radiographs with sonography is helpful to differentiate simple from unbalanced SBOs, if both examinations are performed by the same, experienced radiologist.

In simple SBO, plain films may show dilated loops with multiple, thin valvulae conniventes proximal to the point of obstruction ("transition zone") and collapsed loops distal to the site of obstruction. Enteric stasis in the dilated loops may be gaseous, liquid, or mixed.

Unbalanced SBO is characterized by the presence of dilated loops with thin walls and a more represented fluid stasis. Ultrasound may demonstrate these findings and fluid between the loops and in peritoneal cavity.[65] Plain film radiographs and ultrasound are of little assistance in differentiating simple from complicated SBOs, however.

Multidetector CT

The study of the "bowel-mesentery" complex is the field in which CT finds its true role! CT scanning is useful in making an early diagnosis of complicated SBOs and in delineating the myriad other causes of acute abdominal pain.[66]

The CT examination should be performed after administration of intravenous contrast medium using a biphasic (arterial and portal) acquisition.

In complicated SBO, findings include increased, normal, or decreased enhancement of the bowel wall associated with haziness or thickening of the supporting mesentery (**Fig. 15**). In this case, fluid may have high attenuation values, or it can be definitely hemorrhagic.[67] If surgery is not undertaken

promptly in these patients, bowel loops and their mesentery become necrotic, leading to bowel perforation and peritonitis.[68]

CT scanning is about 90% sensitive and specific in detecting SBO. CT also has proved useful in distinguishing extrinsic causes of SBO, such as adhesions and hernia, from intrinsic causes, such as neoplasms or Crohn's disease. It also differentiates these extrinsic and intrinsic causes from intraluminal causes such as bezoars or gallstone ileus. Multiplanar reformations improve the sensitivity and accuracy of CT by demonstrating the spatial details of the bowel and the mesenteric complex and revealing the transition zone.[69] In the context of acute SBO, however, CT should not be used universally, for every patient, but should be reserved for selected cases in which clinical and radiographic findings are inconclusive.[70]

REFERENCES

1. Bartz S. Gastrointestinal disorders in the elderly Anals of Long Term Care: Clinical Care and Aging 2003;11(7):33–9.
2. Grassi R. Diagnostic imaging of deglutition and continence-defecation disorders. Radiol Med 2003; 106(3 Suppl 1):90–3.
3. Bryan D. Abdominal pain in elderly persons. Updated October 5, 2006. Available at: http://www. emedicine.com/EMERG/topic931.htm. Accessed June 2, 2008.
4. Amjad N. Acute abdomen in the elderly—a diagnostic dilemma. Available at: http://www.e-imj.com/Vol2-No1/Vol2-No2-E1.htm.
5. Jones B, Donner MW. Examination of the patient with dysphagia. Radiology 1988;167:319–26 [Erratum in Radiology 1991;179:881].
6. Ott DJ, Pikna LA. Clinical and videofluoroscopic evaluation of swallowing disorders. AJR Am J Roentgenol 1993;161:507–13.
7. Lind CD. Dysphagia: evaluation and treatment. Gastroenterol Clin North Am 2003;32:553–75.
8. Chaundhry V, Umapathi T, Ravich WJ. Neuromusclar diseases and disorders of the alimentary system. Muscle Nerve 2002;25(6):768–84.
9. Barbiera F, Iacono G, Carroccio A, et al. Digital cineradiographic study of swallowing in infants with neurologic disease. Our experience. Radiol Med 2004;107:286–92.
10. Hamdy S. The diagnosis and management of adult neurogenic dysphagia. Nurs Times 2004;100:52–4.
11. Kendall KA, Leonard RJ. Videofluoroscopic upper esophageal sphincter function in elderly dysphagic patients. Laryngoscope 2002;112:332–7.
12. Feinberg MJ, Ekberg O. Deglutition after near-fatal choking episode: radiologic evaluation. Radiology 1990;176(3):637–40.

13. Tracy JF, Logemann JA, Kahrilas PJ, et al. Preliminary observations on the effects of age on oropharyngeal deglutition. Dysphagia 1989;4(2):90–4.

14. Feinberg MJ, Ekberg O. Videofluoroscopy in elderly patients with aspiration: importance of evaluating both oral and pharyngeal stages of deglutition. AJR Am J Roentgenol 1991;156(2):293–6.

15. Jones B, Donner MW. Normal and abnormal swallowing. New York: Springer Verlag; 1991. p. 77–8.

16. Dodds WJ, Stewart ET, Logemann JA. Physiology and radiology of the normal oral and pharyngeal phases of swallowing. AJR Am J Roentgenol 1990; 154(5):953–63.

17. Olsson R, Castell J, Johnston B, et al. Combined videomanometric identification of abnormalities related to pharyngeal retention. Acad Radiol 1997; 4(5):349–54.

18. Feinberg MJ, Ekberg O, Segall L, et al. Deglutition in elderly patients with dementia: findings of videofluorographic evaluation and impact on staging and management. Radiology 1992;183(3):811–4.

19. Barbiera F, Fiorentino E, D'agostino T, et al. Digital cineradiographic swallow study: our experience. Radiol Med (Torino) 2002;104(3):125–33.

20. Ekberg O, Feinberg MJ. Altered swallowing function in elderly patients without dysphagia: radiologic findings in 56 cases. AJR Am J Roentgenol 1991; 156(6):1181–4.

21. Chen MY, Ott DJ, Peele VN, et al. Oropharynx in patients with cerebrovascular disease: evaluation with videofluoroscopy. Radiology 1990;176:641–3.

22. Dodds WJ, Taylor AJ, Stewart ET, et al. Tipper and dipper types of oral swallows. AJR Am J Roentgenol 1989;153(6):1197–9.

23. Ekberg O. Epiglottic dysfunction during deglutition in patients with dysphagia. Arch Otolaryngol 1983; 109(6):376–80.

24. Schmidt J, Holas M, Halvorson K, et al. Videofluoroscopic evidence of aspiration predicts pneumonia and death but not dehydration following stroke. Dysphagia 1994;9:7–11.

25. Pikus L, Levine MS, Yang YX, et al. Videofluoroscopic studies of swallowing dysfunction and the relative risk of pneumonia. AJR Am J Roentgenol 2003;180:1613–6.

26. Horner J, Massey EW, Riski JE, et al. Aspiration following stroke: clinical correlates and outcome. Neurology 1988;38:1359–62.

27. Paciaroni M, Mazzotta G, Corea F, et al. Dysphagia following stroke. Eur Neurol 2004;51:162–7.

28. Upadya A, Thorevska N, Sena KN, et al. Predictors and consequences of pneumonia in critically ill patients with stroke. J Crit Care 2004;19:16–22.

29. Curtis DJ, Hudson T. Laryngotracheal aspiration: analysis of specific neuromuscular factors. Radiology 1983;149:517–22.

30. Rasley A, Logemann JA, Kahrilas PJ, et al. Prevention of barium aspiration during videofluoroscopic swallowing studies: value of change in posture. AJR Am J Roentgenol 1993;160:1005–9.

31. Ekberg O, Nylander G. Dysfunction of the cricopharyngeal muscle. A cineradiographic study of patients with dysphagia. Radiology 1982;143:481–6.

32. Maglinte DD, Kelvin FM, Fitzgerald K, et al. Association of compartments defects in pelvic floor dysfunction. AJR Am J Roentgenol 1999;172:439–44.

33. Stoker J, Halligan S, Bartram CI. Pelvic floor. Imaging Radiol 2001;218(3):621–41.

34. Frudinger A, Bartram CI, Halligan S, et al. Examination techniques for endosonography of the anal canal. Abdom Imaging 1998;23:301–3.

35. Mahieu P, Pringot J, Bodart P. Defecography: I. Description of a new procedure and results in normal patients. Gastrointest Radiol 1984;9:247–51.

36. Mahieu P, Pringot J, Bodart P. Defecography: II. Contribution to the diagnosis of defecation disorders. Gastrointest Radiol 1984;9:253–61.

37. Berthoux A, Bory S, Huguier M, et al. Une technique radiologique d'exploration des prolapsus genitaux et des incontinences d'urine:le colpocystogramme. Ann Radiologie 1965;8:809–12.

38. Mondot L, Novellas S, Senni M, et al. Pelvic prolapse: static and dynamic MRI. Abdom Imaging 2007;32(6):775–83.

39. Grassi R, Catalano O, Salzano A, et al. Disordini funzionali ano-rettali: reperti defecografici associati e loro corrispondenza con la sitomatologia. Radiol Med 1994;88:56–62 [in Italian].

40. Grassi R, Pomerri F, Habib FI, et al. Defecography study of outpouchings of the external wall of the rectum: posterior rectocele and ischio-rectal hernia. Radiol Med 1995;90:44–8.

41. Cavallo G, Salzano A, Grassi R, et al. Rectocele in males: clinical defecographic and CT study of singular cases. Dis Colon Rectum 1991;34:964–6.

42. Grassi R, Romano S, Micera O, et al. Radiographic findings of post-operative double stapled trans anal rectal resection (STARR) in patient with obstructed defecation syndrome (ODS). Eur J Radiol 2005;53:410–6.

43. Scaglione M, Grassi R, Pinto A, et al. Positive predictive value and negative predictive value of spiral CT in the diagnosis of closed loop obstruction complicated by intestinal ischemia. Radiol Med 2004;107:69–77.

44. Ruotolo RA, Evans SR. Mesenteric ischemia in the elderly. Clin Geriatr Med 1999;15(3):527–57.

45. Scholz FJ. Ischemic bowel disease. Radiol Clin North Am 1993;31:1197–218.

46. Boley SJ, Brandt LJ, Sammartano RJ. History of mesenteric ischemia. The evolution of a diagnosis and management. Surg Clin North Am 1997;77(2):275–88.

47. Brandt LJ, Boley SJ. AGA technical review on intestinal ischemia. American Gastrointestinal Association. Gastroenterology 2000;118(5):954–68.
48. Fink S, Chaudhuri TK, Davis HH. Acute mesenteric ischemia and malpractice claims. South Med J 2000;93(2):210–4.
49. Mansour MA. Management of acute mesenteric ischemia. Arch Surg 1999;134(3):328–30 [discussion: 331].
50. Rosenblum JD, Boyle CM, Schwartz LB. The mesenteric circulation. Anatomy and physiology. Surg Clin North Am 1997;77(2):289–306.
51. Romano S, Lassandro F, Scaglione M, et al. Ischemia and infarction of the small bowel and colon: spectrum of imaging findings. Abdom Imaging 2006;31(3):277–92.
52. Bassiouny HS. Nonocclusive mesenteric ischemia. Surg Clin North Am 1997;77(2):319–26.
53. Herbert GS, Steele SR. Acute and chronic mesenteric ischemia. Surg Clin North Am 2007;87(5): 1115–34.
54. Dang C, Wade J, Mandal A. Acute mesenteric ischemia. Available at: http://www.emedicine.com/med/TOPIC2627.htm.
55. Jacobs JE, Birnbaum BA, Maglinte DDT. Vascular disorders of the small intestine. In: Herlinger H, Maglinte DDT, Birnbaum BA, editors. Clinical imaging of the small intestine. 2nd edition. New York: Springer-Verlag; 1999. p. 439–65.
56. Grassi R, Di Mizio R, Pinto A, et al. Serial plain abdominal film findings in the assessment of acute abdomen: spastic ileus, hypotonic ileus, mechanical ileus and paralytic ileus. Radiol Med 2004;108: 56–70.
57. Nicoloff AD, Williamson WK, Moneta GL, et al. Duplex ultrasonography in evaluation of splanchnic artery stenosis. Surg Clin North Am 1997;77(2): 339–55.
58. Chou CK, Mak CW, Tzeng WS, et al. CT of small bowel ischemia. Abdom Imaging 2004;29:18–22.
59. Gore RM, Miller FH, Pereles FS, et al. Helical CT in the evaluation of the acute abdomen. AJR Am J Roentgenol 2000;174:901–13.
60. Romano S, Romano L, Grassi R. Multidetector row computed tomography findings from ischemia to infarction of the large bowel. Eur J Radiol 2007; 61(3):433–41.
61. Di Mizio R, Scaglione M, editors. Small-bowel obstruction: CT features with plain film and US correlations. Springer Verlag; 2007.
62. Di Mizio R. Occlusione meccanica dell'intestino tenue: radiologia-ecografia. In: Romano L, editor. L'addome acuto radiologico. Naples (Italy): Idelson Gnocchi; 2000. p. 113–8.
63. Maglinte DDT, Heitkamp DE, Howard TJ, et al. Current concepts in imaging of small bowel obstruction. Radiol Clin North Am 2003;41:263–83.
64. Maglinte DD, Kelvin FM, Sandrasegaran K, et al. Radiology of small bowel obstruction: contemporary approach and controversies. Abdom Imaging 2005;30(2):160–78.
65. Grassi R, Romano S, D'Amario F, et al. The relevance of free fluid between intestinal loops detected by sonography in the clinical assessment of small bowel obstruction in adults. Eur J Radiol 2004;50: 5–14.
66. Balthazar EJ, Birnbaum BA, Megibow AJ, et al. Closet-loop and strangulating intestinal obstruction: CT signs. Radiology 1992;185:769–75.
67. Chou CK. CT manifestations of bowel ischemia. AJR Am J Roentgenol 2002;178:87–91.
68. Zalcman M, Sy M, Donckier V, et al. Helical CT signs in the diagnosis of intestinal ischemia in small bowel obstruction. AJR Roentgenol 2000;175:1601–7.
69. Aufort S, Charra L, Lesnik A, et al. Multidetector CT of bowel obstruction: value of post-processing. Eur Radiol 2005;15:2323–9.
70. Scaglione M, Romano S, Pinto F, et al. Helical CT diagnosis of small bowel obstruction in the acute clinical setting. Eur J Radiol 2004;50:15–22.

Imaging Findings of Genitourinary Tumors in the Elderly

Roberto Pozzi-Mucelli, MD*, Niccolò Faccioli, MD, Riccardo Manfredi, MD

KEYWORDS
- Kidney • Renal tumor
- Genitourinary tumor • Elderly • Geriatric

Aging induces in the kidney a progressive, functional, and anatomic decay that does not have, however, a particular clinical impact. The kidney is more vulnerable when other pathologies occur, altering the omeostasis of the renal parenchyma, in particular the hemodynamic and hydrosaline equilibrium.[1] Aging-correlated pathologies are atherosclerosis, arterial hypertension, diabetes mellitus, bacterial infections, and malnutrition. The progressive impairment of renal function is the cause of the drug-induced renal pathologies: direct damage induced by nephrotoxic drugs (nonsteroidal anti-inflammatory agents, aminoglicosides, or contrast media) or indirect damage induced by decreased renal excretion of serum molecules.[1,2]

The most important morphologic alterations of the aged kidney are represented by a volume reduction, approximately 20% to 30% in 80-year-old men, and a loss of weight that decreases from 250 to 270 g to 180 to 200 g after age 65.[2] Moreover, the kidney increases in consistency and often shows a pseudolobular appearance. The renal capsule becomes thickened and there is an increase of the perirenal fatty tissue, in particular at the hilum (**Figs. 1** and **2**). A decrease in the number and size of the glomerular portion occurs in the cortex. Retention cysts probably develop because of inflammatory reactions and infections that occur in the distal tract of the tubuli. The functional alterations of the aged kidney are characterized principally by a progressive reduction of the renal plasmatic flux, from 600 mLl per minute to 300 mL per minute, and of the glomerular filtration,

from 130 mL per minute to 60 to 80 mL per minute, compared with that in young adults.[2,3] In the elderly, an increase of different pathologies occurs in the genitourinary tract. Among these pathologies, there is an increase in neoplastic disorders, as in other organs (eg, lungs and digestive tract); at the same time, several non-neoplastic pathologies are more frequent in old patients. This article has two sections, considering first the neoplastic genitourinary pathologies and second the non-neoplastic genitourinary pathologies.

NEOPLASTIC GENITOURINARY PATHOLOGIES

Renal tumors have a higher incidence in the elderly: the most common histologic type is renal adenocarcinoma, responsible for 85% to 90% of all cases. The median age at presentation is 66 years, and 25% of all diagnoses are performed in patients over age 75.[1–4]

A comprehensive approach to renal tumors in the elderly must consider the clinical, diagnostic, and therapeutic points of view.

Occasional findings of renal tumors are increasing; at the same time, there is a reduction in size of the discovered tumors, depending on their early diagnosis.

Renal cell carcinoma is a tumor derived from the renal tubular epithelium and accounts for 3% of all malignancies, with a peak incidence in the seventh decade. Because the tumor is located in the retroperitoneum, it can become large before clinical detection. In elderly patients, many carcinomas present insidiously, often in a background of

Department of Radiology, G.B. Rossi Hospital, University of Verona, Piazzale Scuro 10, 37134 Verona, Italy
* Corresponding author.
E-mail address: roberto.pozzimucelli@univr.it (R. Pozzi-Mucelli).

Radiol Clin N Am 46 (2008) 773–784
doi:10.1016/j.rcl.2008.04.008

radiologic.theclinics.com

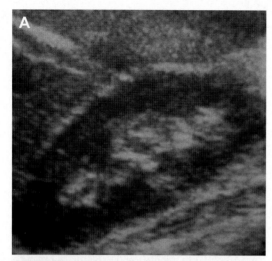

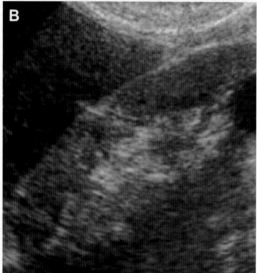

Fig. 1. Echostructural changes correlated with aging: (*A*) parenchymal echogenicity lower than liver and spleen in young adult man; (*B*) parenchynal echogenicity greater than liver and spleen in an elderly patient.

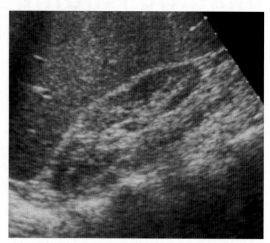

Fig. 2. Right small renal kidney in an elderly patient who had mild renal failure. The kidney shows a reduction of the longitudinal diameter; the parenchymal echogenicity is the same or mildly superior to that of the liver.

co-existing disease, and are not diagnosed until the disease is advanced.[2–4]

Nowadays, however, most tumors are completely asymptomatic and found incidentally in elderly patients during imaging of the upper abdomen, mainly with ultrasound (US) or CT. In the authors' experience, during CT examinations of the upper abdomen, 75% of the incidental findings in the renal area are renal tumors equal to or below 3 cm that do not have symptomatology.

In the elderly, imaging of the renal tumors is not different from that in patients of other ages: at US, these tumors have a "solid" echostructure, varying from hyperechoic to isoechoic to hypoechoic.

Hyperechoic masses are more common than iso-hypoechoic masses. In general, the degree of hyperecogenicity is mild, so that these lesions easily can be differentiated from angiomyolipomas, which tend to be more hyperechogenic. Isoechoic masses can be difficult to visualize, because they have the same echostructure of the renal parenchyma and can be recognized if they modify the renal profile. Color and power Doppler US can be useful for improving the detection of these small renal masses.[5] CT is effective in the detection and characterization of these small renal tumors. Multidetector CT has expanded the possibilities of CT in the detection of the small renal masses. At CT, small renal tumors appear as a round, sharply demarcated renal mass, which, depending on the size, can be totally intrarenal or partially intrarenal and extrarenal. Small renal tumors present soft tissue density, with variable degrees of contrast enhancement. The density is homogenenous but heterogeneous areas also are common. MR imaging also has good sensitivity for these lesions although only a few cases are detected initially with this imaging modality because of the limited use of MR imaging in the abdomen.[6]

When facing elderly patients who have renal tumors, mainly if small in size, special attention should be given to the growth rate of the tumor, the tumor diameter, the tumoral grading, and the impact on the therapy.

The growth rate of small renal lesions in the elderly is low in a series of small renal tumors[7]: the medium growth rate time was 0.35 cm per year, with a range of 0 to 10 cm. The same studies demonstrated a great variance of growth rate with the majority of small renal tumors characterized by a slow growth potential, with a low incidence of distant metastasis. Conversely the majority ofmedium- and large-sized tumors usually are characterized by local invasiveness and distant metastases.[6,7]

Small renal tumors usually have a low grading, between grade I–II; tumors greater than 3 cm have a high grading, usually grade II–III.[6]

The regularity of the margins, round or oval, seems the most suggestive aspect correlated to a low growth rate (**Fig. 3**).

Evolution in imaging techniques has led to an increase of the detection of incidental lesions, generating new questions related to therapeutic approaches: Which tumors must be resected? What kind of surgical technique must be used? And, finally, in which cases can watchful waiting be considered a reasonable option? According to guidelines, watchful waiting is suitable in cases of small lesions in old patients who have high risks correlated to surgical resection; a follow-up every 3 months is recommended in the first year after diagnosis.[8] Recently, less invasive therapies with the potential to avoid open surgery and better preserve renal function have been investigated. These techniques include advanced therapeutic techniques, such as cryoablation[9–11], radiofrequency

ablation[12–14], and ablation using high-intensity focused US.[15]

The most important clinical sign in the suspicion of renal or urinary tract pathology is hematuria, requiring assessment of the entire urothelium and the renal parenchyma for tumor and of the urinary tract. The standard workup for these patients is urinalysis and cytologic analysis, cystoscopy, and US.[16,17] Excretory urography (EU) has shown significant limitations in assessing renal parenchyma. Currently, MDCT urography is the preferred imaging method for assessing patients who have hematuria, offering superior detection of renal parenchymal masses, and, in some studies, improved detection of urothelial lesions.[17,18] MR imaging, including MR angiography and MR urography, also is used, particularly in patients who cannot tolerate iodinated contrast material and in whom multiplanar, vascular, and collecting system imaging is required.

Partial or total nephrectomy is the therapeutic approach usually used in renal carcinoma. Nevertheless, in cases of small tumors, which rarely develop metastasis, and in particular in the elderly, a valid therapeutic alternative is represented by noninvasive techniques, such as percutaneous thermal ablation with US radiofrequencies, CT, or MR imaging–guided intervention. Recently in the literature, many investigators have reported valid

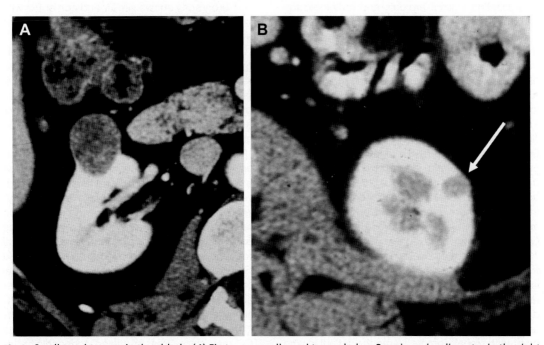

Fig. 3. Small renal tumors in the elderly. (*A*) First case: small renal tumor below 3 cm in major diameter in the right kidney with intrarenal and extrarenal extension. The lesion is inhomogeneous, with sharp margins. (*B*) Second case: very small renal tumor (1.5 cm in diameter) with homogeneous soft tissue density and sharp margins (*arrow*).

therapeutic results with the use of the percutaneous treatment of renal tumors of maximum size less than 3 cm with radiofrequencies; they obtained areas of complete coagulative necrosis with no hypervascular neoplastic residue in the short and long follow-up (3–12 months) by CT or in the histologic evaluation of patients who underwent nephrectomy. The principal advantages of this therapy are lower morbidity rate, inferior costs, and higher patient compliance.[12–14,19]

Urothelial (transitional cell) cancer (TCC) is the most common urinary tract cancer, with a stable incidence in men over the past 2 decades but a slight increase in women.[20,21] Also this is a disease of older patients, most older than 65 years, and is more common in men than in women. The 5-year survival rate currently is 82% overall.[20,21] The most common presenting symptom is gross hematuria, although microscopic hematuria may be detected at urinalysis. Patients also may experience voiding symptoms, such as frequency, dysuria, and pelvic pain. Upper TCC typically occurs in the sixth and seventh decades of life, with men affected three times more often than women.[21]

Twenty-five percent of upper tract tumors occur in the ureter whereas 60% to 75% are found in the lower third, with no side predominance.[22] Synchronous or metachronous tumor of the ipsilateral or contralateral collecting system also is common, necessitating vigilant urologic and radiologic follow-up.[19]

Besides increasing age and male gender, the most important risk factors are smoking, chemical carcinogens, and cyclophosphamide therapy, and all predispose to synchronous and metachronous tumor development.[18–22] Upper tract TCC is histologically and cytologically similar to bladder TCC. These tumors usually are small at diagnosis, grow slowly, and follow a relatively benign course. Pedunculated or diffusely infiltrating tumor is less common, accounting for approximately 15% of upper tract TCCs, but tends to behave more aggressively and be more advanced at diagnosis. Infiltrating tumors are characterized by thickening and induration of the ureteric or renal pelvic wall. Of patients who have upper tract TCC, 11% to 13% subsequently develop metachronous upper tract tumors. Furthermore, up to 50% of patients initially presenting with upper tract TCC develop metachronous tumors in the bladder, typically developing within 2 years of surgical treatment and seen more commonly with ureteric tumors than with renal tumors. Among patients who have bladder TCC, 2% also have synchronous upper tract tumors at presentation and 6% develop metachronous upper tract disease.[18–22]

The diagnosis of upper tract TCC is made most frequently at EU in patients undergoing investigation for hematuria, but now CT urography is more and more accepted as a primary diagnostic investigation, considered a one-stop diagnostic and staging assessment of suspected urothelial malignancy.[23–25] At EU, renal TCC usually manifests as a filling defect within the contrast-enhanced collecting system, which may be single or multiple and smooth, irregular, or stippled. The stipple sign refers to tracking of contrast material into the interstices of a papillary lesion.[16,20]

Filling defects within dilated calices may occur secondary to tumor obstruction of the infundibulum and may lead to caliceal "amputation." Tumor-filled, distended calices have been called "oncocalices." If these fail to opacify with contrast material, they are known as "phantom calices." Ureteric TCC typically is seen as single or multiple ureteric filling defects with or without surface stippling and proximal ureteric dilatation. Longstanding tumor obstruction of the ureteropelvic junction or ureter may lead to generalized hydronephrosis and poor excretion. This is a major disadvantage of EU compared with CT urography, which allows assessment of nonfunctioning kidneys. Upper tract filling defects may be nonspecific at EU, and obstruction of pelvicaliceal drainage may obscure distal synchronous ureteric tumors.[16,20]

CT urography shows similar findings of EU with the advantage of showing tissue component of the tumor and its extension (**Fig. 4**).[26–28]

CT urography offers single breath-hold coverage of the entire urinary tract, improved resolution, the ability to capture multiple phases of contrast material excretion, and improved diagnostic potential over EU and US in the assessment of patients who have hematuria that results from calculi or tumor.[26–29]

Renal US frequently is requested in the evaluation of patients who have hematuria to assess for renal parenchymal masses. US is not as sensitive as EU and CT urography, however, in identifying or characterizing TCC in the pelvis and ureter.[20–22] US can allow assessment of the degree of hydronephrosis and guide interventional procedures in the setting of acute obstruction. At US, renal pelvic TCC typically appears as a central soft tissue hypoechoic mass in the echogenic renal sinus, with or without hydronephrosis. TCC usually is slightly hyperechoic relative to surrounding renal parenchyma; occasionally, high-grade TCC may show areas of mixed echogenicity. Infundibular tumors may cause focal hydronephrosis. Although lesions may extend into the renal cortex and cause focal contour distortion, typically

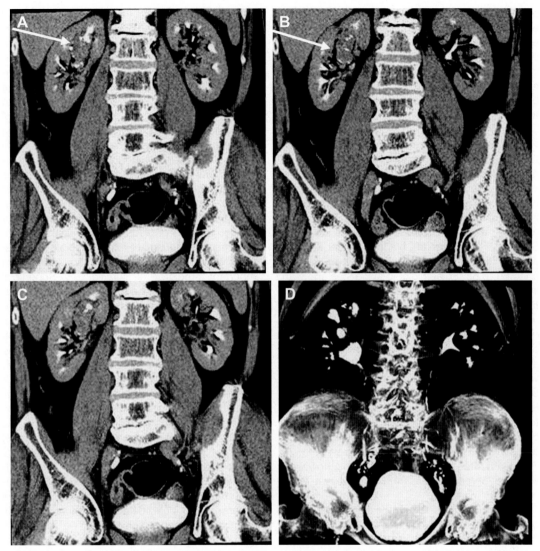

Fig. 4. Urinary tract tumor of the right upper calices and pelvis: CT urography in parenchymal (*A–C*) and urographic phase (*D*) shows a soft tissue mass in the sinus of the right kidney involving and infiltrating the upper calices.

TCC is infiltrative and does not distort the renal contour.[20–22]

MR imaging infrequently is used in the primary assessment of upper tract TCC, and the MR imaging characteristics of this tumor are not welldescribed. In general, MR imaging has not played a leading role in renal tumor imaging because of limitations in image quality, time-consuming sequences, and susceptibility to artifacts. The development of newer fast sequences, however, has led to increasing use and MR imaging is shown to equal CT in the detection and diagnosis of renal masses.[20–22] MR imaging offers inherently high soft tissue contrast and allows multiplanar imaging, which permits direct image acquisition in the

plane of tumor spread. The coronal plane often is advantageous because it allows evaluation of the kidneys, pelvis, ureter, and bladder in a small number of sections. TCC has lower signal intensity than the normally high signal intensity urine on T2-weighted images, permitting good demonstration of tumor in a dilated collecting system. TCC, however, is nearly isointense to renal parenchyma on T1- and T2-weighted images, meaning that gadolinium contrast material is necessary for accurate assessment of tumor extent. Although TCC is a hypovascular tumor, moderate enhancement is seen with gadolinium contrast material, although not to the same degree as renal parenchyma.[20–22] Postcontrast imaging may be performed with 3-D sequences to allow dynamic evaluation of the kidney. MR imaging evaluation of upper tract TCC should include MR imaging urography, which may be static or dynamic byusing gadolinium contrast material.[25] This technique is helpful in patients in whom CT urography cannot be performed because of allergy to iodinated contrast material.

The traditional treatment of upper tract TCC involves total nephroureterectomy with excision of the ipsilateral ureteric orifice and a contiguous cuff of bladder tissue.[25]

Bladder neoplasms account for 2% to 6% of all tumors, with bladder cancer ranked as the fourth most common malignancy in men and eighth in women, with an increase in incidence after 65 years.[30] After age 80, bladder cancer is twice as likely to develop and cause death than in those aged 60 to 65. Epidemiologic evidences show an increase of incidence of bladder cancer, even though there is not a corresponding increase of mortality, probably related to the most accurate diagnostic and therapeutic solutions. Bladder cancer is more common in men than in women, with a male-to-female ratio of 3–4:1; however, in women it is diagnosed at a more advanced stage and has a higher mortality rate than in men. Survival of female patients at 5 years is 78%, equal to the 10-year survival for men. Although urothelial cancer is less than half as common in black men, they have a higher mortality rate than white men. The death rate is declining in all groups, however, with the 5-year survival rate currently at 82% overall.[30,31]

The pathogenesis for urothelial tumors in the bladder is the direct prolonged contact of the urothelium with urine containing excreted carcinogens. Other risk factors include bladder stones, chronic infection and irritation, and drugs. Bladder diverticula have an increased risk (2%–10%) for developing cancer because of stasis. Most urothelial tumors are located on the bladder base (80% at initial diagnosis), 60% are single, and more than 50% measure less than 2.5 cm at cystoscopy. They can be papillary, sessile, or nodular. Sessile lesions include reactive urothelial hyperplasia, atypia, dysplasia, and carcinoma in situ.[32] Sessile lesions are more likely to invade muscle; however, the prognosis correlates more with tumor grade than with morphology (ie, papillary versus flat). Most invasive tumors are high-grade carcinoma.[33] Papillary lesions include papilloma, inverted papilloma, papillary urothelial neoplasm of low malignant potential, and low-grade and high-grade papillary urothelial carcinoma. Seventy percent of patients have superficial papillary tumors, which have a "frond-like" appearance at cystoscopy.

The majority have a prolonged clinical course with multiple recurrences responding to local resection, without progression to malignancy. Twenty percent of tumors are aggressive and invasive de novo, and 10% are metastatic at presentation. Twenty percent of patients who initially have noninvasive tumors develop progression, and 12% die of bladder cancer.[31–33] Predictors of behavior include depth of invasion, multiplicity, history of prior tumors, tumor size, and grade in decreasing order of importance. Urothelial carcinoma tends to be multicentric with synchronous and metachronous bladder and upper tract tumors. Multicentric bladder tumors occur in up to 30% to 40% of cases. Upper tract tumors occur in 2.6% to 4.5% of bladder tumor cases and are seen most frequently when multiple bladder lesions are present. Pathologic stage is the most important predictor of survival.[32,33] Superficial bladder cancer is confined to the mucosa and lamina propria. Once extension occurs into the detrusor muscle layer, the tumor is considered invasive. Invasion may progress to involve local organs, including the prostate, vagina, uterus, and pelvic wall. Tumors metastasize most commonly to pelvic lymph nodes; then, distant metastases occur in the lung, liver, and bone in decreasing order of frequency. The standard imaging workup for gross hematuria and suspected urothelial tumor has shifted from EU to cross-sectional modalities, such as US, CT, and MR imaging. Cystoscopy and biopsy are the standard of reference for bladder evaluation, but imaging is important for accurate staging and treatment planning. Superficial tumors may not be evident with any imaging study and are not staged radiologically.

To perform an accurate clinical staging of invasive urothelial tumors, however, detection of pelvic wall invasion or lymphadenopathy is critical.

Furthermore, complete evaluation of the urothelial tract (upper and lower) is indicated because of the propensity for multicentric disease. US may be used for initial evaluation of hematuria but rarely is the definitive test, given its limitations in the demonstration of muscle invasion and lymph node status. Most tumors appear as a papillary, hypoechoic mass or area of focal wall thickening. Doppler imaging shows flow within a mass, aiding in differentiation of tumor from blood clot. At CT or CT urography, urothelial carcinoma appears as an intraluminal papillary or nodular mass or focal wall thickening (**Fig. 5**). Lesions may be missed without adequate bladder distention, especially small, flat tumors. Bladder tumors enhance early, approximately 60 seconds from injection. The presence of ureteral obstruction strongly suggests the presence of muscle invasion. Once a tumor

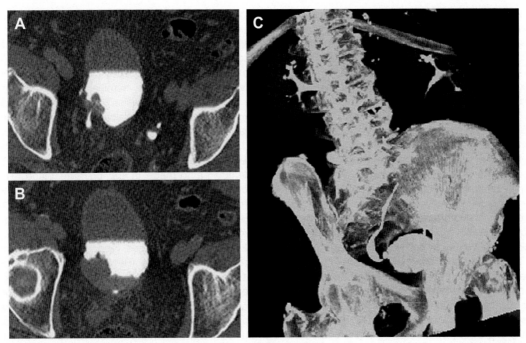

Fig. 5. Bladder tumor. CT urography shows a large tumor inside the bladder (*A, B*), at the posterior and right lateral wall. The tumor shows extension outside the bladder with infiltration of the right distal ureter. The 3-D volume rendered image (*C*) in an oblique view shows the narrowing of the right distal ureter in proximity to the bladder and mild dilatation of the pelvic tract of the ureter.

extends into the perivesical fat, increased attenuation or infiltration is noted in fatty tissue. Accuracy in staging a primary tumor with CT has ranged from 40% to 85%.[31] Technical improvements in MR imaging, such as surface coils, 3-D sequences, and fast dynamic imaging have improved spatial and temporal resolution and MR accuracy. The high intrinsic contrast of MR imaging allows distinction of bladder wall layers. On T1-weighted images, urine is dark; the bladder wall and tumor are intermediate in signal intensity. As fat is high in signal intensity, T1-weighted sequences are optimal for detection of extravesical infiltration, nodes, and bone metastases. Tumor is intermediate in signal intensity on T2-weighted images, contrasting with the high signal intensity of urine and low signal intensity of muscle. T2-weighted sequences are optimal for evaluation of tumor depth and differentiating tumor from fibrosis and for detection of invasion of surrounding organs and bone marrow metastases. With fast dynamic contrast-enhanced imaging, bladder cancer enhances more avidly and earlier than other tissues, such as normal bladder and post-biopsy changes. This may enable differentiation of tumor from fibrosis or edema, although this is still difficult soon after transurethral resection.

MR imaging has a reported staging accuracy of 72% to 96% for the primary tumor and is superior to CT for differentiation of superficial versus deep muscle invasion.[30] As with CT, however, inflammation can mimic perivesical fat invasion and result in overstaging. Superficial tumors are treated with cystoscopic resection followed by close monitoring for recurrences. Recurrent tumors are treated with intravesical agents. Radical cystectomy and urinary diversion are reserved for invasive cancer.[30–33]

Prostate carcinoma is the most frequently diagnosed visceral cancer and the second most common cause of cancer death among American men.[34] In the United States, African American men have a higher incidence of and more than twice the death rate from prostate cancer as whites. Fortunately, death rates from prostate cancer are declining. Established risk factors include age, ethnicity, and family history, the last a contributor in only 5% to 10% of cases.[35] Environmental factors, including diets high in saturated fat, may increase risk, and obesity may increase the risk for dying from the disease. The incidence of this tumor is high because of the progressive increase of the average age and screening programs. Many lesions, however, are not diagnosed in life because of their slow growth rate, and are classified as "latent" prostate carcinoma, diagnosed at pathologic examination after death that has occurred from other causes. The 5-year survival is effectively 100% when the disease is local or regional but drops to 34% if distant metastases are present at diagnosis. For all stages, survival is 99% at 5 years, 92% at 10 years, and 61% at 15 years. At presentation, early prostate cancer is commonly asymptomatic. When present, local symptoms include difficulty starting or stopping the urine flow; painful, weak, or interrupted urine flow; increased frequency of urination; and hematuria. Back, pelvis, or thigh pain may indicate metastasis. Unfortunately, these symptoms are not specific to prostate cancer and can be mimicked by a variety of benign conditions.

Prostate adenocarcinoma originates from the peripheral zone of the gland (lateral and posterior lobes). The "incidental" prostate carcinomas frequently are diagnosed with biopsy in elderly asymptomatic patients who have a high serum level of prostate-specific antigen (PSA) at screening. The histologic grading evaluation is based on the Gleason score. In contrast to the monofocal counterpart, the plurifocal variant is characterized by a more frequent intraglandular and local invasion. Moreover, carcinoma not associated with a significant hypertrophy of the gland usually is diagnosed in a late and advanced phase, with frequent distant metastases.

Cancers diagnosed at imaging essentially are adenocarcinomas that develop in the peripheral zone.

Imaging plays an important role in an integrative approach to patients who have prostate cancer. The contributions from imaging have expanded from characterizing locally advanced or metastatic disease to including intra- and extraprostatic tumor delineation. In cases of prostate carcinoma in the elderly, the appropriate clinicotherapeutic algorithm considers the age of a patient, the clinical status, the values of the PSA, and the need versus no need to perform a biopsy; MR imaging usually is not necessary. The first imaging technique used for clinically suspected prostate carcinomas is endorectal sonography for directing biopsies. Using a high-frequency transducer, US can delineate zonal anatomy but cannot reliably differentiate between benign and malignant prostate tissue. Tumors have varying appearances on US: approximately 40% to 50% are hypoechoic, 40% are isoechoic, and others are hyperechoic. Confounding lesions, such as prostatitis, atrophy, prostatic epithelial neoplasia, and ductal ectasia, also can present as hypoechoic lesions.[34] Color or power Doppler sonography may show lesions not visualized by conventional US; however, such findings are not specific, and the new techniques do not perform as well as a systematic biopsy in diagnosing prostate cancer.[34–39] Extraprostatic disease is defined on MR imaging as extracapsular extension, seminal vesicle invasion, or lymph node metastasis. The efficacy of gadolinium-enhanced or dynamic imaging is controversial, and these techniques are not used routinely. T1-weighted axial images are used to screen the pelvic nodes and bones for metastasis and to identify hemorrhage in the prostate gland. The zonal anatomy is seen best on T2- weighted images but cannot be distinguished on T1-weighted images. The central zone typically is heterogeneous and predominantly hypointense on T2- weighted images, because of benign prostatic hyperplasia (BPH), and isointense on T1-weighted images. It is difficult to separate cancer in the central zone from BPH that invariably occurs in this age group. Normally, the peripheral zone is relatively homogeneous and hyperintense on T2-weighted images and isointense on T1-weighted images (Fig. 6). The neurovascular bundles are recognized as oval in axial and linear in long-axis, hypointense structures surrounded by hyperintense fat on T1-weighted images. Prostate tumors usually are located in the peripheral zone and are hypointense on T2-weighted images and isointense on T1-weighted images. Low

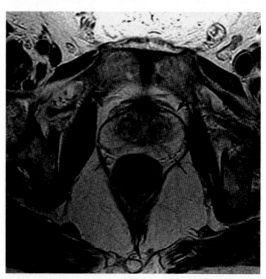

Fig. 6. Anatomy of the prostate: T2-weighted images. On axial T2-weighted images, rapid acquisition with relaxation enhancement (RARE) the central zone appears relatively hypointense on T2-weighted images, whereas the peripheral zone is hyperintense on T2-weighted images. The capsule appears hypointense on T2-weighted images, all around the gland (*arrows*).

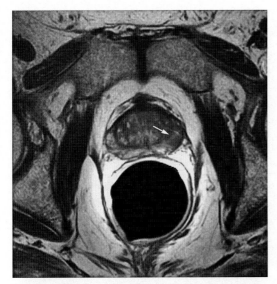

Fig. 7. Localized prostate cancer: T2-weighted images. Axial T2-weighted images (RARE) show a hypointense lesion in the left peripheral zone adjacent to the prostate capsule (*arrow*). The left prostate capsule is intact and there is no extension of the lesion to the periprostatic fat.

T2-weighted signal, however, is not specific for cancer. Underlying hemorrhage resulting from biopsy, prostatitis, atrophy, or post-treatment change can present with low signal intensity. In general, MR imaging is performed at least 3 weeks after prostate biopsy to allow resolution of hemorrhage, which has become more problematic with the extended numbers of core biopsies. Fortunately, hemorrhage can be identified as an area of high signal on T1-weighted images. Magnetic resonance spectroscopic imaging (MRSI) with an endorectal coil has been used to improve tumor detection. The most commonly studied markers for prostate cancer include choline, creatine, and citrate; others include polyamines, lipids, and lysine.[39] Most commonly, prostate cancer is identified by increased choline, a product of increased cell membrane metabolism, and decreased citrate, a normal product of prostate metabolism. In conjunction with endorectal MR imaging, MRSI has been reported to provide sensitivity and specificity for prostate cancer as high as 95% and 91%, respectively, and to provide accuracy similar to that of sextant biopsy for intraprostatic tumor localization, except at the apex, where MR imaging with MRSI was more accurate than biopsy. Drawbacks of MRSI include poor spatial resolution, technical demand, artifacts, inability to directly depict the periprostatic area, and requirements of specialized software and expertise in acquiring and interpreting the data.

Currently, the main role of MR imaging of the prostate is local staging of tumors in patients who have an intermediate risk for treatment failure (**Figs. 7** and **8**).[38,39]

The range of radiologic techniques, including endorectal sonography, MR imaging, CT, and nuclear medicine studies, allows an integrative approach to prostate cancer. The results of imaging studies performed in the appropriate laboratory and clinical context can contribute essential information that enhances the capacity to provide individualized risk stratification, a suitable treatment strategy, and monitoring of patients who have prostate cancer.

NON-NEOPLASTIC GENITOURINARY PATHOLOGIES
Acute and Chronic Renal Impairment

Renal or extrarenal diseases that are able to affect the glomerular filtrate can facilitate an acute renal impairment. Chronic renal impairment in the elderly is approximately ten times more frequent than in adulthood, and the causes are predominantly diabetes and amiloidosis.

The clinical presentation of nephropathies of the elderly is nonspecific. The most valuable imaging technique for these pathologic entities is US: the increase of the echogenicity of the parenchyma and, in particular, the medullary part, is typical in the elderly. As a result, the normal corticomedullary differentiation is lost (see **Fig. 2**; **Fig. 9**).

These two features are not universally codified because of the diversity of the US devices, habitus of patients, and radiologist experience. The most objective comparison between organs' echogenicity is to compare the renal parenchymal echogenicity with that of the spleen because of the difficulty of making a comparison with the liver in cases of steatosis.

Correlation of clinical and laboratory data is of fundamental importance in the management of each nephropathy.

In the study of the vascular disease of the kidney, color Doppler also has an important role because it allows evaluation of the morphologic and functional features.[1–3]

Urinary Tract Infections

After the seventh decade, 30% to 50% of women and 10% of men have a bacteriuria, often asymptomatic and the result of obstruction of the urinary flux and abundant postmicturial residue.

The agent responsible of the infection often is *Escherichia coli*, but *Klebsiella*, *Enterococcus*, and *Pseudomonas* also are frequent, in some cases as a result of invasive procedures.

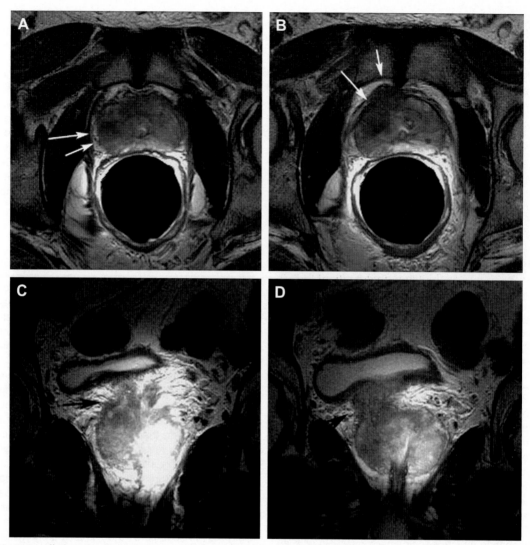

Fig. 8. Locally invasive prostate cancer: axial and coronal T2-weighted images. Axial T2-weighted images (RARE) show shows a hypointense neoplasm in the right peripheral zone infiltrating the prostate capsule and the periprostatic fat (*arrow*) (*A*); the lesion extends to the central zone (*arrow*) (*B*). On coronal T2-weighted images (RARE), the neoplasm infiltrates the prostate capsule obliterating the fat plane between the prostate and the ejaculatory ducts (*arrow*) (*C*); furthermore, the tumor infiltrates the right seminal vesicles (*arrow*) (*D*).

A predisposing factor in the elderly is diabetes, which occurs with greater incidence in old patients.

Imaging of acute renal infections is based on US and CT. Contrast-enhanced CT is the imaging of choice for the detection and characterization of renal infections, which may include acute diffuse and focal pyelonephritis, renal abscesses, and pyonephrosis.[2,3,23]

Recently, CT has assumed an important role in the definition of the acute pielonephritis, often misdiagnosed at US. The most common findings at CT are hypodense inhomogeneous wedge-shaped areas from the papilla to the cortex, not enhancing after contrast material administration,

with or without swelling that results from interstitial edema, ischemia, and mechanical obstruction from inflammatory tissue. Moreover, linear hypo- or hyperdense bands can be recognized parallel to the tubular axes. The hypodense areas can be absorbed or turn to abscesses.

In the most severe cases, the inflammatory process extends into the perirenal and pararenal spaces. CT detects fluid collections and thickening of the renal fasciae in these cases.

Urolithiasis

In the elderly, metabolic changes causing ossaluria and hypercalciuria may increase the incidence

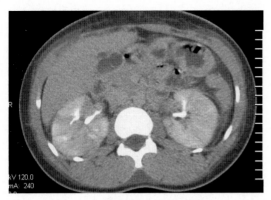

Fig. 9. Acute pyelonephritis. Both kidneys are enlarged and present diffuse inhomogeneities with low densities areas diffusely involving the parenchyma. The parenchymal thickness is increased and the sinus is reduced in size. The calyces and pelvis are compressed.

of urolithiasis. Also, urinary stasis (for instance, in patients who have prostatic hypertrophy), decreased fluid intake, and prolonged immobilization causing re-absorption of calcium from bones may cause stones formation in the urinary tract.

The role of different imaging modalities has changed with the evolution of US and CT. X-ray plain film of the abdomen still is used but its sensitivity is much lower than that of unenhanced CT. US is a valid modality to detect stones in the kidney and bladder; stones also can be detected in the distal tract of the ureter but not in the lumbar and pelvic tract. US is useful for detecting hydronephrosis and for follow-up. Unenhanced CT is the most sensitive technique for renal stones in the kidney, ureter, and bladder. Also, hydronephrosis can be demonstrated easily. Limitations of high doses are not a concern in elderly patients.[1–3]

Benign Prostatic Hyperplasia

BPH is a common disease; its prevalence increases with patient age, reaching approximately 80% of men over age 75, but it is not an indication for imaging. An enlarged median lobe of the prostate that bulges into the base of the bladder, however, may be incidentally seen and needs to be distinguished from an intrinsic bladder mass.

The diagnostic imaging of patients who have symptoms related to BPH is based on US. The US examination usually is performed with a transrectal probe to define the size of the gland, which is measured on the vertical, axial, and anteroposterior diameters (anteroposterior × transverse × cephalocaudal × 0.52).

The US examination also should evaluate the walls of the bladder, in particular for the thickness

and the presence of diverticuli and the postmicturition residue, conventionally considered pathologic when greater than 50 cm^3. In some cases, the prostatic hypertrophy may be so large as to simulate a bladder mass at US or eventually at CT: the site of origin of the mass located in the central part of the gland is helpful for the differential diagnosis. At MR imaging, BPH has a characteristic appearance, consisting of round nodules of varying sizes that have high signal intensity with T2-weighted sequences and a variable amount of low signal intensity fibrosis in the central portion of the gland.[40] The relative proportion of nodules to stromal reaction depends on the degree of stromal versus glandular hyperplasia.

REFERENCES

1. Davison AM. Renal disease in the elderly. Nephron 1998;80(1):6–16.
2. Mulder WJ, Hillen HF. Renal function and renal disease in the elderly: part II. Eur J Intern Med 2001;12(4):327–33.
3. Mulder WJ, Hillen HF. Renal function and renal disease in the elderly: part I. Eur J Intern Med 2001;12(2):86–97.
4. Doherty JG, Rüfer A, Bartholomew P, et al. The presentation, treatment and outcome of renal cell carcinoma in old age. Age Ageing 1999;28(4):359–62.
5. Pallwein L, Mitterberger M, Aigner F, et al. Small renal masses: the value of contrast-enhanced colour Doppler imaging. BJU Int 2007;99(3):579–85.
6. Silverman SG, Mortele KJ, Tuncali K, et al. Hyperattenuating renal masses: etiologies, pathogenesis, and imaging evaluation. Radiographics 2007;27(4):1131–43.
7. Bosniak MA, Birnbaum BA, Krinsky GA, et al. Small renal parenchymal neoplasms: further observations on growth. Radiology 1995;197(3):589–97.
8. Davidson AJ, Hartman DS, Choyke PL, et al. Radiologic assessment of renal masses: implications for patient care. Radiology 1997;202(2):297–305.
9. Lee JM, Han JK, Choi SH, et al. Comparison of renal ablation with monopolar radiofrequency and hypertonic-saline-augmented bipolar radiofrequency: in vitro and in vivo experimental studies. AJR Am J Roentgenol 2005;184(3):897–905.
10. Rodriguez R, Chan DY, Bishoff JT, et al. Renal ablative cryosurgery in selected patient with peripheral renal masses. Urology 2000;55:25–30.
11. Gill IS, Novick AC, Meraney AM, et al. Laparoscopic renal cryoablation in 32 patients. Urology 2000;56:748–53.
12. Gervais DA, McGovern FJ, Wood BJ, et al. Radiofrequency ablation of renal cell carcinoma: early clinical experience. Radiology 2000;217:665–72.

13. Ogan K, Jacomides L, Dolmatch BL, et al. Percutaneous radiofrequency ablation of renal tumors: technique, limitations, and morbidity. Urology 2002; 60:954–8.

14. Farrel MA, Charboneau WJ, DiMarco DS, et al. Imaging-guided radiofrequency ablation of solid renal tumors. AJR Am J Roentgenol 2003;180:1509–13.

15. Wu F, Wang ZB, Chen WZ, et al. Preliminary experience using high intensity focused ultrasound for the treatment of patients with advanced stage renal malignancy. J Urol 2003;170:2237–40.

16. Dyer RB, Chen MY, Zagoria RJ. Classic signs in uroradiology. Radiographics 2004;24(Suppl 1): S247–80.

17. Gray Sears CL, Ward JF, Sears ST, et al. Prospective comparison of computerized tomography and excretory urography in the initial evaluation of asymptomatic microhematuria. J Urol 2002;168:2457–60.

18. Grossfeld GD, Carroll PR. Evaluation of asymptomatic microscopic hematuria. Urol Clin North Am 1998;25:661–76.

19. Rehman J, Landman J, Lee D, et al. Needle-based ablation of renal parenchyma using microwave, cryoablation, impedance- and temperature-based monopolar and bipolar radiofrequency, and liquid and gel chemoablation: laboratory studies and review of the literature. J Endourol 2004;18(1):83–104.

20. Yousem DM, Gatewood OM, Goldman SM, et al. Synchronous and metachronous transitional cell carcinoma of the urinary tract: prevalence, incidence, and radiographic detection. Radiology 1988;167(3):613–8.

21. Wong-You-Cheong JJ, Wagner BJ, Davis CJ Jr. Transitional cell carcinoma of the urinary tract: radiologic-pathologic correlation. Radiographics 1998;18(1):123–42.

22. Melamed MR, Reuter VE. Pathology and staging of urothelial tumors of the kidney and ureter. Urol Clin North Am 1993;20:333–47.

23. Dalla Palma L, Morra A, Grotto M. CT-Urography. Radiol Med (Torino) 2005;110(3):170–8.

24. Maher MM, Kalra MK, Rizzo S, et al. Multidetector CT urography in imaging of the urinary tract in patients with hematuria. Korean J Radiol 2004;5:1–10.

25. Kawashima A, Glockner JF, King BF Jr. CT urography and MR urography. Radiol Clin North Am 2003;41:945–61.

26. Perlman ES, Rosenfield AT, Wexler JS, et al. CT urography in the evaluation of urinary tract disease. J Comput Assist Tomogr 1996;20:620–6.

27. Joffe SA, Servaes S, Okon S, et al. Multi–detector row CT urography in the evaluation of hematuria. Radiographics 2003;23:1441–55.

28. Hall MC, Womack S, Sagalowsky AI, et al. Prognostic factors, recurrence, and survival in transitional cell carcinoma of the upper urinary tract: a 30-year experience in 252 patients. Urology 1998;52: 594–601.

29. Kirkali Z, Tuzel E. Transitional cell carcinoma of the ureter and renal pelvis. Crit Rev Oncol Hematol 2003;47:155–69.

30. Wong-You-Cheong JJ, Woodward PJ, Manning MA, et al. From the archives of the AFIP: neoplasms of the urinary bladder: radiologic-pathologic correlation. Radiographics 2006; 26(2):553–80.

31. Wong-You-Cheong JJ, Woodward PJ, Manning MA, et al. From the archives of the AFIP: inflammatory and nonneoplastic bladder masses: radiologic-pathologic correlation. Radiographics 2006;26(6): 1847–68.

32. Barentsz JO, Jager GJ, Witjes JA, et al. Primary staging of urinary bladder carcinoma: the role of MRI and a comparison with CT. Eur Radiol 1996;6: 129–33.

33. Pashos CL, Botteman MF, Laskin BL, et al. Bladder cancer: epidemiology, diagnosis, and management. Cancer Pract 2002;10:311–22.

34. Kundra V, Silverman PM, Matin SF, et al. Imaging in oncology from the University of Texas M.D. Anderson Cancer Center: diagnosis, staging, and surveillance of prostate cancer. AJR Am J Roentgenol 2007;189(4):830–44.

35. Padhani AR, Gapinski CJ, Macvicar DA, et al. Dynamic contrast-enhanced MRI of prostate cancer: correlation with morphology and tumour stage, histological grade and PSA. Clin Radiol 2000;55: 99–109.

36. Kozlowski P, Chang SD, Jones EC, et al. Combined diffusion weighted and dynamic contrast-enhanced MRI for prostate cancer diagnosis: correlation with biopsy and histopathology. J Magn Reson Imaging 2006;24:108–13.

37. Futterer JJ, Heijmink SW, Scheenen TW, et al. Prostate cancer localization with dynamic contrast-enhanced MR imaging and proton MR spectroscopic imaging. Radiology 2006;241:449–58.

38. Futterer JJ, Engelbrecht MR, Huisman HJ, et al. Staging prostate cancer with dynamic contrast-enhanced endorectal MR imaging prior to radical prostatectomy: experienced versus less xperienced readers. Radiology 2005;237:541–9.

39. Costouros NG, Coakley FV, Westphalen AC, et al. Diagnosis of prostate cancer in patients with an elevated prostate-specific antigen level: role of endorectal MRI and MR spectroscopic imaging. AJR Am J Roentgenol 2007;188:812–6.

40. Gozzi G, Conti G, Peroni R, et al. Consensus conference about imaging of benign prostatic hypertrophy. Radiol Med 2005;110(3):179–89.

Oncohaematologic Disorders Affecting the Skeleton in the Elderly

Andrea Baur-Melnyk, MD*, Maximilian Reiser, MD

KEYWORDS

• Oncohaematologic disorders • Bone marrow imaging
• MRI • MDCT

MULTIPLE MYELOMA

Multiple myeloma is a characteristic hemato-oncologic disease in the elderly population with a peak incidence in the eighth decade. The black population has a significantly higher incidence (55 per 100,000 women and 70 per 100,000 men) than the white population (25 per 100,000 women and 45 per 100,000 men).

Multiple myeloma represents a malignant bone marrow neoplasia in which a monoclonal strain of atypical plasma cells proliferates and typically secretes paraproteins. The atypical plasma cells are distributed in the bone marrow, either focally or in a diffuse distribution, and they may result in bone destruction. Bone marrow aspirates or, preferably, bone marrow biopsy are indispensable for the diagnosis. Because of various therapeutic options and the wide variations in survival, the sensitive detection of myeloma involvement of the skeleton is mandatory for an accurate staging. The most widely used clinical staging system described, by Durie and Salmon[1] (Table 1), is based upon laboratory parameters and X-rays of the whole skeleton. This includes radiograms of the spine, the pelvis, the skull, the upper arms, and the upper thighs.

Radiography

Predilection sites for multiple myeloma manifestations are the axial skeleton (spine and pelvis), and also the ribs, the shoulder region, the skull, and the proximal femur. The appearance of multiple myeloma in X-rays is either focally circumscribed "punched out" bone destructions or diffuse inhomogeneous osteopenia, especially in the spine. In the skull, multiple osteolytic lesions of similar size are found. In the long bones, the osteolytic lesions are often, but not exclusively, centrally located. With increasing size, they lead to endosteal scalloping of the cortex. Large lesions may penetrate the cortex and extend into the soft-tissues. Intraosseous enlargement of the tumor may lead to apparent expansion of bone with a soap bubble appearance. Affection of the ribs usually manifests as osteolyses, or an inhomogeneous appearance of the spongiosa in combination with a circumscribed expansion of the bone. Differentiation of multiple myeloma from metastatic skeletal disease can be very challenging without the knowledge of laboratory parameters. Most important discriminating features of myeloma versus metastases are: osteolytic rather than the combination of osteolytic and sclerotic lesions; diffuse osteopenia; well defined lesions that are uniform in size; and cortical scalloping rather than cortical destruction.

Sclerotic or osteolytic lesions with a sclerotic rim are rarely seen in myeloma.[2] Primary diffuse sclerosis of the skeleton is also rare (< 3% of cases), and appears more often after therapy. Differential diagnoses in those cases include osteoblastic metastases, myelofibrosis, lymphoma, renal osteodystrophy, and mastocytosis.

Diffuse osteopenia because of myelomatous infiltration and tumor-induced osteoclast activity is difficult to distinguish from postmenopausal or senile osteoporosis. This is also true for vertebral fractures. Both osteoporotic fractures as well as neoplastic fractures are common in this patient group.[3] In addition, the combination of the advanced age of the patients suffering from multiple

Department of Clinical Radiology, University of Munich, Grosshadern, Germany
* Corresponding author.
E-mail address: andrea.baur@med.uni-muenchen.de (A. Baur-Melnyk).

Radiol Clin N Am 46 (2008) 785–798
doi:10.1016/j.rcl.2008.05.002
0033-8389/08/$ – see front matter. Published by Elsevier Inc.

Table 1
Durie and Salmon staging system for multiple myeloma (1975)

Stage	Criteria
I	All crtieria need to be fulfilled:
	Hemoglobin >10 g/dL
	Serum Ca < 12 mg/dL
	X-ray: normal bony structure or single osteolytic lesions
	M- Gradient IgG < 5 g/dL
	IgA < 3 g/dL
	Bence-Jones protein uric-excretion < 4g/24 Std.
II	Neither fitting to stage I nor stage III
III	One criteria need to be accomplished at minimum:
	Hemoglobin < 8.5 g/dL
	Serum Ca > 12 mg/dL
	X-ray: progressive osteolytic lesions
	M- Gradient IgG > 7 g/dL
	IgA > 5 g/dL
	Bence-Jones protein uric-excretion > 12 g/24 Std.

myeloma and cortisone therapy favors bone loss. In these situations MR imaging can help in differential diagnosis.[4–6]

Multislice Computed Tomography

Multisclice computed tomography (MSCT) is more sensitive than radiography in detecting myeloma.[7]

Scanners with 16 and more detector rows are suitable for this kind of whole body multidetector computer tomography (MDCT) (**Fig. 1**). Because of the high contrast of bone to soft tissue, a low-dose protocol can be used (approximately 100 mAs, 120 KV) so that radiation dose can be limited (approximately 4 mSv). Raw data sets should be

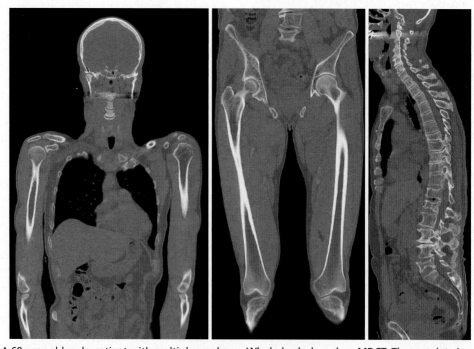

Fig. 1. A 69-year-old male patient with multiple myeloma. Whole-body, low-dose MDCT. The raw data images are reconstructed in 3-mm axial slices, coronal slices for the upper and lower parts, and sagittal slices for the spine. 100 mAs are usually sufficient (120 KV) to image bony structures in detail.

reconstructed in 3-mm to 4-mm axial slices, sagittal slices of the spine, and coronal slices for the whole body, separately for the upper (skull, thorax, arms) and the lower parts (pelvis, legs).[8]

Bony destructions in multiple myeloma are usually well circumscribed and have a narrow zone of transition. The most common site of involvement is the spine (**Fig. 2**). Focal osteolyses or vertebral body destruction and vertebral fractures may be encountered. They usually have Hounsfield units (HU) of soft-tissue density (approximately 40 HU– 80 HU). The bony destruction in multiple myeloma involves the trabecular first, then growth on the cortex, and eventually by soft-tissue expansion. In the skull the osteolyses manifest as punched-out lesions that are situated within the tabula externa and interna (**Fig. 3**). Differential diagnosis includes choroid plexus enlargement; however, those show up with contiguity to the subarachnoidal space. Rib lesions are often overlooked in MDCT because the ribs are small structures and signs of involvement may be subtle (**Fig. 4**). Focal enlargement of a particular rib with soft tissue density within the lesion is indicative of myeloma involvement. The cortex may be normal or thinned. If the tumor continues to grow, a pathologic rib fracture may result. In the diaphyses of the long tubular bones where only sparse trabecular bone

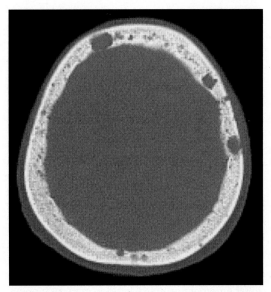

Fig. 3. A 66-year-old female with multiple myeloma and typical punched out osteolyses within the skull. They are typically located within the tabula interna and externa.

is present, early osteolyses may be missed when only looking at the bone window. Circumscribed areas with soft-tissue density (> 30 HU–40 HU) within the normal fatty marrow (negative HU values) are highly suspicious for myeloma manifestations. Comparison with the contralateral side may be helpful. Cortical scalloping in the long bones may be visible on axial or reformatted images.

In cases with diffuse bone marrow infiltration, inhomogeneous osteoporosis can be detected with MDCT in the spine. However, as in radiograms, this is often hard to distinguish from senile

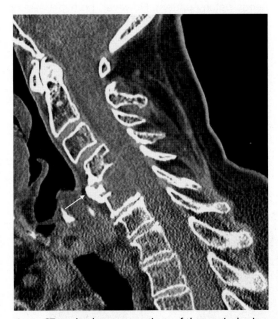

Fig. 2. CT, sagittal reconstructions of the cervical spine. An 82-year-old female with osseous destruction of the fourth to sixth cervical vertebral body filled with soft tissue. The fifth cervical vertebral body is completely destructed and only visible in the anterior parts (*arrow*). These were the sole manifestations of multiple myeloma.

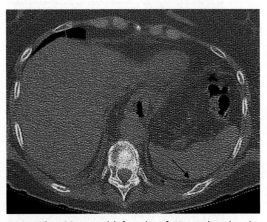

Fig. 4. The 66-year-old female of **Fig. 3** showing involvement of the rib. Circumscribed enlargement with soft-tissue density.

or perimenopausal osteoporosis. In those cases, MR imaging should be performed, which can demonstrate diffuse neoplastic bone marrow infiltration in the absence of bony destruction.[9] In the long tubular bones and in the pelvis, where only sparse trabecular bone is present, diffuse infiltration can be detected in the soft-tissue window. The fatty marrow is replaced by tissue with soft-tissue density (**Fig. 5**).

MR Imaging

In patients suffering from multiple myeloma, the pattern and degree of bone marrow infiltration can directly be displayed with the use of MR imaging. Five different infiltration patterns can be differentiated in MR imaging.[10] First, a normal looking bone marrow signal is found in patients with low-grade interstitial infiltration with plasma cells (< 20 volume percent or Vol % in bone marrow biopsy). Therefore, a normal bone marrow signal in MR imaging does not exclude the diagnosis of multiple myeloma. However, those patients are eligible for a watch-and-wait strategy.

Second, focal myeloma infiltration can be found in about 30% of cases. Circumscribed areas of high signal intensity can be identified on fat saturated sequences, such as short inversion time inversion recovery (STIR) images, which are best for depicting focal lesions.[11] They correspond to areas of low-signal intensity on unenhanced T1-weighted spin echo (SE) images. In a few cases isointense signal is found on T1-weighted SE images. Because of the high signal intensity of normal fat-containing marrow, T2-weighted turbo spin echo sequences (because of J-Coupling) usually provide no sufficient contrast (**Fig. 6**).

Third, diffuse bone marrow infiltration is characterized by a homogeneous decrease of signal on T1-weighted SE images and increased signal intensity on fat-suppressed T2-weighted images (**Fig. 7**). In cases of high-grade diffuse involvement (>50 Vol % in bone marrow biopsy), the signal intensity is nearly equal to the signal intensity of the intervertebral disc on T1-weighted SE images because of the increase of water and decrease of fatty components. In cases of intermediate grade of involvement in biopsy (20 Vol %–50 Vol %) the signal reduction is only moderate and often hard to diagnose. In those cases, intravenous injection of gadolinium-chelates is recommended to verify diffuse involvement. If the percentage increase of signal enhancement exceeds the limit of 40%, this can be considered pathologic.[12]

Fourth, a combined focal and diffuse infiltration pattern can be found. On T1-weighted SE images the bone marrow signal intensity is diffusely decreased with additional foci of decreased signal interspersed. Those foci are often better demarked on fat saturated sequences.

Fifth, in a few cases, a so-called "salt-and-pepper" pattern can be found. On T1-weighted SE images, but also on T2-weighted SE sequences, the bone marrow presents a very inhomogeneous patchy pattern. However, no hyperintense areas are demarcated in fat saturated sequences. In histology this corresponds to bone marrow with circumscribed fat islands beside normal bone marrow with a minor infiltration of plasma cells (<20 Vol %). In the early stage of multiple

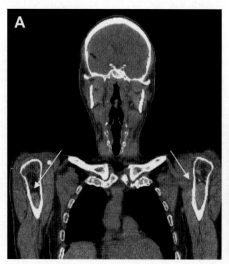
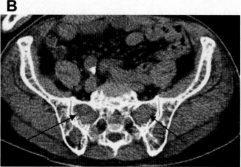

Fig. 5. CT of a 66-year-old male with recurrent myeloma 2 years after allogenic bone marrow transplant (*A, B*). CT shows diffuse hyperintensity within the marrow cavities with coarse osteoporosis (*white arrows, A; black arrows, B*).

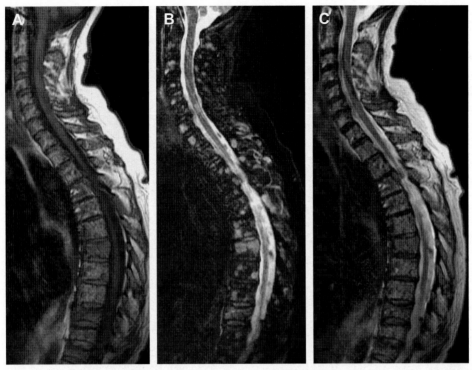

Fig. 6. MR image of the spine. Focal involvement in a 66-year-old female with multiple myeloma, stage III. Focal hypointensities on T1-weighted SE images (*A*) correspond to focal hyperintensities on STIR images (*B*). On T2-weighted turbo-spin echo sequences, the myeloma foci are not well displayed (*C*).

myeloma, this special pattern is thought to be initiated by a hematopoesis-inhibiting factor. Enhancement of bone marrow does not exceed 40%. These patients are usually stage I disease and do not require therapy.

When radiographs are compared with MR imaging, high false-negative rates between 29% to 90% have been reported for radiographs in patients with multiple myeloma.[13,14] Even in asymptomatic patients (stage I, according to staging criteria of Durie and Salmon) with normal radiographs, MR depicted diffuse or focal tumor infiltration in 29% to 50% of patients.[15,16] Approximately one third of patients is understaged if MR is not used.[17]

Current MR techniques allow a time-effective comprehensive whole-body examination of the bone marrow using fast T1-weighted SE and STIR sequences in combination with dedicated receiver-coil elements, such as the total imaging matrix function in combination with parallel imaging. Thus, the entire bone marrow can be displayed, without patient repositioning, within approximately 35 minutes.[9]

Positron Emission Tomography-CT

Schirrmeister and colleagues[18] examined 28 patients with multiple myeloma and 15 patients with solitary plasmacytoma of bone. They observed increased tracer uptake in 38 out of 41 known osteolytic bone lesions. Another 71 bone lesions were detected that were negative on radiographs. As a result of F-18 fluorodeoxyglucose (FDG)-positron emission tomography (PET) imaging, clinical management was influenced in five patients. In a study of Durie and colleagues[19], 16 previously untreated subjects with multiple myeloma had positive FDG scans, either focally or diffuse. Four of them had negative radiographs and in another four subjects extramedullary disease was detected. In another prospective study published by Zamagni and colleagues[20], PET-CT was compared with MR imaging (spine and pelvis) and radiography in 46 newly diagnosed subjects. PET-CT proved to be significantly superior to plain radiographs. However, in 30% of subjects, PET-CT failed to show myeloma infiltration when compared with MR imaging.

Prognosis

The time of survival in patients with multiple myeloma can significantly vary between courses of a few months or more than 10 years, the so called "smoldering myeloma." Because of the possibility of detecting tumor infiltrations earlier with MR imaging than using conventional X-rays, the value

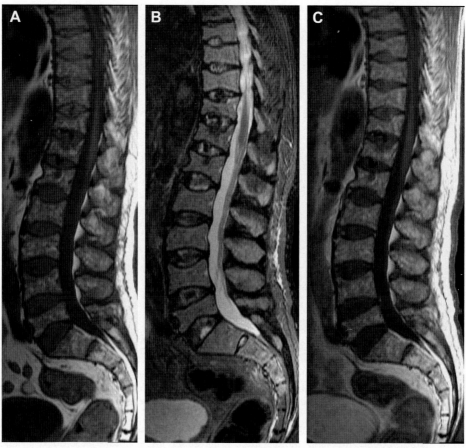

Fig. 7. A 66-year old male patient with intermediate grade of diffuse infiltration. Note diffuse lowering of signal on T1-weighted SE images (A). In contrast to high-grade diffuse infiltration, there is still a notable signal difference to the intervertebral disc. Diffuse increased signal is on STIR images (B). There is marked enhancement after gadolinium application of 45% (C).

of MR imaging with respect to patients' prognosis was analyzed in patients defined as stage I disease according to Durie and Salmon.[1] In a patient group of 24 examined by Vande Berg and colleagues[15] and 38 examined by Moulopoulos and colleagues[21], and suffering from multiple myeloma stage I, patients with pathologic MR imaging findings had a significantly earlier progression of disease compared with patients with normal MR imaging findings. Dimopoulos and colleagues[16] examined 23 patients in stage I disease and found 7 out of 23 patients with definite myeloma infiltrates in MR imaging, despite normal X-rays. A disease progression was noted after an average of 11 months in patients with infiltrates versus 44 months, without evidence of involvement in MR imaging. Kusumoto and colleagues[22] reported about 61 patients in different stages of the disease and had similar results. Patients showing pathologic MR imaging scans presented a 5-year survival rate of 30%, while patients with

normal MR imaging had a 5-year survival rate of 80%.

In a survival analysis in 77 patients with newly diagnosed multiple myeloma, the authors showed for the first time that MR imaging of the spine had significant prognostic impact, not only concerning the time to progression but also concerning the survival of patients. Twenty-five out of 77 patients would have been understaged according to the established staging system of Durie and Salmon, which includes only radiography as an imaging method. MR imaging staging represented an independent prognostic parameter and the inclusion of MR imaging in the staging system of Durie and Salmon improved the discrimination of the three risk groups (low, intermediate, and high). Concerning the infiltration patterns, a significantly longer survival time was found in patients with normal looking bone marrow and also in patients presenting a salt-and-pepper pattern.[17] Patients with diffuse or focal infiltrates did not differ significantly in survival time. The extent of infiltration was much more important.

Staging

A current issue of debate is the choice of adequate imaging modalities in patients with multiple myeloma on a routine basis. Radiographs are associated with a high rate of false negatives and, therefore, in many institutions whole body MR imaging, or whole body MDCT is performed for primary diagnosis and for follow-up. Because the importance of MR imaging for sensitive detection and the prognostic significance of bone marrow infiltratation were demonstrated, recently Durie and colleagues proposed the Durie and Salmon[23] PLUS staging system. In a consensus conference, new myeloma management guidelines have been agreed upon. Concerning diagnostic imaging, MR imaging and FDG-PET were included in staging of patients with multiple myeloma (**Table 2**).

Monitoring Response or Disease Progression

According to the European Bone Marrow Transplantation/International Bone Marrow Transplantation registry criteria, a definite increase in size of bone destructions or soft-tissue manifestations, as well as the development of new skeletal lesions, are imaging criteria indicative of progressive disease. New compression fractures are not recognized as criteria of progressive disease, as they are often caused by osteoporosis.

Only a few MR imaging studies have addressed bone marrow signal changes in patients with multiple myeloma with regard to response to therapy. Moulopoulos and colleagues[24] examined 20 patients before and after chemotherapy, including high-dosed cortisone medication. Patients with clinical complete response showed either a normalization of bone marrow signal in MR imaging or an absent or only peripheral enhancement of the lesions. However, those changes were not detected in all patients with clinical response to therapy in terms of complete remission. Patients with partial response to therapy showed an overall decrease of bone marrow alterations, with an increase in signal on T1-weighted SE images because of an increase of fat cells. In those patients, focal and diffuse pathologic contrast media uptake was still present. Despite clinical remission, new compression fractures occurred in the spine of 10 patients, despite normalization of the bone marrow MR imaging signal. Those vertebral fractures were assumed to result from progressive osteoporosis, which is regularly observed in multiple myeloma because of the combination of senile and corticosteroid induced osteoporosis. In patients with a diffuse infiltration pattern, who responded to therapy, the bone marrow signal shows an increase on T1-weighted SE images, indicating restitution of fat cells.

Early results in small patient cohorts indicate that F18-FDG-PET might be a good method in monitoring relapse or response to therapy. Negative PET scans reliably predicted stable MGUS. The development of new FDG-positive sites in the skeleton after therapy indicated relapse and poor prognosis.[19] Decreased tracer uptake has been reported in patients with good response.[25] The largest cohort was examined by Zamagni and colleagues[20] with MR imaging and FDG-PET-CT. They examined 23 patients before and 3 months after autologous stem cell transplantation. Response could be detected in FDG-PET-CT as decreased standard uptake value or decrease in the number and sites of myeloma lesions after successful therapy, with partial or complete response in all patients. In MR imaging, nine patients showed no change despite good clinical response. Therefore, FDG-PET-CT seems to be superior to MR imaging in evaluating response to therapy. However, it is mandatory to perform an FDG-PET-CT scan before therapy so that a comparison can be made.

Table 2 Durie and Salmon PLUS staging system	
Classification	**Whole Body MR Imaging and/or FDG-PET**
MGUS	All negative
Stage I A	Normal skeletal survey or single lesion (smoldering)
Stage I B	< 5 focal lesions or mild diffuse disease
Stage II A/B	5–20 focal lesions or moderate diffuse disease
Stage III A/B	> 20 focal lesions or severe diffuse disease

Abbreviations: MGUS, monoclonal gammopathy of unknown significance. (Subclassification in stages II and III: A, normal renal fct.; B, abnormal renal fct.) Stage = predictive of survival.

METASTASES

Skeletal metastases represent the most common malignant bone tumor and are the third most common location for distant metastases. They occur predominantly in adults, especially in the elderly population. Most frequently, skeletal metastases originate from prostate cancer in men and from breast cancer in women. Other frequent primaries are cancers of the lung, kidney, thyroid, alimentary tract, bladder, and skin.

Radiography

Plain radiography remains the first imaging technique for the evaluation of skeletal tumors and metastases. On the other hand, X-rays might be false-negative in the detection of bone destructions. In experimental studies of the spine, Edelstyn and colleagues[26] showed that 50% to 75% of cancellous bone in the beam axis of the vertebral body must be destroyed before it can be seen on lateral radiographs. The detection rate was even less accurate on a-p radiographs. A small break in the cortex was much more readily apparent, especially when it is positioned tangential to the X-ray beam.

Multislice Computer Tomography

MSCT is the modality of choice for showing the osteolytic or osteoblastic components and for fracture risk assessment in bony metastases. It allows one to exactly demonstrate the extent of osseous destruction of the trabecular network and the cortex. It is mandatory for preoperative planning of surgery. With the multislice CT, especially 16-row and 64-row scanners, a very thin collimation of approximately 0.7 mm became possible. Therefore, small details and especially the trabecular network can be visualized. The images can be reconstructed in three orthogonal planes, as well as oblique and curved planes, so that MSCT can now be seen as a real multiplanar modality. The measurement of Hounsfield units permits to differentiate solid (30 HU–100 HU) and cystic lesions (approximately 0 HU–10 HU), as well as calcifications (approximately 250 HU–1,000 HU).

Fracture risk assessment

MDCT is most useful in the precise assessment of the extent of bony destructions and thereby in the prediction of fracture risk. A vertebral body is at risk for fracture in the thoracic spine if more than 50% of the vertebral body is missing or if more than 25% osseous destruction of the vertebral body is combined with a destruction of the costovertebral joint. In the lumbar spine, a vertebral body is at risk of fracture if more than 35% of the body is destroyed or if more than 20% destruction of the body is combined with involvement of the posterior elements and pedicles (**Box 1**).[27]

Numerous studies have been undertaken to identify metastatic lesions in tubular bones that are at risk of fracture. However, most of these studies lack a sound statistical analysis. One of the most reliable risk analyses for fractures of the tubular bones was performed by Mirels[28], who proposed a classification system including four risk factors: location, lesion type, pain, and lesion size. To every risk factor, one to three points are allotted. Scores range from 4 to 12 points. When a score of seven or less is obtained, the probability of a fracture is low (5%). Such a lesion can be treated conservatively. In patients with a score of nine and more, prophylactic surgery is recommended. If the sum is eight, individual decisions should be made.

Van der Linden and colleagues[29] emphasized the importance of cortical involvement in femoral metastases. This is best done using MSCT. Cortical involvement of more than 3 cm (in head feet direction) and greater than 50% circumferential cortical involvement (on axial slices) was predictive of fracture. It has to be mentioned that in all cases, individual circumstances have to be considered before prophylactic surgery is performed in order not to over treat patients with only limited life expectancy. Radiologic parameters can effectively support therapeutic decisions.

MR Imaging

MR imaging is superior in precisely visualizing the extent of a metastatic tumor spread within in the soft-tissues or within the marrow cavity (**Fig. 8**). The relationship to neural and vascular structures, as well as the precise assessment of the extent of the metastases, is of utmost importance for determining resectability and planning radiation therapy.

MR imaging is most sensitive for the detection of metastases. It is superior to X-rays as well as to

---

Box 1
Fracture risk assessment in vertebral bodies

> 50% destruction of thoracic (Th1-10) vertebral bodies (vb)

> 25% destruction of thoracic vb + costovertebral destruction

> 35% destruction of thoracolumbar (Th11-L5) vb

> 20% destruction of thoracolumbar (Th11-L5) + pedicle/posterior elements

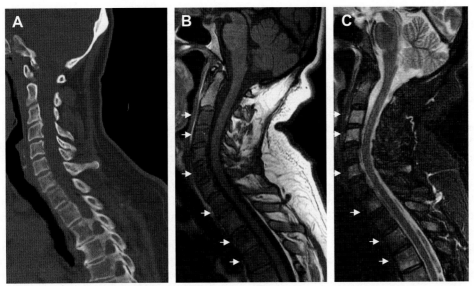

Fig. 8. A 52-year-old female with breast cancer and pain in the spine. CT (*A*) did not demonstrate any osteolytic or osteoblastic metastases to the cervical spine. MR imaging of (*B*) T1-weighted SE plus (*C*) STIR detected multiple metastases to the spine (*arrows*).

MSCT.[30] Metastases have no specific signal intensity when compared with myeloma or lymphoma. They usually appear as foci of hypointense signal on T1-weighted SE images corresponding to high signal intensity on fat-saturated sequences. Pure osteoblastic metastases are usually hypointense in T1-weighted and T2-weighted sequences. On fat saturated sequences, they may be missed as they are usually isointense. Contrast uptake is usually low or missing in osteoblastic metastases. In mixed osteolytic and osteoblastic metastases, they yield mostly slight hyperintense signal on fat-saturated sequences, dependent on the proportion of neoplastic cells and fatty marrow components.

Sometimes nontumoral lesions, such as stress fractures, may mimic metastases in MR imaging in which extensive bone marrow edema and contrast enhancement may be misleading. In those cases, CT may demonstrate subtle cortical fracture lines, which allow exclusion of a malignant bone tumor. Another differential diagnosis includes the differentiation of acute benign (usually osteoporotic) versus metastatic vertebral compression fractures. Both entities occur in elderly individuals and exhibit similar signal intensities: for example, low signal on T1-weighted SE images and high signal on fat-suppressed sequences, such as STIR. Both fracture types result in contrast enhancement. A band-like bone marrow signal change along the fractured end-plates or residual hyperintense fatty marrow within the fractured vertebral body indicates the benign nature of

a fracture. Homogeneous low-signal intensity within the whole vertebral body is usually associated with tumor. Diffusion-weighted imaging can assist differentiation between metastatic vertebral fractures and acute osteoporotic vertebral fractures with bone marrow edema.[6]

CHRONIC LYMPHATIC LEUKEMIA

Chronic lymphatic leukemia (CCL) is a typical malignancy of the elderly patient with a peak incidence of 30 per 100,000 at greater than 80 years of age. Two thirds of patients are older than 60 years of age. Chronic lymphatic leukemia is the most common variety of chronic leukemia. It is a type of low-grade lymphocytic non-Hodgkin-lymphoma. The etiology is still unclear. CLL is characterized by an accumulation of mature monoclonal B- or, more rarely, T-lymphocytes in the bone marrow, the blood, the spleen, and lymph nodes. Therefore, the spleen and lymph nodes may be enlarged. In the bone marrow, the atypical cells displace the normal three cell rows (erythrocytopoeisis, thrombopoesis, and lymphopoesis). In the later stages myelofibrosis occurs. In the early stages of the disease the patients are often asymptomatic for many years. With progression of disease, weakness and recurrent infections are the most common signs.

Radiography and MSCT

Marrow hyperplasia may result in diffuse osteopenia, which is unspecific. Multiple small osteolytic lesions are observed in less than 3% of patients, especially in the femur and humerus. Soft-tissue accumulation of masses of leukemic cells (chloromas) may produce osseous erosions. It can also affect the small bones of the hand, which is termed "leukemic acropachy." Bone destructions, clubbing, and soft-tissue edema can occur, especially in the metacarpals and the terminal phalanges. Arthritis is noted in approximately 12% of patients with CLL. It is usually polyarticular, affecting most frequently the knee, the shoulder, and the ankle. Radiographic findings are limited to osteopenia and soft-tissue swelling. Gout, osteonecrosis because of corticosteroid therapy, and osteomyelitis are secondary complications of CLL.

MR Imaging

In MR imaging, the marrow infiltration with mature lymphocytes produces an unspecific diffuse infiltration form (**Fig. 9**). In the axial skeleton, the signal intensity on T1-weighted SE images is diffusely markedly decreased because of the decrease of fat cells and the increase of cell-bound water. In fat-suppressed images, the signal intensity is diffusely increased and there is marked enhancement after gadolinium application. In the peripheral skeleton, a reconversion of the fatty bone marrow to hematopoietic bone marrow is noted.

Only a few studies have dealt with CLL and MR imaging. Lecouvet and colleagues[31] examined changes in bone marrow composition and distribution by quantitative MR imaging. Twelve out of 29 patients showed normal bone marrow in the spine and femur. Twelve out of 29 patients had an abnormal prolongation of T1-relaxation times within the vertebral marrow of the lumbar spine, and 16 out of 29 had an increased proportion of nonfatty marrow in the femur. Patients with abnormal marrow composition or distribution had significantly higher blood and marrow lymphocytosis than those without these features. In patients

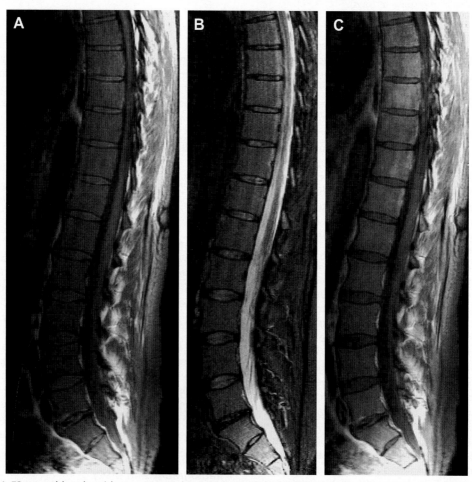

Fig. 9. A 53-year-old male with CLL. T1-weighted SE images show diffuse marked hypointensity (*A*) within the whole bone marrow, indicating low fat content. STIR shows diffuse marked hyperintensity (*B*), indicating hypercellularity. After gadolinium application, marked enhancement is noted (*C*).

with early stages of CLL and abnormal MR imaging with a prolongation of T1-relaxation times, the course of disease was more severe and required earlier therapy.[32]

APLASTIC ANEMIA

Aplastic anemia is a hematologic disorder characterized by pancytopenia, bone marrow hypoplasia, and lack of extramedullary hematopoiesis. Incidence is low (3–6: 1 Mio). There are two peaks of age, a first in childhood (10–25 years of age) and a second one in the elderly around 65 years of age. It is differentiated into a primary hereditary form (Fanconi anemia), which develops in early childhood, and a secondary form. The etiology of the secondary form is often unknown (>70%) or associated with radiation, virus infections, and drugs.[33]

Radiography and MSCT

As of yet, no characteristic findings of aplastic anemia have been described in radiography and MSCT.

MR Imaging

MR imaging appears to have a potential in the initial diagnosis and as a method of monitoring the therapeutic response. In MR imaging, three patterns have been described.[34] First is a homogenous high signal on T1-weighted SE and opposed-phase T1-weighted radio frequency (RF)-spoiled gradient echo (GE), and low signal on STIR sequences, representing diffuse pancytopenia with markedly diffuse increase of fat cells within the marrow cavity. Second is a more patchy pattern with low signal intensity on T1-weighted SE and opposed-phase T1-weighted RF-spoiled GE, and high signal on STIR. Third is a pattern with low signal on T1-weighted SE and high on STIR, and opposed-phase T1-weighted RF-spoiled GE. MR spectroscopy showed that the ratio of water-to-fat was significantly decreased. In the marrow type 3 it was increased when compared with normals, consistent with reactive hypercellular marrow. The focal areas in marrow type 2 showed no differences in ratio of water-to-fat when compared with normals. In biopsy, these areas represented residual normal hematopoesis.[35] No fat signals specific for aplastic anemia were found with MR spectroscopy. MR imaging may also be a noninvasive means of investigating bone marrow after treatment.[36]

OSTEOMYELOFIBROSIS AND SCLEROSIS

Osteomyelofibrosis and sclerosis (OMF/OMS) is a chronic myeloproliferative disease of the elderly with a peak incidence in the sixth and seventh decade of life. OMF/OMS can be either primary or secondary in association with other malignant bone marrow diseases, such as leukemias, lymphomas, or multiple myeloma. In the early stages of the disease it is characterized in histology by hyperplastic marrow, with an increase of all three cell rows and clusters of large dysplastic megacaryocytes. Fat is reduced. This is followed by excessive marrow fibrosis and sclerosis and a hypocellular stage. Fat is also reduced in this stage (**Fig. 10**). Typically, extramedullary hematopoesis (paravertebral masses) and hepatosplenomegaly is found in patients suffering from osteomyelofibrosis and osteomyelosclerosis. Clinical symptoms are often unspecific and include fatigue, weakness, and weight loss. The peripheral blood demonstrates normocytic anemia.

Radiography and MSCT

In 30% to 70% of patients, a homogeneous osteosclerosis of the skeleton, especially the central skeleton, can be found. In the long bones, enosteal sclerosis can lead to cortical thickening. In the spine, sclerosis is mostly homogeneous but can be end-plate accentuated (sandwich vertebrae). In case that the new built osteoid is not yet calcified, the typical sclerosis is missing. Bone and ankle pain are common in those patients. A polyarthritis simulating rheumatoid arthritis has been described. Hemarthrosis can be the initial manifestation of the disease. Impaired platelet function presumably contributes to the bleeding. Secondary gout occurs in 5% to 20% of patients and may antedate the diagnosis. The differential diagnosis includes osteopetrosis, diffuse osteoplastic metastatic disease (especially in prostate cancer and breast cancer), mastocytosis, and renal osteodystrophy.[37]

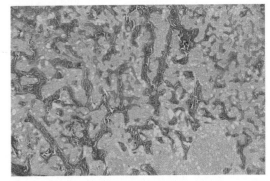

Fig. 10. BMBS plastic. Histology of a patient with osteomyelofibrosis/sclerosis. Ladewig stain, highlighting component of osteoid (*pink*) in osteosclerotic bone. Increased fibrosis and sclerosis of bone. Note also strong reduction in fat cell component.

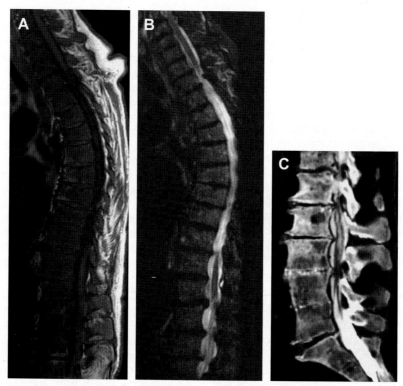

Fig. 11. MR imaging of the spine (*A, B*). An 84-year-old female with osteomyelofibrosis/sclerosis. On T1-weighted SE images (*A*) as well as on STIR images (*B*) diffuse hypointensity is noted. This is because of fibrosis and sclerosis of the bone marrow, accompanied by a decreased fat content. Post-myelo-CT (*C*) of the lumbar spine shows the typical sclerosis of the vertebral bodies. Note also fusion of L3 to L5.

MR Imaging

In MR imaging, diffuse marrow changes can be detected, which are dependent on the stage of disease.[38] The signal intensity is markedly reduced on T1-weighted and T2-weighted SE sequences because of the increase in cells and reduction in fat cells in the early stages, or because of fibrosis in the late stages (**Fig. 11**). Small residual areas of fatty marrow can be interspersed. On fat saturated images, such as STIR, the signal can be bright in the early stages or low in the later stages. Because of abnormal increase in capillaries, widened sinusoids, and an increase of permeability of the vessels, a strong enhancement in the bone marrow is detected in many patients.[39] Non-enhancing regions can occur and correspond to areas of marrow ischemia.[40] Differential diagnosis includes myeloma and leukemia in the early stages and hemosiderosis and diffuse osteoplastic metastases in the late stages.

REFERENCES

1. Durie BG, Salmon SE. A clinical staging system for multiple myeloma: correlation of measured myeloma cell mass with presenting clinical features, response to treatment and survival. Cancer 1975; 36:842–54.

2. Hall FM, Gore SM. Osteosclerotic myeloma variants. Skeletal Radiol 1988;17:101–5.

3. Lecouvet FE, Van de Berg BC, Michaux L, et al. Development of vertebral fractures in patients with multiple myeloma: does MRI enable recognition of vertebrae that will collapse? J Comput Assist Tomogr 1998;22:430–6.

4. Cuenod CA, Laredo JD, Chevret S, et al. Acute vertebral collapse due to osteoporosis or malignancy: appearance on unenhanced and gadolinium enhanced MR images. Radiology 1996;199:541–9.

5. Baur A, Stäbler A, Arbogast S, et al. The fluid sign in acute osteoporotic and neoplastic vertebral compression fractures. Radiology 2002;225:730–5.

6. Baur A, Stäbler A, Brüning R, et al. Diffusion-weighted MR imaging of bone marrow: differentiation of benign versus pathologic vertebral compression fractures. Radiology 1998;207:349–56.

7. Mahnken AH, Wildberger JE, Gehbauer G. Multidetector CT of the spine in multiple myeloma: comparison with MR imaging and radiography. Am J Roentgenol 2002;178:1429–36.

8. Baur-Melnyk A, Buhmann S, Dürr HR, et al. Role of MRI for the diagnosis and prognosis of multiple myeloma. Eur J Radiol 2005;55:56–64.

9. Baur-Melnyk A, Buhmann S, Becker C, et al. Whole body MRI versus whole body MDCT for the staging of patients with multiple myeloma. Am J Roentgenol 2008;190:1097–104.

10. Stäbler A, Baur A, Bartl R, et al. Contrast enhancement and quantitative signal analysis in MRI of multiple myeloma: assessment of focal and diffuse growth patterns in marrow correlated with biopsies and survival rates. Am J Roentgenol 1996;167:1029–36.

11. Rahmouni A, Divine M, Mathieu D, et al. Detection of multiple myeloma involving the spine: efficacy of fat suppression and contrast-enhanced MRI. Am J Roentgenol 1993;160:1049–52.

12. Baur A, Bartl R, Pellengahr C, et al. Neovascularization of bone marrow in patients with diffuse multiple myeloma: a correlative study of MR-imaging and histopathologic findings. Cancer 2004;101:2599–604.

13. Tertti R, Alanen A, Remes K. The value of MRI in screening myeloma lesions of the lumbar spine. Br J Haematol 1995;91:658–60.

14. Lecouvet F, Malghem J, Michaux L, et al. Skeletal survey in advanced multiple myeloma: radiographic versus MRI survey. Br J Haematol 1999;106:35–9.

15. Van de Berg B, Lecouvet F, Michaux L, et al. Stage I multiple myeloma: value of MRI of the bone marrow in the determination of prognosis. Radiology 1996;201:243–6.

16. Dimopoulos MA, Moulopoulos A, Smith TL, et al. Risk of disease progression in asymptomatic multiple myeloma. Am J Med 1993;94:57–61.

17. Baur A, Stäbler A, Nagel D, et al. Magnetic resonance imaging as a supplement for the clinical staging system of Durie and Salmon? Cancer 2002;95:1334–45.

18. Schirrmeister H, Bommer M, Buck AK, et al. Initial results in the assessment of multiple myeloma using F18-FDG PET. Eur J Nucl Med Mol Imaging 2002;29:361–6.

19. Durie BG, Waxman AD, DAgnolo A, et al. Whole body F18-FDG PET identifies high risk myeloma. J Nucl Med 2002;43:1457–63.

20. Zamagni E, Nanni C, Patriarca F, et al. A prospective comparison of 18F-fluorodeoxyglucose positron emission computer tomography, magnetic resonance imaging and whole body planar radiographs in the assessment of bone disease in newly diagnosed multiple myeloma. Haematologica 2007;92:50–5.

21. Moulopoulos LA, Dimopoulos MA, Smith TL, et al. Prognostic significance of magnetic resonance imaging in patients with asymptomatic multiple myeloma. J Clin Oncol 1995;13:251–6.

22. Kusumoto S, Jinnai I, Itoh K, et al. Magnetic resonance imaging patterns in patients with multiple myeloma. Br J Haematol 1997;99:649–55.

23. Durie BG, Salmon SE. Myeloma management guidelines: a consensus report from the Scientific Advisors of the International Myeloma Foundation. Hematol J 2003;4:379–98.

24. Moulopoulos LA, Dimopoulos MA, Alexanian R, et al. Multiple myeloma: MR patterns of response to treatment. Radiology 1994;193:441–6.

25. Bredella MA, Steinbach L, Caputo G, et al. Value of FDG PET in the assessment of patients with multiple myeloma. Am J Roentgenol 2005;184:1199–204.

26. Edelstyn GA, Gillespie PJ, Grebbell FS. The radiological demonstration of osseous metastases. Experimental observations. Clin Radiol 1967;18:158–62.

27. Taneichi H, Kaneda K, Takeda N, et al. Risk factors and probability of vertebral body collapse in metastases of the spine. Spine 1997;22:239–45.

28. Mirels H. Metastatic disease in long bones. A proposed scoring system for diagnosing impending pathologic fractures. Clin Orthop Relat Res 2003;415:4–13 [reprint].

29. Van der Linden YM, Dijkstra PD, Kroon HM, et al. Comparative analysis of risk factors for pathological fracture with femoral metastases. J Bone Joint Surg Br 2004;86:566–73.

30. Buhmann-Kirchhoff S, Becker C, Duerr HR, et al. Detection of osseous metastases of the spine: comparison of high resolution multi-detector CT with MRI. Eur J Radiol 2008 [Epub ahead of print].

31. Lecouvet FE, Van de Berg BC, Michaux L. Chronic lymphocytic leukemia: changes in bone marrow composition and distribution assessed with quantitative MRI. J Magn Reson Imaging 1998;8:733–9.

32. Lecouvet FE, Van de Berg BC, Michaux L, et al. Early chronic lymphocytic leukemia: prognostic value of quantitative bone marrow MR imaging findings and correlation with hematologic variables. Radiology 1997;204:813–8.

33. Lee GR, Bithell TC, Foerster J, et al. Clinical haematology. 9th edition. Philadelphia: Lee & Febinger; 1993:911–31.

34. Amano Y, Kumazaki T. Proton MR imaging and spectroscopy evaluation of aplastic anemia: three bone marrow patterns. J Comput Assist Tomogr 1997;21:286–92.

35. Kaplan PA, Asleson RJ, Klassen LW, et al. Bone marrow patterns in aplastic anemia: observations with 1.5-T MR imaging. Radiology 1997;164:441–4.

36. McKinstry CS, Steiner RE, Young AT, et al. Bone marrow in leukaemia and aplastic anemia: MR imaging before, during and after treatment. Radiology 1987;162:701–7.

37. Resnick D. Bone and joint disorders. Chapter: Lymphoproliferative and myeloproliferative disorders. 4th edition. Philadelphia: Saunders. 2002. p. 2332–7.

38. Guermazi A, de Kerviler E, Cazals-Hatem D, et al. Imaging findings in patients with myelofibrosis. Eur Radiol 1999;9:1366–75.

39. Amano Y, Onda M, Amano M, et al. Magnetic resonance imaging of myelofibrosis. Clin Imaging 1997;21:264–8.

40. Van de Berg B, Malghem J, Labaisse A, et al. Apparent focal bone marrow ischemia in patients with arrow disorders: MR studies. J Comput Assist Tomogr 1993;17:792–7.

Neurodegenerative Diseases

Massimo Gallucci, MD[a],[*], Nicola Limbucci, MD[a],
Alessia Catalucci, MD[a], Massimo Caulo, MD, PhD[b]

KEYWORDS
- Neurodegenerative diseases • Normal aging
- Alzheimer disease • Parkinson disease • MR imaging

NORMAL BRAIN AGING

Normal brain aging can be defined as a normal biologic process of the elderly characterized by relative cerebral atrophy without severe compromising of normal cognitive and motor performances. The aging brain shows volumetric decrease, usually associated with diffuse or focal white-matter signal abnormalities. A clear clinical or pathologic cut-off between physiologic and abnormal aging in the brain does not exist, however.

Diffuse Cerebral Atrophy

Aging causes volume loss in the cortex and white matter with secondary enlargement of the cerebral sulci, cisterns, and ventricles. These findings are common in asymptomatic persons more than 70 years of age, and there is a significant overlap between physiologic volume loss and the atrophy seen in neurodegenerative diseases. The expression "diffuse cerebral atrophy" should be reserved for cases when serial studies have shown longitudinal persistent volumetric reduction, with widening of ventricular and cortical ventricular spaces. "Focal atrophy" is defined as brain volume loss limited to specific areas in the context of normal brain, such as in hippocampal atrophy.[1] Volumetric indexes are used to quantify and compare atrophy. Usually indexes remain relatively stable over time in normal aging, but they progressively become impaired in Alzheimer's disease (AD) and some other types of degenerative atrophy.[2,3] The clinical role of volumetric indexes is only ancillary to neurologic and psychiatric assessment, however, because of the wide overlap between the pathologically and the normally aging brain.

Advanced MR imaging techniques have shown subtle changes in the normal-appearing white matter in the normally aging brain.[4] Spectroscopy revealed reductions in N-acetyl aspartate (NAA), and in the NAA:choline and NAA:creatinine ratios and increases in the ratios of choline and creatinine in the cortical, semi-oval, and temporal regions. Moreover, NAA and choline ratios seemed to be decreased significantly in the hippocampal and cortical regions, respectively.[5] Another study with 3 years of follow-up demonstrated that most metabolites were stable in elderly persons, although mioinositol showed an increase that was not correlated with any change in neurocognitive function during aging.[6]

Diffusion tensor imaging also has been used to investigate the normal aging process.[7] Some studies have shown that aging leads to a slight but significant increase in the apparent diffusion coefficient (ADC), whereas fractional anisotropy is progressively reduced; a correlation between diffusion tensor imaging and spectroscopy findings was found.[8]

Focal Abnormalities

MR imaging examinations of elderly persons often show small, well-defined, hyperintense foci on T2-weighted sequences. They usually are

[a] Department of Neuroradiology, S. Salvatore Hospital, University of L'Aquila, 67100 Loc. Coppito, L'Aquila, Italy
[b] Itab and Department of Clinical Science and Bioimaging, University of Chieti, via dei Vestini 31, Chieti, viale Pindaro 42, Pescara, Partita IVA 01335970693, Italy
* Corresponding author.
E-mail address: massimo.gallucci@cc.univaq.it (M. Gallucci).

Radiol Clin N Am 46 (2008) 799–817
doi:10.1016/j.rcl.2008.06.002
0033-8389/08/$ – see front matter © 2008 Elsevier Inc. All rights reserved.

nonspecific, and their interpretation requires careful evaluation of their number, signal, dimensions, site, and clinical significance. In more than 50% of cases these abnormalities are areas of reparative gliosis and thus are the result of microinfarctions caused by microcirculation failure. More than 40% of the hyperintense foci are dilated perivascular (Virchow-Robin) spaces.[9]

Subcortical white-matter nonspecific focal lesions do not correlate with impairment in cognitive function. Patchy, often confluent, areas can be observed in the deep white matter, especially in the watershed zones, and are associated with history of hypertension, diabetes, and cardiovascular diseases.[9,10]

Dilated perivascular spaces are observed more frequently in elderly persons than in young people because diffuse atrophy causes widening of subarachnoid spaces and congruous widening of perivascular spaces also.[11,12] Moreover, the reduction in the diameter of the arterioles caused by arteriolosclerosis causes a relative increase of fluid in the perivascular spaces. In extreme cases, defined as "status cribrosus," tiny and very abundant dilated perivascular spaces are observed in the basal ganglia (**Fig. 1**). Perivascular spaces can be found in any white-matter location, however. Distinguishing nonspecific gliosis from perivascular spaces is simple, because the former shows hyperintensity on proton-density-weighted and fluid-attenuated inversion recovery (FLAIR) sequences, and the latter usually have the same signal as cerebrospinal fluid (CSF) on all sequences, including FLAIR.[9]

Many periventricular abnormalities are observed in the elderly. Periventricular round or triangular signal abnormalities also are very common in the normally aging brain. They usually are observed in the white matter surrounding the frontal horns of the lateral ventricles or in the paratrigonal areas (**Fig. 2**). In patients who have a history of hypertension, nonspecific patchy focal periventricular lesions are common. Moreover, a thin periventricular rim on T2-weighted images is a common finding caused by subependymal gliosis and loss of ependymal lining (see **Fig. 2**); this finding has no pathologic significance. Hyperintense caps around the frontal horns of the lateral ventricles also can be found in patients of any age. This finding is related to ependimitis granularis and is not pathologic.

PRIMARY DEGENERATIVE DEMENTIAS

The diagnosis of dementia is based on clinical criteria. Therefore, neuroradiology has a supportive role in the diagnosis of dementia, but it has an important role in ruling out causes of the cognitive impairment. Although there is a significant overlap between the clinical aspects of normal aging and the various type of dementia, MR imaging can identify correctly and discriminate among most forms of dementia. One of the most important roles of MR imaging is to rule out secondary dementias, because in most of these cases specific treatments exist. Finally, advanced MR imaging techniques are an interesting adjunct in studying the pathogenesis of various dementias.

Alzheimer's Disease

AD is the most common acquired degenerative disease of the brain, accounting for about 75% of all dementias. In the United States more than 14% of individuals older than 65 years of age and more than 50% of persons older than 85 years

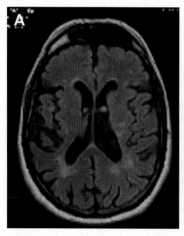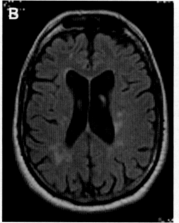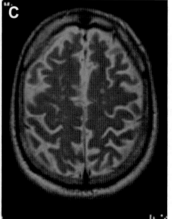

Fig. 1. In a normal aging brain, FLAIR imaging shows multiple focal white-matter abnormalities (*A*) in the paratrigonal areas and (*B*) in the subcortical white matter, with a thin, hyperintense periventricular rim. (*C*) Fast spin-echo T2-weighted image shows punctate gliotic foci in the deep white matter.

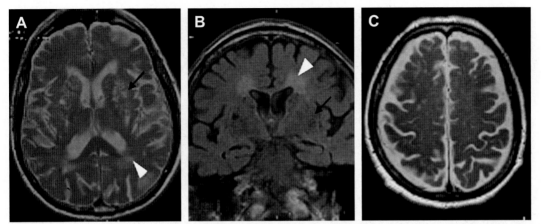

Fig. 2. Dilated perivascular spaces. (*A*) The fast spin-echo T2-weighted image shows several dilated perivascular spaces (*black arrow*) in the basal ganglia (status cribrosus). (*B*) Spaces become hypointense on the FLAIR image. Paratrigonal white-matter abnormalities (*arrowheads*) are observed also. (*C*) At a more cranial level multiple thin perivascular spaces appear perpendicular to brain surface.

of age have AD. Most cases are sporadic, but familial autosomal dominant forms are possible.[13] The genetic basis of AD is complex, but some mutations that could be responsible for AD have been identified. It has been postulated that mutations alter the metabolism of the amyloid precursor protein, leading to the deposition and fibrillar aggregation of its residue, beta-amyloid. This peptide is thought to have neurotoxic properties.[14]

Onset typically occurs after 65 years of age, although it usually is earlier in familial forms. About 10% of elderly patients who have mild cognitive impairment develop AD each year. The course of the disease is progressive, and death usually occurs 5 to 10 years after onset.[13]

In typical cases, subtle memory disturbances are the only symptoms in the early stages. Later, signs of impairment of other brain functions usually occur. In some cases, aphasia, apraxia, or agnosia may precede memory impairment. Sensory and motor function, hearing, and visual function are normal until the late stage of the disease. Gait disturbance, sphincteric incontinence, and bradykinesia occur in advanced forms. Progressive cognitive impairment takes place, and many patients sink into a state of akinesia and mutism and lose the ability to stand and walk.

The main pathologic features are neuronal loss with gliosis in the temporal cortex, neurofibrillary tangles formed by tau protein aggregates, granulovacuolar degeneration of neurons, senile plaques, and amyloid angiopathy mainly formed by beta-amyloid deposits.

The diagnosis of AD relies on clinical findings and neuropsychiatric tests, and the main role of neuroradiology is to exclude secondary causes

of dementia. CT typically shows enlargement of the temporal horn of the lateral ventricles and the sylvian scissure (**Fig. 3**). Since CT was introduced into clinical practice, several studies have attempted to find correlations between cognitive impairment and neuroimaging assessment of cerebral atrophy. Early CT studies demonstrated relatively weak correlations between ventricular and sulcal enlargement and cognitive impairment. Studies of CT brain attenuation values were not able to establish a difference between demented patients and normal subjects. MR imaging is more sensitive in visualizing the temporal lobe changes that are thought to be the early manifestation of AD and in discriminating AD from normal aging.[15,16] These changes, which often are asymmetrical, are hyperintensity of the hippocampus on proton-density and T2-weighted images associated with hippocampal thinning and consequent enlargement of temporal horn and choroidal-hippocampal fissure (**Fig. 4**). FLAIR sequences demonstrated very high sensitivity in detecting these subtle signal changes. Nonspecific gliotic areas in the subcortical and deep white matter often are observed in AD; the clinical value of these areas is difficult to assess, but one must remember that many patients have mixed forms of dementia, with both AD and vascular dementia.

The measurement of temporal atrophy is highly subjective and is based on many indices.[17] For instance, the interuncal distance has been proposed as a measure for hippocampal atrophy in AD, but its real diagnostic value is still debated because of the wide overlap observed in measurements of the brain in AD and the normal aging brain.[18] Longitudinal studies showed that temporal lobe

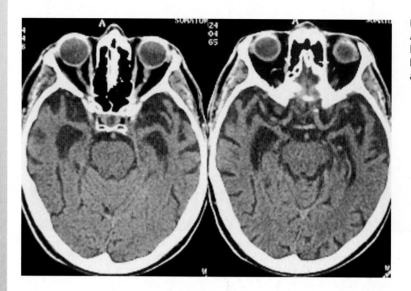

Fig. 3. CT in a patient who has Alzheimer's disease shows enlargement of the temporal horns of the lateral ventricles and temporal lobe atrophy.

changes are progressive in patients who have worsening symptoms. With disease progression, diffuse ventricular enlargement and cortical atrophy become more evident. Recently, voxel-based morphometric techniques have been developed to reduce bias in the subjective selection of anatomic regions of interest and operator dependency.

Some studies have shown that the earliest pathologic abnormalities involve the entorhinal cortex before the hippocampus.[19] Therefore, volumetric sequences have been developed to obtain accurate and reproducible measurement of the volume of this area. These sequences rarely are used in clinical practice,[20] although hippocampal atrophy correlates with clinical worsening.[21] Some recent studies showed that the rate of atrophy was higher in the entorhinal cortex than in the hippocampus, but routine measurement of the hippocampus seems to be more feasible in clinical practice.[22] Voxel-based morphometry studies showed that atrophy beyond the medial temporal lobe is

characteristic of patients who have mild cognitive impairment who will progress to dementia.[23]

Nuclear medicine is less accurate than MR imaging for identifying atrophy or structural abnormalities, but single proton emission computed tomography (SPECT) and positron emission tomography (PET) are very sensitive for the identification of perfusional and metabolic alterations in AD.[24] Nevertheless, SPECT is considered an optional study and is not mandatory for the routine work-up of patients who have typical clinical presentations. SPECT is more useful in selected cases with atypical presentations that may be confused with other forms of dementia. When positive, SPECT shows hypoperfusion in the temporoparietal regions. The severity of this finding has been correlated with the degree of clinical abnormalities.

Fluorodeoxyglucose (FDG)-PET is an effective tool for early diagnosis and for differentiating AD from other types of dementia, although it usually is reserved for complex diagnostic cases or for

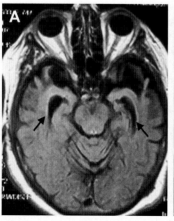
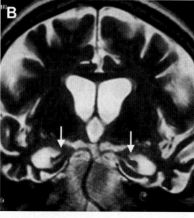

Fig. 4. MR imaging in Alzheimer's disease. (*A*) Axial FLAIR and (*B*) coronal fast spin-echo T2-weighted images clearly show selective hippocampal atrophy with enlargement of the temporal horns (*black arrows*) and the choroidal fissures (*white arrows*).

selected patients at risk for AD before the onset of symptoms.

PET typically shows temporoparietal glucose hypometabolism, which is correlated with the severity of dementia with sensitivity of 94% and a specificity of 73%.[25] Frontal involvement may be evident in advanced cases. Temporal hypometabolism was observed in patients who had minor cognitive impairment and later developed AD. The predictive value of PET could lead to important changes in the early treatment of AD. Some researches are working to develop a specific ligand for beta-amyloid plaques that might enhance the diagnostic accuracy of PET for early diagnosis of AD.[24]

Advanced MR imaging techniques currently are used for clinical and research purposes in patients who have AD.[26] Perfusional MR imaging techniques can provide information similar to that provided by SPECT and PET with the advantage of simultaneous morphologic and structural evaluation. Some studies showed significant correlation between dynamic susceptibility contrast perfusion-weighted imaging (PWI) and FDG-PET in demonstrating reductions in cerebral blood volume (CBV) in patients who had AD.[27] One PWI study comparing patients who had AD and normal age-matched controls showed CBV reductions of 18% in the temporoparietal regions and of 8% to 9% in the sensorimotor areas.[28,29] These results correlated positively with those of SPECT examinations. Another study showed that PWI MR imaging with dynamic susceptibility using temporoparietal regional CBV has a sensitivity of 96% and a specificity of 93% in identifying patients who have possible or probable AD. PWI had low sensitivity and specificity in the evaluation of sensorimotor areas.[30] Arterial spin-labeling PWI also has been used in patients who have AD. This technique provides results similar to those of dynamic susceptibility contrast PWI, but it does not require the administration of a contrast agent.

Diffusion-weighted imaging has been suggested for identifying early structural abnormalities in the normal-appearing white matter. In patients who have early or mild symptoms of AD, an increase in the ADC and a decrease in fractional anisotropy values have been reported in temporal lobe, hippocampus, posterior white matter, and corpus callosum.[26] Moreover, correlation has been observed among ADC and fractional anisotropy values and neuropsychiatric impairment. There is, however, some variability and overlapping of ADC values among AD and normal subjects, preventing the wide clinical application of these studies.

MR imaging spectroscopy rarely is performed to study patients who have AD. Typical metabolic changes are decreased NAA and increased mioinositol. The NAA:mioinositol ratio could become an interesting tool for diagnostic and staging purposes.

Lewy Body Dementia

Clinical features of Lewy body dementia (LBD) include extrapyramidal symptoms, fluctuating cognitive deficit, hallucinations, depression, and agitation. LBD must be differentiated from AD, because patients who have LBD can develop irreversible extrapyramidal symptoms after the uptake of antidopaminergic and anticholinergic neuroleptic therapies used to treat dementia-associated psychosis.[31] The histopathologic hallmark of this disease is the presence of intraneuronal aggregates (Lewy bodies). MR imaging features are not specific, because LBD usually manifests with diffuse atrophy that is not as severe as in AD (**Fig. 5**).[15] An useful differential aspect is putaminal atrophy, which often is observed in LBD but not in AD.

Frontotemporal Degeneration

Frontotemporal degeneration includes various forms of dementia that share some clinical aspects and are characterized by prevalent atrophy of the frontal and anterior temporal lobes. It is estimated that this frontotemporal degeneration is the third most common cause of primary dementia.[32] About 12% of patients who experience the onset of dementia before the age of 65 years suffer from frontotemporal degeneration. The classification of frontotemporal degeneration is complex and not unique.

Pick's disease

Pick's disease is the most common form of dementia included in the category of frontotemporal degeneration. The onset usually occurs in the sixth decade, earlier than that of AD. The course is progressive, and the main symptoms are aphasia and behavioral disturbances. Memory loss is less pronounced in the early stages. In some cases the signs and symptoms are similar to those of AD. Atrophy of the frontal and temporal lobes is observed, and the findings are asymmetric in 60% of patients (**Fig. 6**). Neuronal loss leads to the loss of subcortical myelinated fibers (lobar atrophy). Spared neurones show cytoplasmic argentophilic inclusions known as "Pick bodies."

Both CT and MR imaging show anterior frontal and temporal atrophy with typical sparing of the posterior aspect of the second temporal gyrus and with sulcal and ventricular enlargement prevalent on the frontal and temporal horns (**Fig. 7**). The

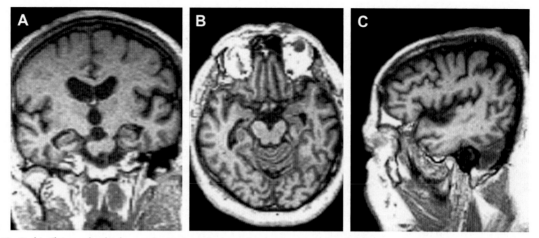

Fig. 5. (A–C) Lewy body dementia. Fast spoiled gradient echo T1-weighted images show mild nonselective atrophy, without specific features.

parietal and occipital lobes are relatively spared. No significant hippocampal involvement is found. Small focal hyperintense areas can be observed on T2-weighted images in the deep white matter of frontal and temporal lobes. Imaging findings can be asymmetrical.

Primary progressive aphasia

There are two main kinds of progressive aphasia: nonfluent progressive aphasia (NFPA) and fluent progressive aphasia (FPA), also known as "semantic dementia". NFPA is characterized clinically by impairment of the grammatical organization of language with preservation of verbal comprehension. Typical symptoms are severe disruption of conversational speech, speech dysfluency, and phonologic errors. In the late stage the disease may progress to mutism. Behavioral changes are not observed in typical cases, although a variant

with associated cognitive and behavioral impairment has been described.[33]

CT and MR imaging findings are not specific. Usually atrophy is found in the perisylvian regions of the frontal and temporal lobes; abnormalities typically are more severe on the left side. A recent study comparing patients who had NFPA, FPA, and normal controls reported that in NFPA significant atrophy can been observed in the pars opercularis, in the pars triangularis (corresponding to the Broca's area), and in a small region of the pars orbitalis of the left inferior frontal gyrus. Atrophy also involved the left precentral gyrus of the insula, the inferior precentral sulcus and gyrus, and the caudate nucleus.[34]

Nuclear medicine and proton-weighted MR imaging studies usually show reduced CBF in the left frontal and temporal lobes (Fig. 8), whereas bilateral hypoperfusion is found only in 30% of cases.

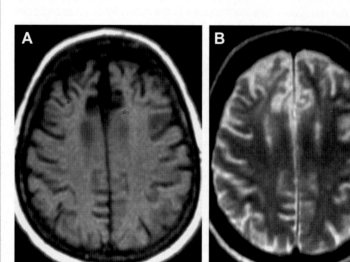

Fig. 6. MRI in a patient who has Pick's disease. (A) T1-weighted and (B) T2-weighted fast spin-echo images show selective frontal atrophy, more apparent on the right side.

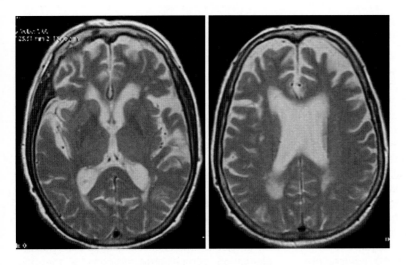

Fig. 7. MR imaging in a different patient who has Pick's disease. Fast spin-echo T2-weighted images show mild frontotemporal atrophy with sparing of the parietal lobes.

FPA typically manifests with progressive anomia, aphasia, and impaired understanding of word meaning, while other cognitive functions are spared. In the later stages the patient also may develop other behavioral and cognitive features of frontotemporal degeneration. Imaging findings are not specific, and bilateral anterior temporal atrophy has been observed. Other studies reported predominantly left temporal atrophy.

Recently, a new variant called "logopenic progressive aphasia" has been described.[34] In this form, patients present with a slow rate of speech output and word-finding pauses, without severe agrammatism and articulation deficits. In the logopenic type of progressive aphasia, the atrophic areas are more posterior than in the other variants, because the atrophy involves the angular gyrus, the posterior third of the middle temporal gyrus, and the superior temporal sulcus.

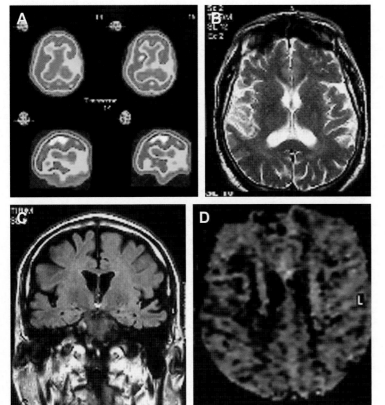

Fig. 8. Nonfluent primary progressive aphasia. (A) SPECT clearly shows reduced uptake in the left temporal lobe. Structural MR imaging with (B) T2-weighted and (C) FLAIR images is unremarkable apart from minimal symmetric sylvian fissure enlargement. (D) Proton-weighted MR imaging in the same patient reveals mild reduction of cerebral blood flow in the left frontotemporal region (L).

EXTRAPYRAMIDAL SYSTEM DISEASES
Neurodegeneration with Brain Iron Accumulation

The term "neurodegeneration with brain iron accumulation" (NBIA) has been introduced recently to describe a heterogeneous group of progressive extrapyramidal disorders characterized by neurodegeneration and excessive focal iron accumulation in the basal ganglia. Hallervorden-Spatz disease is included in this category.[35] NIBA can have a classic infantile onset, which is rapidly progressive, or an atypical late onset characterized by slowly progressive disease. Clinical findings include progressive gait failure, loss of tendon reflexes, and progressive involvement of all cerebral functions at a later stage.

Most forms of NBIA are caused by autosomal recessive mutations in the PANK2 gene that encodes a pantothenate kinase that is important in the biosynthesis of coenzyme A from vitamin B_5. PANK2 is mutated in all cases of classic NBIA and in one third of the cases of atypical disease. Pathology is characterized by spheroid neuronal degeneration caused by the storage of proteins in neuron bodies and axons, prevalent in the gray matter of the basal ganglia, the brain stem, and the dorsal columns of the spinal cord. Storage of lipids and pigment also is detected in the globus pallidus and the pars reticularis of the substantia nigra.

CT shows inconstant calcium deposits in the globi pallidi. Iron deposits in the globus pallidus and substantia nigra appear as low-density areas in these structures.

MR imaging findings are much more specific and in typical cases can be pathognomonic.[36–39] In very early cases MR imaging can show pallidal high intensity in T2-weighted images caused by spheroids. More commonly, MR imaging shows the "tiger-eye" sign, which is thought to indicate a later stage of the disease and to be caused by the degeneration of spheroids and subsequent accumulation of iron. On T2- and T2*-weighted sequences, this pattern consists of an area of high signal intensity in the center of the globus pallidus surrounded by a hypointense rim caused by iron and pseudo-calcium deposits. Rarely, only pallidal low signal with no central hyperintensity can be detected. Iron accumulation also can be observed in the substantia nigra.

Recently, an absolute correlation has been demonstrated between the presence of a mutation in PANK2 and the classical tiger-eye sign; this sign was not observed in any patient negative for the mutation.[40] Moreover, no specific MR imaging findings were observed in the subjects who did not have the mutation, and an higher association

with cerebral and cerebellar atrophy was found. This evidence confirms that NBIA is a heterogeneous group of diseases and that varieties caused by the PANK2 mutation can be identified by means of MR imaging.

Idiopathic Parkinson Disease

Parkinson disease (PD) is a common degenerative disease with an incidence of 1/1000 per year in the population over the age of 50 years and a prevalence of 1% among people older than 65 years. Disease onset usually occurs between the ages of 40 and 70 years. The peak age of onset is in the sixth decade. PD is slightly more common in men.

Pathologic characteristics include the loss of pigmented dopaminergic neurons of the pars compacta of the substantia nigra and the loss of pigmented cells of the locus ceruleus and the dorsal motor nucleus of the vagus. Reactive astrocytosis and intraneuronal aggregations of Lewy bodies in the pars compacta are present as well. Many studies suggest that PD and LBD share a common ethiopathogenesis and should be considered different expressions of the same disease rather than distinct disorders.

Classic clinical features of PD are resting tremor, rigidity, and bradykinesia. The symptoms are variably dominant at onset and during the course of the disease. Approximately 30% to 80% of patients who have PD develop dementia. The clinical features of dementia in PD are similar to those of LBD; they mainly are attention deficits and impairment in executive functions, and memory impairment may be minimal. Depression, agitation, and visual hallucinations also may be present.

The role of neuroradiology in patients who have clinical parkinsonism is mainly to exclude multisystem atrophy and any possible cause of secondary parkinsonism (including vascular disorders, hydrocephalus, and neoplasms). CT and MR imaging usually are unremarkable or unspecific. In some patients who have longstanding disease and who are imaged with high-field-strength MR imaging units, narrowing of the pars compacta of the substantia nigra can be observed. This finding is not constant, and right/left asymmetry of the pars compacta may be an earlier feature of the disease, especially in patients who have hemiparkinsonism symptoms (Fig. 9).[41,42] The normal width of the pars compacta has been reported to be 4 mm, whereas in PD the average width is 2.7 mm.[43] Other authors reported reduction or absence of the usual hypointense signal on T2-weighted images in the pars reticulata of the substantia nigra with microlacunar aspects related

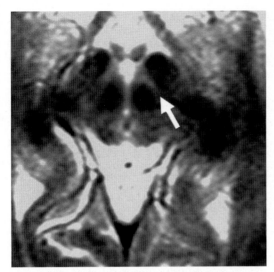

Fig. 9. MR imaging in a patient who has Parkinson disease with predominantly right-sided symptoms. Narrowing of the pars compacta of the substantia nigra is more evident on the left side (*arrow*).

to selective neuronal loss.[44] Mild, nonspecific cortical and subcortical volume loss can observed in a some patients, but structural MR imaging does not show significant differences between patients who have PD with dementia and those who have PD without dementia.[45] Diffusion tensor MR imaging studies have found a significant reduction of fractional anisotropy in the bilateral posterior cingulate bundles of patients who have PD with dementia compared with patients who have PD without dementia.[46] Fractional anisotropy reduction of cortical and white matter of the frontal lobes has been observed in patients who have no morphologic abnormalities. Spectroscopy rarely is used in the clinical practice, but NAA in the occipital lobes was significantly reduced in patients who had PD and dementia compared with patients who did not have cognitive impairment.[47]

Nuclear medicine has a major role in the differential diagnosis of PD and secondary parkinsonism. SPECT imaging of the dopamine transporter can be performed with special radiolabeled ligands, such as TRODAT-1. The reduced uptake of dopamine transporter ligands can be observed very early in the course of the disease. PET also can be useful in selected cases, because it shows reduced 18F-dopa uptake in the putamina, reflecting the reduced transport of 18F-dopa into dopamine neurons.

Secondary Parkinsonism

Secondary parkinsonism can be posttraumatic, metabolic (after osmotic myelinolysis), neoplastic,

toxic (from exposure to carbon monoxide, methanol, neuroleptic drugs, and other toxic agents), or vascular. The vascular form has a rapid onset and a stable course if it is caused by lacunar infarctions of the basal ganglia or frontal infarctions. When vascular Parkinsonism is caused by infarctions of the deep white matter of the semiovales centers, its course can be more subtle and progressive.

Multisystem Atrophy

The terms "multisystem atrophy" and "Parkinson-plus syndromes" include a heterogeneous group of syndromes characterized by the association of Parkinson-like symptoms (indicative of extrapyramidal system involvement) and symptoms indicative of other system dysfunction. Multisystem atrophy affects 25% of patients who have parkinsonism and is poorly responsive to dopamine-replacement therapy. MR imaging is useful for the diagnosis, because the pattern of selective atrophy of involved structures and the storage of paramagnetic substances can be quite specific. When an extrapyramidal disease is suspected, fast spin-echo T2-weighted sequences should be avoided, and standard spin-echoT2- and T2*-weighted sequences should be preferred, because they are more sensitive to the paramagnetic effects of iron or other pigments.[48]

Striatonigral degeneration
Apart from less evidence of rigidity and resistance to levodopa, striatonigral degeneration is clinically undistinguishable from PD. The typical pathologic feature is selective atrophy and neuronal loss of the putamen; atrophy of the pars compacta of the substantia nigra is often present too, but without evidence of Lewy bodies. MR imaging shows atrophy of the putamina, best seen on inversion-recovery coronal sequences, and putaminal hypointense signal is seen on T2-weighted sequences. Rarely, thin hyperintense bands can be seen lateral to the putamina (**Fig. 10**). Narrowing and hypointensity of the pars compacta of the substantia nigra can be observed also, sometimes giving the appearance of fusion between pars reticularis and red nucleus.

Autonomic degeneration (Shy-Drager disease)
Autonomic degeneration is a complex syndrome characterized by extrapyramidal dysfunction associated with autonomic system impairment. The onset occurs in the fifth decade, and the course of the disease is more severe than PD. Typical symptoms are orthostatic hypotension, urinary incontinence, inability to sweat, and extrapyramidal and cerebellar disturbances. As in striatonigral

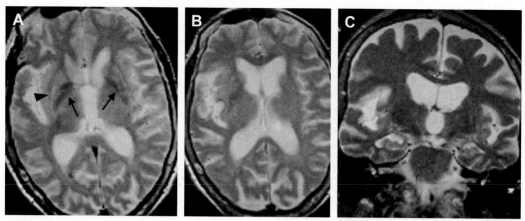

Fig. 10. MR imaging in a patient who has striatonigral degeneration. (A) T2-weighted images show bilateral selective atrophy of the putamina that appears hypointense (arrows). A thin hyperintense band can be seen lateral to the right putamen (arrowhead). (B) A more cranial T2-weighted image confirms caudate atrophy. (C) Coronal T2-weighted image shows mild frontal atrophy is associated with enlargement of the ventricular system.

degeneration, MR imaging shows putaminal hypointensity on T2-weighted images related to iron deposits that are associated with cell degeneration.[49]

Olivopontocerebellar degeneration

Olivopontocerebellar degeneration can occur either alone or together with parkinsonian syndrome within the Parkinson-plus group. The disease can be autosomal dominant or sporadic, its onset usually is during the fifth decade, and it is characterized clinically by progressive ataxia and bulbar symptoms. Typical pathologic features are primary degeneration of pontine neurons with secondary

anterograde loss of pontine transverse and pontocerebellar fibers.

MR imaging shows small olives and medulla with atrophy of the pons and of the cerebellar hemispheres and relative sparing of the vermis. Hyperintensity of the transverse pontine fibers, brachium pontis, middle cerebellar peduncles, and bulbar olives usually is detected on proton density–weighted and T2-weighted images (Fig. 11).[50] Olive hyperintensity is related to transsynaptic degeneration. The atrophy is progressive, and in later stages MR imaging demonstrates loss of the bulbo-protuberential sulcus and flattening of the anterior surface of the pons (Fig. 12). When olivopontocerebellar degeneration is seen in the

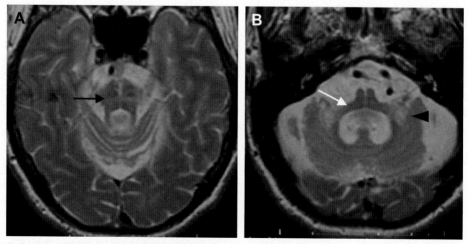

Fig. 11. MR imaging in olivopontocerebellar degeneration. (A) Hyperintensity of the transverse pontine fibers with a "cross" aspect is evident (black arrow). (B) There is atrophy of the pons, the middle cerebellar peduncles (white arrow), and the cerebellar hemispheres, with relative sparing of the vermis. The fourth ventricle is enlarged. Demyelination of the middle cerebellar peduncles is present (arrowhead).

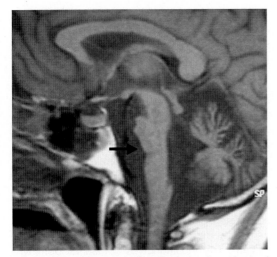

Fig. 12. Olivopontocerebellar degeneration. Sagittal T1-weighted image shows flattening of the anterior surface of the pons and the disappearance of the bulbo-protuberential sulcus (*arrow*).

context of a multisystem atrophy, T2-weighted images frequently show hypointensity of the putamen, globus pallidus, and substantia nigra.

Progressive Supranuclear Palsy

The onset of progressive supranuclear palsy (Steele-Richardson-Olzsewsky disease) occurs in late adulthood. Typical symptoms include axial rigidity without tremor, pseudobulbar signs, supranuclear gaze palsy, and extrapyramidal signs. Dementia is mild and appears late in the disease.

MR imaging shows severe progressive atrophy in the midbrain, tectum, and superior cerebellar peduncles and, in later stages, in the thalami and caudate nuclei. On sagittal images, the superior surface of the midbrain has a concave profile (**Fig. 13**).[15] Midbrain atrophy results in enlargement of the third ventricle with slope toward the aqueduct and widening of the quadrigeminal and interpeduncular fossa.[51] Hyperintense rim on T2-weighted sequences can be found in the periaqueductal gray matter. Atrophy of the midbrain correlates with motor dysfunction. Frontal lobe atrophy has been described, and its degree has been demonstrated to correlate with behavioral disturbance.[52]

Corticobasal Degeneration

Corticobasal degeneration manifests in late adulthood with extrapyramidal signs, apraxia, and agnosia. Characteristic symptoms are asymmetric limb apraxia and alien limb phenomenon. Severe depression and cognitive decline often are observed. No response to L-dopa is present. Clinical diagnosis is difficult because there is evident overlap with other forms of dementia and

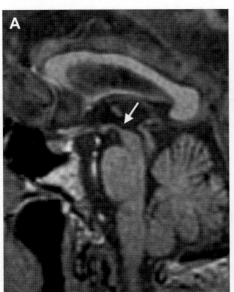
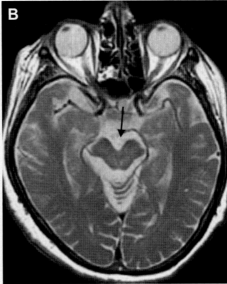

Fig. 13. Early progressive supranuclear palsy. (*A*) Sagittal T1-weighted image shows mild atrophy in the midbrain and the tectum. The superior surface of the midbrain has a concave profile (*white arrow*), and the third ventricle appears slightly enlarged. (*B*) Fast spin-echo T2-weighted image shows widening of the interpeduncular fossa (*black arrow*).

extrapyramidal disorders, such as Pick disease, AD, multisystem atrophy, and progressive supranuclear palsy. MR imaging findings are variable and not specific. Severe and progressive atrophy of the frontal and parietal lobes has been described. Atrophy can be very asymmetric involving the cerebral hemisphere contralateral to the clinically affected side (**Fig. 14**).[53,54] Bilateral atrophy of the putamina and the nuclei caudati, atrophy of the corpus callosum, and hyperintensity in the lentiform nuclei on T2-weighted sequences also have been described.

Wilson Disease

Wilson disease, or epatolenticular degeneration, is a metabolic disorder transmitted by autosomal recessive inheritance. The mutation leads to a defect in the incorporation of copper into ceruloplasmin, with secondary storage of copper in liver, brain, cornea, bone, and kidney. The onset usually is during adolescence, although late onset has been observed. Patients usually present with motor disturbances consisting of slowly progressive tremor at rest or with action, choreoathetoid movements, and dystonia. Mental deterioration may occur. In late stages of the disease a Keiser-Fleischer corneal ring is a typical finding. Neuropathologic studies report symmetric spongiform degeneration involving putamina, thalami, caudate nuclei, pontine and mesencephalic nuclei, and dentate nuclei. Subcortical white matter can be involved in an asymmetrical pattern.

CT usually shows symmetric hypodensity of the lenticular nuclei; thalami are involved less frequently. MR imaging shows high signal in the thalami, putamina, dentate nuclei, and brainstem on T2-weighted images.[55,56] High-field-strength MR imaging sometimes can show typical low T2 signal bands in the involved structures because of copper storage. Cystic necrosis cavities, presenting as very low density on CT and as fluid-like high signal on T2-weighted images, are a less frequent finding. Asymmetrical involvement of subcortical white matter usually is seen as hyperintensity on T2-weighted images, prevalent on the frontal gyri. In some cases both CT and MR imaging are normal or show only mild generalized atrophy.

Huntington Disease (Chorea Major)

Huntington disease is one of the most common hereditary degenerative diseases of the nervous system. The inheritance is autosomal dominant with complete penetrance, but rare sporadic forms exist. Onset occurs in mid-adulthood, although a rare juvenile form has been described. The disease is progressive and leads to death 5 to 15 years from onset.

The classical clinical feature is movement disorder (choreoathetosis), subtle at first but slowly becoming more pronounced and involving the entire musculature. Patients also present with psychiatric disorders, such as depression or psychosis, that may precede the development of chorea. Progressive cognitive deficit and dementia often develop after the onset of choreoathetosis.

MR imaging shows atrophy of the caudati nuclei and the putamina; the atrophy sometimes can be asymmetric. Caudate atrophy particularly involves the head of the caudate nuclei, leading to enlargement of the frontal horns of the lateral ventricles (**Fig. 15**). Some authors describe gray-matter atrophy in the opercular cortex, right paracentral

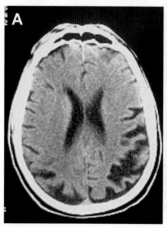 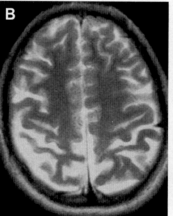 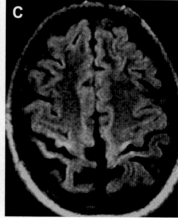

Fig. 14. (*A*) CT in a patient who has corticobasal degeneration shows asymmetric atrophy of the parietal lobes that is more severe on the left side. (*B*) Fast spin-echo T2-weighted and (*C*) FLAIR images in another patient show symmetric parietal atrophy.

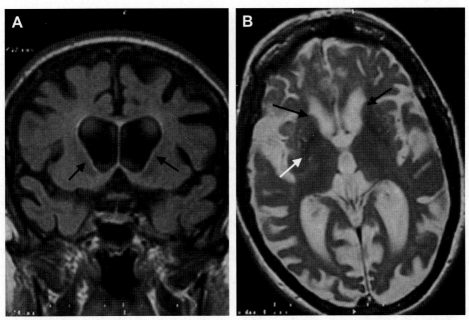

Fig. 15. Huntington disease. (*A*) Coronal FLAIR and (*B*) axial T2-weighed images reveal atrophy of the head of the caudati nuclei (*black arrows in A and B*), more evident on the left side, with enlargement of the frontal horns of the lateral ventricles. The right putamen is slightly atrophic (*white arrow in B*). Mild nonselective cortical atrophy can be observed.

lobule, and hypothalamus. Diffuse cerebral atrophy, more pronounced in the frontal lobes, is observed in the late stages in demented patients. MR imaging signal abnormalities usually are not found in Huntington disease, although hypointensity in the caudate and putamen has been observed on T2-weighted images; hyperintensity in the same structures has been reported in patients who have the juvenile form of Huntington disease.[57]

The loss of brain volume is accompanied by an increase in ADC values,[58] and diffusion tensor imaging studies have shown that even before the onset of manifest Huntington disease, regional fractional anisotropy reduction occurs in the putamina and in the anterior parts of the corpus callosum.[59]

Amyotrophic Lateral Sclerosis

Amyotrophic lateral sclerosis (ALS) is the most common form of degenerative motor neuron disease and is caused by the degeneration of both corticospinal tracts and second moto-neurons.

The disease usually is sporadic, although an hereditary autosomal dominant form accounts for 5% of cases. The annual incidence of ALS is between 0.4 and 1.7/100,000 , and its prevalence today is approximately 46% higher than it was in the 1960s.[60] The onset usually is in middle to late adulthood, and the course of the disease is

progressive, with death occurring 3 to 5 years after onset. Three clinical subtypes are recognized. Classic ALS affects both upper and lower motor neurons and presents as slowly progressive atrophic weakness of the upper limbs, spasticity of the lower limbs, and hyperreflexia. In the upper motor neuron type only central motor neurons are affected, and signs of pyramidal tract impairment are dominant. In the lower motor neuron type signs of peripheral motor involvement are dominant.

The microscopic findings consist of loss of pyramidal and Betz cells in the motor cortex with gliosis of the subcortical white matter. Similar findings are evident in the spinal cord with loss of motor neurons and gliosis of the anterior horns prevalent at the cervical and lumbar levels.

CT findings usually are normal in ALS. MR imaging shows varying hyperintensity of the corticospinal tract on T2- and proton density–weighted images because of anterograde neuronal degeneration. In typical cases the signal abnormality can be followed from the precentral gyrus through the posterior limb of the internal capsule extending downwards to the medulla (**Fig. 16**).[61] FLAIR sequences are much more sensitive than spin-echo ones in depicting signal abnormalities. In some patients a symmetric hypointense band can be observed in the prefrontal cortex, especially if high-field-strength units and T2*-weighted

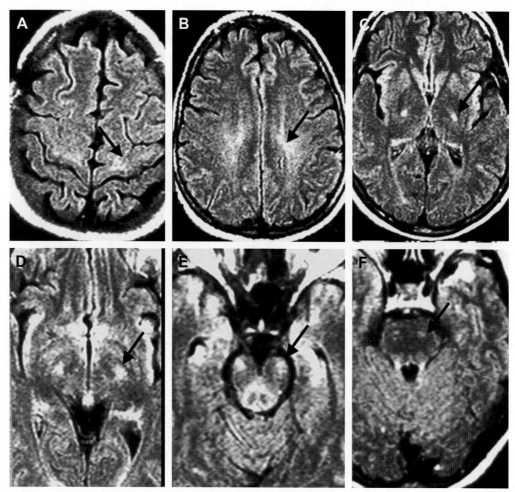

Fig. 16. Amyotrophic lateral sclerosis. (*A–F*) FLAIR images reveal symmetrical hyperintensity of both corticospinal tracts along their entire course. The black arrows indicate the left tract.

sequences are used.[62] These changes may be caused by the deposition of ferric iron in glial cells within the motor cortex, by free radicals, or by increased lipofuscin granules in neurons of the motor cortex. MR imaging of the medulla can show hypotrophy of its anterolateral aspects.[63]

Recently, the presence of whole-brain and regional frontotemporal atrophy in ASL has been demonstrated in a structural MR imaging study comparing ASL patients and normal subjects.[64]

Perfusion-weighted MR imaging can show hypoperfusion in frontal and temporal areas correlated with the impairment of neuropsychologic functions. MR spectroscopy has shown decreased NAA in the primary motor cortex as well as in the frontal lobe, the primary sensory cortex, the superior parietal gyrus, and the anterior cingulate gyrus. Assessment of ALS by diffusion tensor imaging has provided useful information in recent studies. Volumetric analysis of the corticospinal

tracts by using diffusion tensor imaging–based color maps showed significantly reduced volumes in patients who had ALS, compared with normal subjects in both the affected and the nonaffected hemispheres. No significant correlation was found between corticospinal tract volumes and any of the clinical parameters, however.[65] Other authors investigated fractional anisotropy in corticospinal tracts in patients who had ALS and observed that fractional anisotropy along the corticospinal tracts decreases significantly with the worsening of symptoms, reflecting the functional abnormality of the intracranial corticospinal tracts (**Fig. 17**).[66]

VASCULAR DEMENTIA
Multi-Infarction Dementia

Multi-infarction dementia accounts for 10% to 30% of all cases of dementia, although combined

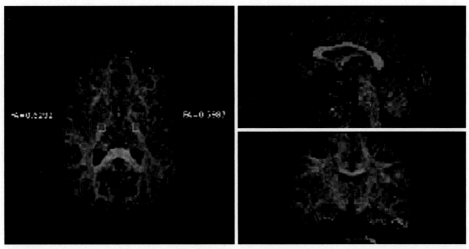

Fig. 17. Diffusion tensor imaging of a patient who has amyotrophic lateral sclerosis. Fractional anisotropy is reduced, especially on the left side.

forms of multi-infarction dementia and AD are very common.

The most important risk factors for vascular dementia are hypertension, diabetes, hyperlipidemia, recurrent stroke, coronary artery disease, and smoking. The course of the disease is characterized by recurrent ischemic episodes. The cognitive deficit correlates directly with the quantity of brain tissue damaged by ischemic events; focal sensory-motor symptoms and extrapyramidal symptoms often are present also. In multi-infarction dementia, ischemic events are related mainly to thromboembolic vascular disease.

CT and MR imaging show multiple focal or confluent lesions with the typical features of encephalomalacic ischemic areas, hypodense on CT and relatively hyperintense on T2-weighted images. Oldest lesions can have a poroencephalic aspect. Diffusion-weighted imaging can be useful in identifying new acute lesions. Ischemic foci can be observed in the cortex, in the basal ganglia, in the pons, and in the superficial and deep white matter. The distribution of the largest lesions corresponds to specific vascular territories or watershed areas.[67]

Binswanger's Subcortical Chronic Encephalopathy

Binswanger's disease or subcortical chronic encephalopathy is considered a variant of multi-infarction dementia. The typical pathologic alteration is atherosclerosis of the long penetrating arteries in patients who have hypertension. This alteration leads to chronic hypoperfusion and ischemia mainly involving periventricular regions and semi-oval centers. Clinical findings are dementia, motor deficit, and, sometimes, pseudobulbar paralysis. CT shows diffuse hypodensity in the periventricular white matter, volume loss with ventricular enlargement, and eventually focal hypodense areas. MR imaging findings are similar[68]; the corpus callosum usually is spared (Fig. 18).

Amyloid Angiopathy

Cerebral amyloid angiopathy is an underestimated entity resulting from the accumulation of beta-amyloid peptide in the media and adventitia of the vessels of the leptomeninges and the cortex of the brain. This pathologic feature typically is observed in patients who have AD, but isolated involvement of the vessels is characteristic of amyloid angiopathy.

Clinical findings include ictal onset resulting from hemorrhage and subacute progressive cognitive dementia. Patients often experience multiple hemorrhagic episodes, and dementia is observed in 40% of patients.[69] The disease is one of the most common causes of spontaneous intracranial hemorrhage, accounting for 15% to 20% of all cases in persons more than 60 years of age.

CT is useful in the acute phases to detect acute hematomas, and it also can show signs of old hemorrhages. MR imaging can show acute lobar hematomas in acute patients, but more often it shows signs of previous hemorrhages with MR imaging features depending on the age of the bleeding.[70] Hemosiderin staining is very common. In 70% of cases patchy confluent areas of white matter are observed on T2-weighted sequences. T2*-weighted sequences are very useful because they often show multifocal punctate hypointense areas

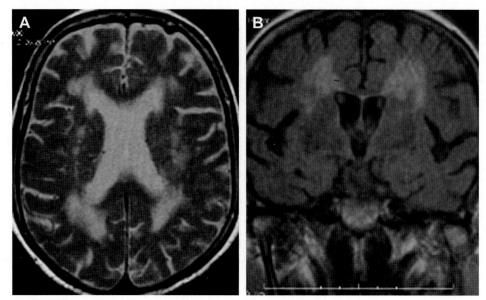

Fig. 18. Vascular dementia with clinical and imaging features of Binswanger disease. (*A*) Axial fast spin-echo T2-weighted and (*B*) coronal FLAIR images show hypodensity in the semi-oval centers and in the periventricular white matter with mild ventricular enlargement.

in the subcortical white matter and in the territory of the deep perforating arteries. These lesions are considered a consequence of remote microhemorrhages; therefore the use of T2*-weighted sequences has been suggested in elderly patients.[71] In the late stage, general brain atrophy often occurs. Distinguishing cerebral amyloid angiopathy from hypertensive encephalopathy with multiple microhemorrhages can be difficult; in cerebral amyloid angiopathy, hemorrhages are localized more frequently in the basal ganglia and in the thalami than in the subcortical white matter.

Normal Pressure Hydrocephalus or Chronic Adult Hydrocephalus

Normal pressure hydrocephalus is a common form of subcortical dementia involving 0.5% to 1% of the population over 65 years of age. The classic triad of symptoms is memory loss, gait disturbances, and urinary incontinence. Gait disturbances usually mark the onset of symptoms.

Normal pressure hydrocephalus may be primary or secondary (usually after subarachnoid hemorrhage and impaired resorption of CSF). The

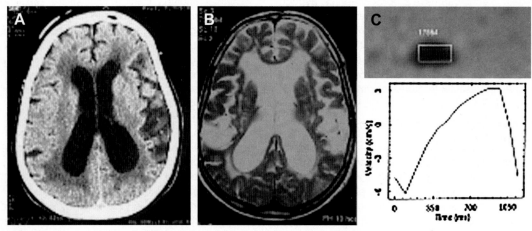

Fig. 19. Normal pressure hydrocephalus. (*A*) CT and (*B*) T2-weighted MR imaging show an enlarged ventricular system with relatively spared superficial sulci. (*C*) The phase-contrast sequence can be useful to observe flow turbulences and to measure CSF flow.

pathogenesis of idiopathic forms is complex and probably depends on abnormal CSF dynamics with normal pressure, but it still is not explained completely. The radiologic diagnosis of normal pressure hydrocephalus is important because ventricular shunting may improve the symptoms; however, the diagnosis is difficult because there is a wide overlap between the features of normal pressure hydrocephalus and those of other degenerative paraphysiologic conditions.[72–74]

The classic radiologic hallmark of normal pressure hydrocephalus is disproportional dilation of the ventricular system with relatively normal-appearing cortical sulci (**Fig. 19**). The evidence of sulcal enlargement together with dilatation of the ventricles indicates the presence of concomitant atrophy and is considered a sign of worse prognosis after treatment. The frontal and temporal horns usually are widened without signs of hippocampal atrophy and with sparing of the parahippocampal fissure.[75] Other structural findings include thinning and convexity of the corpus callosum and scattered areas of T2 hyperintensity deep in the white matter. Increased flow void within the aqueductus is a sign of altered CSF flow, but the significance of this sign is controversial.[74] More recently, directional flow studies performed using cardiac-gated time-of-flight or phase-contrast techniques have shown inversion of flow direction in the aqueduct and can be useful in selecting surgical candidates.[76] Measurement of CSF "stroke volume" in the aqueductus has been proposed as well. These techniques seem to be more sensitive than CT cysternography in differentiating atrophy from normal pressure hydrocephalus. CT cysternography is performed by introducing iodinated contrast agent into the subarachnoid space and performing serial cerebral CT scans within 24 hours. In normal subjects, the contrast agent is found in the basal cisterns after 6 hours, and after 8 to 12 hours it reaches the subarachnoid spaces of the vault. At 24 hours it is absorbed completely and no longer is evident. In chronic adult hydrocephalus, inversion of CSF flow, delay in absorption, or both can occur. This technique is considered less specific than CSF pressure monitoring, however. Radioisotopic cisternography also can be used and offers similar results.

REFERENCES

1. Scheltens P, Pasquier F, Weerts JG, et al. Qualitative assessment of cerebral atrophy on MRI: inter- and intra-observer reproducibility in dementia and normal aging. Eur Neurol 1997;37(2):95–9.

2. Yue NC, Arnold AM, Longstreth WT, et al. Sulcal, ventricular, and white matter changes at MR imaging in the aging brain: data from the cardiovascular health study. Radiology 1997;202(1):33–9.

3. Fox NC, Freeborough PA, Rossor MN. Visualisation and quantification of rates of atrophy in Alzheimer's disease. Lancet 1996;348(9020):94–7.

4. Minati L, Grisoli M, Bruzzone MG. MR spectroscopy, functional MRI, and diffusion-tensor imaging in the aging brain: a conceptual review. J Geriatr Psychiatry Neurol 2007;20:3–21.

5. Angelie E, Bonmartin A, Boudraa A, et al. Regional differences and metabolic changes in normal aging of the human brain: proton MR spectroscopic imaging study. AJNR Am J Neuroradiol 2001;22:119–27.

6. Ross AJ, Sachdev PS, Wen W, et al. Longitudinal changes during aging using proton magnetic resonance spectroscopy. J Gerontol A Biol Sci Med Sci 2006;61:291–8.

7. Nusbaum AO, Tang CY, Buchsbaum MS, et al. Regional and global changes in cerebral diffusion with normal aging. AJNR Am J Neuroradiol 2001; 22:136–42.

8. Charlton RA, Barrick TR, McIntyre DJ, et al. White matter damage on diffusion tensor imaging correlates with age-related cognitive decline. Neurology 2006;66:217–22.

9. Gallucci M, Bozzao A, Splendiani A, et al. Le alterazioni del segnale RM nell'encefalo dell'anziano: correlazioni anatomo-patologiche. Riv Neurorad 1990; 3:193–202.

10. Challa VR. White matter lesions in MR imaging of elderly subjects. Radiology 1987;164:874.

11. Braffman BH, Zimmerman RA, Trijanowsky JQ, et al. Brain MR: pathologic correlation with gross and histopathology. I. Lacunar infarction and Wirchow-Robin spaces. AJNR Am J Neuroradiol 1988;9:621–8.

12. Jungreis CA, Kanal E, Hirsch WL, et al. Normal perivascular spaces mimicking lacunar infarction: MR imaging. Radiology 1988;169:101–4.

13. Husain MM, Garrett RK. Clinical diagnosis and management of Alzheimer's disease. Neuroimaging Clin N Am 2005;15:767–77.

14. Mott RY, Hulette CM. Neuropathology of Alzheimer's disease. Neuroimaging Clin N Am 2005;15:755–65.

15. Keyserling H, Mukundan S. The role of conventional MR and CT in the work-up of dementia patients. Magn Reson Imaging Clin N Am 2006;14:169–82.

16. Sandor T, Jolesz F, Tieman J, et al. Comparative analysis of computed tomographic and magnetic resonance imaging scans in Alzheimer patients and controls. Arch Neurol 1992;49:381–4.

17. Frisoni GB, Beltramello A, Weiss C, et al. Linear measures of atrophy in mild Alzheimer disease. AJNR Am J Neuroradiol 1996;17:913–23.

18. Dahlbeck JW, McCluney KW, Yeakley JW, et al. The interuncal distance: a new MR measurement for hippocampal atrophy in Alzheimer's disease. AJNR Am J Neuroradiol 1991;12:931–2.

19. Minoshima S. Imaging Alzheimer's disease: clinical applications. Neuroimaging Clin N Am 2003;13: 769–80.

20. Bobinski M, de Leon MJ, Convit A, et al. MRI of entorhinal cortex in mild Alzheimer's disease. Lancet 1999;353(9146):38–40.

21. Jack CR Jr, Petersen RC, Xu Y, et al. Rates of hippocampal atrophy correlate with change in clinical status in aging and AD. Neurology 2000;55:484–9.

22. Ramani A, Jensen JH, Helpern JA. Quantitative MR imaging in Alzheimer disease. Radiology 2006;241: 27–44.

23. Karas G, Sluime J, Goekoop R, et al. Amnestic mild cognitive impairment: structural MR imaging findings predictive of conversion to Alzheimer disease. AJNR Am J Neuroradiol 2008;29:944–9.

24. Lascola C. Molecular imaging in Alzheimer's disease. Neuroimaging Clin N Am 2005;15:827–35.

25. Silverman DH, Small GW, Chang CY, et al. Positron emission tomography in evaluation of dementia: regional brain metabolism and long-term outcome. JAMA 2001;286:2120–7.

26. Krishnan S, Talley BD, Slavin MJ, et al. Current status of functional MR imaging, perfusion-weighted imaging, and diffusion-tensor imaging in Alzheimer's disease diagnosis and research. Neuroimaging Clin N Am 2005;12:853–68.

27. Gonzalez RG, Fischman AJ, Guimaraes AR, et al. Functional MR in the evaluation of dementia: correlation of abnormal dynamic cerebral blood volume measurements with changes in cerebral metabolism on positron emission tomography with fluorodeoxyglucose F 18. AJNR Am J Neuroradiol 1995;16: 1763–70.

28. Pearlson GD, Harris GJ, Powers RE, et al. Quantitative changes in mesial temporal volume, regional cerebral blood flow, and cognition in Alzheimer's disease. Arch Gen Psychiatry 1992;49:402–8.

29. Harris GJ, Lewis RF, Satlin A, et al. Dynamic susceptibility contrast MRI of regional cerebral blood volume in Alzheimer's disease. Am J Psychiatry 1996;153:721–4.

30. Harris GJ, Lewis RF, Satlin A, et al. Dynamic susceptibility contrast MR imaging of regional cerebral blood volume in Alzheimer disease: a promising alternative to nuclear medicine. AJNR Am J Neuroradiol 1998;19:1727–32.

31. McKeith IG. Dementia with Lewy bodies. Br J Psychiatry 2002;180:144–7.

32. Kitagaki H, Mori E, Yamaji S, et al. Frontotemporal dementia and Alzheimer disease: evaluation of cortical atrophy with automated hemispheric surface display generated with MR images. Radiology 1998; 208:431–9.

33. Kertesz A, Davidson W, McCabe P, et al. Primary progressive aphasia: diagnosis, varieties, evolution. J Int Neuropsychol Soc 2003;9:710–9.

34. Gorno-Tempini ML, Dronkers NF, Rankin KP, et al. Cognition and anatomy in three variants of primary progressive aphasia. Ann Neurol. 2004;55:335–46.

35. Gregory A, Hayflick SJ. Neurodegeneration with brain iron accumulation. Folia Neuropathol 2005;43:286–96.

36. Gallucci M, Cardona F, Arachi M, et al. Follow-up MR studies in Hallervorden-Spatz disease. J Comput Assist Tomogr 1990;14:118–20.

37. Mutoh K, Okuno T, Ito M, et al. MR imaging of a group I case of Hallervorden-Spatz disease. J Comput Assist Tomogr 1988;12:851–3.

38. Savoiardo M, Halliday WC, Nardocci N, et al. Hallervorden-Spatz disease: MR and pathological findings. AJNR Am J Neuroradiol 1993;14:155–62.

39. Sener RN. Pantothenate kinase-associated neurodegeneration: MR imaging, proton MR spectroscopy, and diffusion MR imaging findings. AJNR Am J Neuroradiol 2003;24:1690–3.

40. Hayflick SJ, Hartman M, Coryell J, et al. Brain MRI in neurodegeneration with brain iron accumulation with and without PANK2 mutations. AJNR Am J Neuroradiol 2006;27:1230–3.

41. Huber SJ, Chakeres DW, Paulson GW, et al. Magnetic resonance imaging in Parkinson's disease. Arch Neurol 1990;47:735–7.

42. Braffman BH, Grossman RI, Goldberg HI, et al. MR imaging in Parkinson disease with spin-echo and gradient-echo sequences. AJNR Am J Neuroradiol 1989;152:159–65.

43. Friehs GM, Ojakangas CL, Pachatz P, et al. Thalamotomy and caudatotomy with the gamma knife as a treatment for parkinsonism with a comment on lesion sizes. Stereotact Funct Neurosurg 1995; 64(Suppl 1):209–21.

44. Braffman BH, Grossman RI, Goldberg HI, et al. MR imaging of Parkinson's disease with spin-echo and gradient echo sequences. AJNR Am J Neuroradiol 1988;9:1093–9.

45. Beyer MK, Larsen JP, Aarsland D. Gray matter atrophy in Parkinson disease with dementia and dementia with Lewy bodies. Neurology 2007;69:747–54.

46. Matsui H, Nishinaka K, Oda M, et al. Dementia in Parkinson's disease: diffusion tensor imaging. Acta Neurol Scand 2007;116:177–81.

47. Summerfield C, Gomez-Anson B, Tolosa E, et al. Dementia in Parkinson disease a proton magnetic resonance spectroscopy study. Arch Neurol 2002; 59:1416–20.

48. Testa D, Savoiardo M, Fetoni V, et al. Multiple system atrophy. Clinical and MR observations on 42 cases. Ital J Neurol Sci 1993;14(3):211–6.

49. Savoiardo M, Strada L, Girotti F, et al. MR imaging in progressive supranuclear palsy and Shy-Drager syndrome. J Comput Assist Tomogr 1989;13:555–60.

50. Savoiardo M, Strada L, Girotti F, et al. Olivopontocerebellar atrophy: MR diagnosis and relationship to multisystem atrophy. Radiology 1990;174:693–6.

51. Righini A, Antonini A, De Notaris R, et al. MR imaging of the superior profile of the midbrain: differential diagnosis between progressive supranuclear palsy and Parkinson disease. AJNR Am J Neuroradiol 2004;25:927–32.

52. Cordato NJ, Duggins AJ, Halliday GM, et al. Clinical deficits correlate with regional cerebral atrophy in progressive supranuclear palsy. Brain 2005;128: 1595–604.

53. Tokamaru AN, O'uchi T, Kuru Y. Corticobasal degeneration: MR with hystopathological comparison. AJNR Am J Neuroradiol 1996;17:1849–52.

54. Gallucci M, Bonamini M, Catalucci A, et al. MRI helps in the early diagnosis of corticobasal degeneration. Riv Neurorad 1998;11(Suppl 2):13–4.

55. Gallucci M, Bozzao A. Patologia metabolica: Wilson, Hallervorden-Spatz, mucopolisaccaridosi. Riv Neurorad 1996;9:781–8.

56. Nazer H, Brismar J, Al-Kawi MZ, et al. Magnetic resonance imaging of the brain in Wilson's disease. Neuroradiology 1993;35:130–3.

57. Simmos JT, Pastakia B, Chase TN, et al. Magnetic resonance imaging in Huntington's disease. AJNR Am J Neuroradiol 1986;7:25–8.

58. Mascalchi M, Francesco F, Della Nave R, et al. Huntington disease: volumetric, diffusion-weighted, and magnetization transfer MR imaging of brain. Radiology 2004;232:867–73.

59. Klöppel S, Draganski B, Golding CV, et al. White matter connections reflect changes in voluntary-guided saccades in pre-symptomatic Huntington's disease. Brain 2008;131:196–204.

60. Worms PM. The epidemiology of motor neuron diseases: a review of recent studies. J Neurol Sci 2001;191:3–9.

61. Cheung G, Gawal MJ, Cooper PW, et al. Amyotrophic lateral sclerosis: correlation of clinical and MR imaging findings. Radiology 1995;194:263–70.

62. Oba H, Araki T, Ohtomo K, et al. Amyotrophic lateral sclerosis: T2 shortening in motor cortex at MR imaging. Radiology 1993;189:843–6.

63. Chan S, Kaufmann P, Shungu DC, et al. Amyotrophic lateral sclerosis and primary lateral sclerosis: evidence-based diagnostic evaluation of the upper motor neuron. Neuroimaging Clin N Am 2003;13: 307–26.

64. Mezzapesa DM, Ceccarelli A, Dicuonzo F, et al. Whole-brain and regional brain atrophy in amyotrophic lateral sclerosis. AJNR Am J Neuroradiol 2007;28:255–9.

65. Wang S, Poptani H, Bilello M, et al. Diffusion tensor imaging in amyotrophic lateral sclerosis: volumetric analysis of the corticospinal tract. AJNR Am J Neuroradiol 2006;27:1234–8.

66. Iwata NK, Aoki S, Okab S, et al. Evaluation of corticospinal tracts in ALS with diffusion tensor MRI and brainstem stimulation. Neurology 2008;70:528–32.

67. Guermazi A, Miaux Y, Rovira-Cañellas A, et al. Neuroradiological findings in vascular dementia. Neuroradiology 2007;49:1–22.

68. Kinkel WR, Jacobs L, Polachini I. Subcortical arteriosclerotic encephalopathy Binswanger's disease: CT, NMR, and clinical correlations. Arch Neurol 1985;42: 951–9.

69. van Straaten EC, Scheltens P, Barkhof F. MRI and CT in the diagnosis of vascular dementia. J Neurol Sci 2004;226:9–12.

70. Smith EE, Gurol ME, Eng JA, et al. White matter lesions, cognition, and recurrent hemorrhage in lobar intracerebral hemorrhage. Neurology 2004; 63:1606–12.

71. Walker DA, Broderick DF, Kotsenas AL, et al. Routine use of gradient-echo MRI to screen for cerebral amyloid angiopathy in elderly patients. AJR Am J Roentgenol 2004;182:1547–50.

72. Bradley WG Jr, Whittemore AR, Watanabe AS, et al. Association of deep white matter infarction with chronic communicating hydrocephalus: implications regarding the possible origin of normal pressure hydrocephalus. AJNR Am J Neuroradiol 1991;12:31–9.

73. Bradley WG. Normal pressure hydrocephalus: new concepts on etiology and diagnosis. AJNR Am J Neuroradiol 2000;21:1586–90.

74. Schroth G, Klose U. Cerebrospinal fluid flow, III: pathological cerebrospinal fluid pulsations. Neuroradiology 1992;35:16–24.

75. Holodny AI, Waxman R, George AE, et al. MR differential diagnosis of normal-pressure hydrocephalus and Alzheimer disease: significance of perihippocampal fissures. AJNR Am J Neuroradiol 1998;19:813–9.

76. Sharma AK, Gaikwad S, Gupta V, et al. Measurement of peak CSF flow velocity at cerebral aqueduct, before and after lumbar CSF drainage, by use of phase-contrast MRI: utility in the management of idiopathic normal pressure hydrocephalus. Clin Neurol Neurosurg 2008;110:363–8.

Neurovascular Emergencies in the Elderly

John B. Weigele, MD, PhD*, Robert W. Hurst, MD

KEYWORDS
- Elderly • Geriatric • Neurovascular • Emergencies
- Stroke • Hemorrhage

Neurovascular diseases are major causes of disability and death in the elderly; many present as medical emergencies. The population over age 65 years in the United States has grown 2% per year, increasing from 12 to 37 million over the period from 1950 to 2005. The elderly population is projected to continue to increase more rapidly than the general population until 2050.[1] With the continuing growth of the geriatric population, there has been increasing interest in the impact of aging on the cerebrovascular system. Recent advances in the clinical neurosciences have demonstrated that neurovascular emergencies in the elderly often are amenable to treatment; neuroimaging plays a critical role in diagnosis and neurointerventional techniques are becoming increasingly important therapeutic options. This article provides an overview of some of the common neurovascular disorders in the elderly that require urgent evaluation and treatment, with an emphasis on the expanding role for interventional neuroradiology in their management.

OVERVIEW: THE AGING BRAIN AND CEREBROVASCULAR SYSTEM

Data from animal models suggest the aging brain is less resistant to physiologic stress.[2] Cerebral blood flow gradually decreases with age.[3] Collateral circulation is impaired, reducing the compensatory response. Vascular autoregulation is less effective.[3] The blood-brain barrier is less efficient.[4] An age-dependent decline in oxidative metabolism occurs in the brain. The damaging excitotoxic response to ischemia may be more pronounced. The abilities to neutralize free radicals, extrude calcium from cells, and synthesize proteins are reduced. Therefore, a comparable ischemic insult may cause more damage in an elderly patient than a younger individual.[3,5]

ACUTE ISCHEMIC STROKE
Epidemiology

The term "stroke" refers to rapidly developing neurologic dysfunction caused by cerebrovascular occlusion (ischemic) or disruption (hemorrhagic).[5] Stroke is the third leading cause of death in the United States surpassed only by cardiac disease and cancer, and it is the leading cause of disability.[6] More than 750,000 new or recurrent strokes occur each year; most (approximately 86%) are ischemic in etiology.[7,8]

Acute ischemic stroke (AIS) is predominately a disease of the elderly. The risk of AIS increases exponentially with age, approximately doubling after age 55 with each successive decade of life; the annual incidence increases from 3 per 1000 in people age 55 to 64 years up to 25 per 1000 in individuals over 85 years old.[7] The incidence of AIS is higher in men up to age 75 years; above this age the incidence is higher in women.

Etiology and Pathophysiology

Ischemic stroke is caused predominantly by temporary or permanent occlusion of a cerebral artery. Common causes include cardioembolism (atrial fibrillation, myocardial infarction, valvular disease,

Department of Radiology, Hospital of the University of Pennsylvania, 2 Dulles-Room 219, 3400 Spruce Street, Philadelphia, PA 19104, USA
* Corresponding author.
E-mail address: john.weigele@uphs.upenn.edu (J.B. Weigele).

Radiol Clin N Am 46 (2008) 819–836
doi:10.1016/j.rcl.2008.04.006

radiologic.theclinics.com

patent foramen ovale); large vessel thromboembolism caused by atherosclerosis (extracranial carotid artery or vertebral artery stenosis, intracranial arterial stenosis); and small vessel occlusion (lacunar infarction). Less common etiologies include arterial dissection (rare in the elderly); prothrombotic and genetic disorders; and vasculitis (temporal arteritis is an uncommon cause of stroke unique to the elderly). No cause can be identified for some strokes (cryptogenic).[5]

Acute cerebral arterial occlusion impairs regional cerebral blood flow. Typically, there is a central core of markedly impaired perfusion surrounded by a peripheral zone of less severely restricted perfusion (ischemic penumbra). Rapid, irreversible infarction occurs in the core when cerebral blood flow drops below 15 mL/100 g/min. In the ischemic penumbra, the cerebral blood flow usually is approximately18 to 20 mL/100 g/min, resulting in nonfunctional but viable neurons that are potentially salvageable for a brief time interval (therapeutic window) before irreversible cell death occurs.[9] The ischemic penumbra represents the target for emergent stroke therapy.

Clinical Outcomes

Elderly patients have a worse prognosis from AIS than younger patients. Mortality increases with age from 10% in individuals less than age 65 years to 40% in those over 85 years old. Functional outcome is also worse in older individuals, even for those with comparable infarcts.[10] The elderly brain may be less capable of recruiting viable neurons for new roles (eg, impaired synaptogenesis), contributing to this poorer prognosis.[5] Ischemic stroke is the leading cause of death in women over age 85 years. Blacks have more than twice the incidence and mortality from AIS than whites at all ages.[11]

Neuroimaging

An emergency unenhanced head CT represents the fundamental neuroimaging examination in AIS to exclude nonischemic causes for the patient's clinical presentation (ischemic stroke mimics, such as tumor, infection, and especially intracranial hemorrhage) before instituting systemic or endovascular thrombolysis.[12] Some thrombolysis trials also have used early CT signs of a large infarction as exclusionary criteria.

Recently, a number of studies have suggested the therapeutic window for systemic thrombolysis can be extended in selected patients using perfusion and diffusion MR imaging to identify those with salvageable ischemic penumbra and also to identify subgroups unlikely to benefit who also have a high risk for symptomatic intracranial

hemorrhage from thrombolysis.[13,14] Similarly, the combination of perfusion CT and CT angiography provides an assessment of the infarct core, ischemic penumbra, arterial occlusion and collaterals that also has the potential to guide therapy.[15]

In contradistinction, other studies have questioned the accuracy of diffusion and perfusion MR imaging in depicting the core infarct and ischemic penumbra; diffusion defects may be reversible and perfusion defects may include regions of relatively mild oligemia not at risk for infarction.[16,17] Although promising, the use of advanced neuroimaging to guide AIS therapy remains experimental and is yet to be validated in prospective, randomized clinical trials.[12,17]

Treatment

The only treatment for AIS currently proved to be clinically effective is reperfusion of the ischemic penumbra before irreversible infarction occurs. Available therapeutic options include systemic (intravenous) administration of a thrombolytic medication and endovascular recanalization techniques. Current evidence suggests advanced age should not be considered a contraindication for active treatment.

Recombinant tissue plasminogen activator is approved by the Food and Drug Administration for systemic thrombolytic treatment of AIS at a total dose of 0.9 mg/kg (maximum dose, 90 mg) administered within 3 hours of symptom onset, primarily as a result of the National Institute of Neurologic Disorders and Stroke study reported in 1995 that demonstrated an 11% to 13% absolute and a 30% to 50% relative increase in favorable clinical outcomes at 3 months despite an increased incidence of symptomatic intracranial hemorrhage.[18] A recent meta-analysis of six major trials confirmed the benefit of systemic tissue plasminogen activator administered within 3 hours. This study also demonstrated that the probability of benefit decreased with increased time to treatment within the 3-hour window and suggested that a smaller therapeutic benefit may extend beyond 3 hours to 4.5 hours from symptom onset, although the risks associated with thrombolysis may be greater.[19]

Considerable concern has been expressed over the safety of systemic thrombolytic therapy for AIS in the very elderly; however, several studies have demonstrated that the benefits are not limited by advanced age. Although overall clinical outcomes are poorer, there still is a significant therapeutic benefit from systemic thrombolysis without an increased incidence of hemorrhage in patients over age 80 years; this therapy should not be withheld from the very elderly.[20–22] Nonetheless, systemic thrombolysis is used less often in very old patients even when they meet eligibility criteria.[23]

In theory, endovascular recanalization techniques hold the potential to achieve more rapid and effective reperfusion, and to extend the therapeutic window. A direct infusion into the thrombus can deliver a much higher local concentration of the thrombolytic agent and may potentially accelerate the rate of thrombolysis while simultaneously limiting the overall systemic dose, presumably decreasing the rate of systemic complications. The addition of mechanical clot disruption using guidewires, snares, and balloon catheters may further accelerate this process. In addition, endovascular devices can be used mechanically to extract the thrombus. Potential disadvantages include the limited availability of these resources, however, and the time delay to perform the procedure.[24]

Despite these promising attributes, only one randomized, controlled phase 3 clinical trial evaluating endovascular recanalization for AIS has been reported, the PROACT II trial. This study randomized 180 patients with AIS less than 6 hours from onset caused by angiographically proved middle cerebral artery occlusion without CT evidence of intracranial hemorrhage or of an infarct involving greater than one third of the middle cerebral artery territory to receive 9 mg intra-arterial prourokinase (r-proUK) infused directly into the thrombus over 2 hours combined with low-dose intravenous heparin or intravenous heparin alone (placebo). At 90-day clinical follow-up, 40% of the r-proUK group had a modified Rankin scale score (mRSS) less than or equal to 2 (functionally independent) versus 25% of the placebo group ($P = .04$). The recanalization rates were 66% for the r-proUK group and 18% for the controls ($P = .001$). Although symptomatic intracranial hemorrhage was more common in the r-proUK group (10% versus 2%, $P = .06$), the mortality rates were not significantly different (25% versus 27%).[25]

On the basis of the PROACT II data, a United States interdisciplinary panel has concluded that intra-arterial thrombolysis is a therapeutic option for selected patients who are not eligible for systemic tissue plasminogen activator (Class I recommendation, level of evidence B).[12] Despite the positive results of PROACT II, no drug currently is approved by the Food and Drug Administration for intra-arterial thrombolysis of AIS.

In addition to the PROACT trial, a number of case series have reported positive results for various chemical and mechanical intra-arterial recanalization techniques for patients with AIS who are not candidates for systemic lytic therapy; most

were treated within the 3- to 6-hour time window.[24] Kim and colleagues[26] recently reported a retrospective review of their experience with intra-arterial thrombolysis for AIS in 33 patients greater than or equal to 80 years old compared with 81 patients less than age 80 years. Recanalization rates (79% versus 68%) and rates of symptomatic intracranial hemorrhage (7% versus 8%) were not significantly different for the two groups. There were, however, lower rates of excellent functional outcomes (mRSS $\leq$1; 26% versus 40%, $P = .02$) and survival (57% versus 80%, $P = .01$) at 90 days in the very elderly. Significantly, severely disabled outcomes were not increased in those greater than or equal to 80 years old. The authors concluded that the endovascular outcomes seem to compare favorably with conservative management; however, a randomized trial is necessary to confirm this impression. This mirrors the present authors' experience that endovascular recanalization techniques performed at a specialized stroke center are safe and probably effective in carefully selected elderly patients with AIS who are not candidates for systemic thrombolytic therapy (**Fig. 1**).

ACUTE HEMORRHAGIC STROKE
Epidemiology

A total of 10% to 15% of all strokes are hemorrhagic, most caused by bleeding into the brain parenchyma (intracerebral hemorrhage [ICH]) or into the cerebrospinal fluid spaces around the brain (subarachnoid hemorrhage [SAH]).[7,8,27] Williams and colleagues[7] analyzed a representative sample of all 1995 United States inpatient discharges; their study estimated there were 682,000 hospitalizations for stroke: 3.4% (23,400) were SAHs; 10.5% (71,600) were ICHs; and 86.1% (587,000) were ischemic strokes.

The incidence of ICH increases exponentially with age; the rate doubles each decade after age 35 years.[28] The mean age is 61 years. Blacks, Hispanics, and Japanese have twice the incidence of ICH. The incidence of SAH is also age-dependent; although the mean age for aneurysmal SAH is lower than for ICH, its incidence increases with age from 1.5 to 2.5 per 100,000 in the third decade of life to 40 to 78 per 100,000 in the eighth decade. The age-adjusted rate is 43% higher for women than men; elderly women have the highest incidence of aneurysmal SAH.[29,30]

Etiology and Pathophysiology

Nontraumatic SAH is caused by a ruptured intracranial aneurysm in 85% of patients; nonaneurysmal perimesencephalic hemorrhage in 10%; and

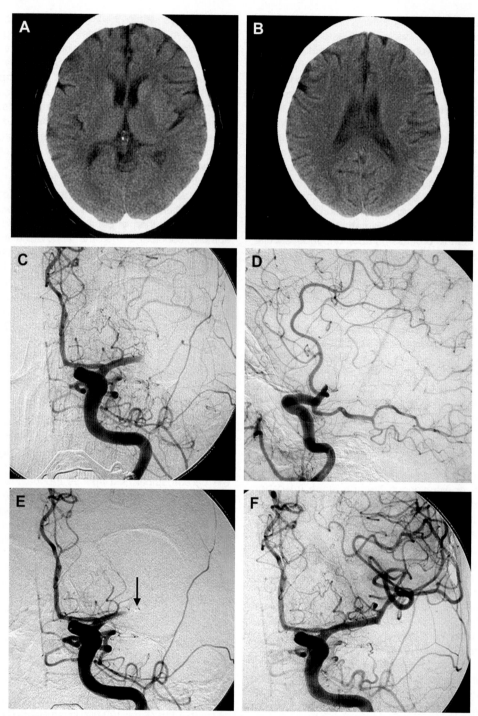

Fig. 1. Acute thromboembolic ischemic stroke in an 82-year-old woman with a 3-hour history of right hemiplegia and aphasia. (*A, B*) The CT appears normal, without early signs of infarction or hemorrhage. (*C*) Anteroposterior (AP) and (*D*) lateral left carotid cerebral angiogram demonstrates complete thromboembolic occlusion of the left middle cerebral artery (MCA) M1 segment, with nonvisualization of the distal MCA branches. (*E*) AP angiogram demonstrates a microcatheter tip (*arrow*) embedded in the proximal aspect of the thromboembolus. (*F*) Completion angiogram after successful chemical and mechanical thrombolysis demonstrates reperfusion of the left MCA territory. The patient made a good clinical recovery.

a variety of rare causes (eg, vasculitis, arterial dissections, tumors, drugs, arteriovenous malformations [AVMs], dural arteriovenous fistulae) in the remaining 5%.[31] Ruptured intracranial aneurysms are associated with high rates of death and disability; contributing factors include rehemorrhage, vasospasm, and hydrocephalus. Nonaneurysmal perimesencephalic hemorrhage is presumably caused by rupture of a perimesencephalic vein; the hemorrhage is typically localized to the interpeduncular and prepontine cisterns, the angiogram is normal, the clinical outcome is invariably good, and rehemorrhage does not occur.

ICH (bleeding into the brain parenchyma) can be classified as primary (no underlying congenital or acquired lesion); secondary (underlying congenital or acquired lesion); or spontaneous (unrelated to trauma or surgery).[28] Chronic hypertension is responsible for 75% of all cases of primary ICH. Cerebral amyloid angiopathy (CAA) is the next most common cause, responsible for more than 20% of ICH in patients over 70 years old. Drugs and coagulopathies are also important causes of primary ICH. Secondary causes of ICH include vascular malformations, aneurysms, tumors, hemorrhagic transformation of AIS, venous infarcts, and moyamoya disease.

It was previously believed that local tissue damage was caused by the mass effect from the hematoma; however, animal models have not confirmed this hypothesis. Currently, it is thought that cerebral edema caused by clot retraction and extrusion of plasma proteins contributes to neurologic deterioration. Thrombin formation may be neurotoxic or damage the blood-brain barrier, exacerbating the vasogenic edema.[28]

Clinical Outcomes

In the elderly, patients with hemorrhagic stroke have a significantly worse prognosis than those with AIS. Lee and colleagues[27] recently analyzed the short- and long-term morbidity and mortality of United States Medicare recipients (>65 years of age) diagnosed with stroke in 1997. Acute mortality rates during hospitalization were 31.9% for SAH, 25.6% for ICH, and 6.8% for AIS. One-year mortality rates were 58.5% for SAH, 51.5% for ICH, and 27.9% for AIS. Factors associated with poor outcomes from ICH include advanced age, blood glucose level, the Glasgow Coma Scale score, hematoma location and volume, and the presence of intraventricular extension of the hemorrhage.[32] In patients with primary ICH, contrast extravasation on CT angiography was an independent predictor for hematoma growth and increased mortality on multivariate analysis.[32]

Specific Causes of Hemorrhagic Stroke

Brain arteriovenous malformations

Brain AVMs are uncommon congenital lesions of the central nervous system that cause intracranial hemorrhage; they are estimated to be responsible for 1% to 2% of all strokes.[33–35] An annual 2% to 4% risk for hemorrhage has been reported in several hospital-based series.[36] In a large prospective study of 166 patients followed over a mean of 23.7 years, Ondra and colleagues[37] reported a 4% annual rate of hemorrhage associated with a 2.7% annual rate of mortality and major morbidity.

The natural history of brain AVMs in the elderly has not received adequate attention and is poorly understood; consequently, their clinical management has been controversial. Despite minimal data, some reports have suggested brain AVMs in the elderly are relatively benign lesions with less risk of bleeding that should be managed conservatively.[38–40]

In contradistinction, other studies have identified an increased incidence of brain AVM hemorrhage with age.[41,42] Crawford and colleagues[42] followed 217 patients with brain AVMs for an average of 10.4 years. Eight of the 11 patients over age 60 years at presentation experienced a hemorrhage during the follow-up period (89% risk at 9 years), whereas the risk of hemorrhage was only 15% in young adults. The increased risk for hemorrhage in older adults was statistically significant ($P<.001$) and independent of the clinical presentation.

In theory, the physiologic changes seen with aging could explain an increased incidence of hemorrhage from brain AVMs in the elderly. Loss of vascular elasticity caused by intimal thickening and fragmentation of the internal elastic lamina may increase the risk for rupture of the vessel wall, especially when subjected to the hemodynamic stress of hypertension.[43] In addition, the incidence of AVM-associated aneurysms increases with age. Sufficient data indicate AVM-associated aneurysms increase the risk for hemorrhage, especially for posterior fossa AVMs (**Fig. 2**).[36]

Two recent case series suggest surgical management of brain AVMs is safe and effective in the elderly. Harbaugh and Harbaugh[43] reported the surgical resection of brain AVMs in six patients age greater than or equal to 65 years who presented with intracranial hemorrhage. No new, persistent postoperative neurologic deficit occurred and four recovered completely neurologically intact. Hashimoto and colleagues[44] retrospectively reviewed surgical treatment of 32 patients over 60 years old with brain AVMs. Most (21 of 32) presented with intracranial hemorrhage. Good to

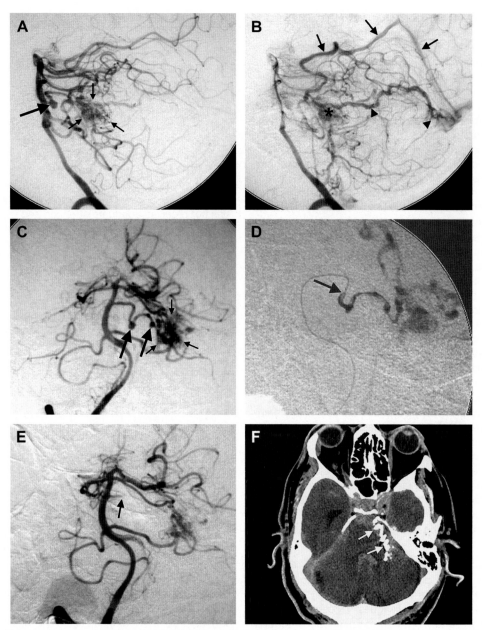

Fig. 2. Pial arteriovenous malformation (AVM) in a 65-year-old man with a headache and subarachnoid hemorrhage (SAH). Early arterial phase of a vertebrobasilar angiogram in lateral (*A*) and AP (*C*) projections demonstrates a left cerebellar AVM (*small arrows*) supplied by a long circumferential arterial feeder containing aneurysms (*large arrows*) that are the likely source of hemorrhage. (*B*) Late arterial lateral view shows early venous drainage from the nidus (*) into the straight sinus (*arrows*) and torcular (*arrowheads*). (*D*) Superselective angiogram by a microcatheter (*arrow*) in the feeder. (*E*) AP angiogram following embolization of the feeder and aneurysms (*arrow*) with *N*-butyl cyanoacrylate. (*F*) Postembolization CT reveals hyperdense *N*-butyl cyanoacrylate in the feeder and the arteriovenous malformation nidus (*arrows*), surrounded by diffuse SAH.

excellent surgical outcomes were achieved in 69.6%. Patients with Spetzler and Martin grade I and II AVMs had significantly better postoperative neurologic scores (*P*<.01), although those with grade III AVMs had poorer postoperative neurologic scores.

These reports have challenged the conventional conservative approach to the management of brain AVMs in the elderly, especially for small, superficial AVMs in noneloquent regions. Some of these patients may be appropriate candidates for surgical resection. Also, some elderly patients who are not surgical candidates because of medical comorbidities, AVM size, or location may benefit from embolization of specific angioarchitectural features, such as aneurysms that represent a high risk for rehemorrhage (see **Fig. 2**).[45] The differential diagnosis of intracranial hemorrhage on a head CT or a brain MR image of an elderly patient should include a ruptured brain AVM. In appropriate patients, conventional angiography may be indicated.

Intracranial aneurysms

Although intracranial aneurysms are the most common cause of nontraumatic SAH, most never rupture. A systematic review of 23 published studies estimated that approximately 2.3% of the population harbor intracranial aneurysms; the prevalence is very low in the first two decades of life and then increases linearly with advancing age. Contrary to a common misperception, intracranial aneurysms are not congenital, but develop during life. The overall risk of aneurysm rupture was estimated to be 1.9% per year. Most aneurysms are less than or equal to 10 mm in diameter; for those the annual rate of rupture is only 0.7%.[46] Similarly, recent prospective data from the International Study of Unruptured Intracranial Aneurysms demonstrated that the risk for aneurysm rupture varies significantly with size (greater risk with increasing size) and location (increased risk for posterior communicating and vertebrobasilar aneurysms), and is very low for small (<7 mm diameter) incidental aneurysms, especially in the anterior circulation.[47] Consequently, as the more frequent use of advanced neuroimaging detects more incidental intracranial aneurysms in aged individuals, the relatively benign natural history for those patients must be carefully weighed against the risks of treatment.

Conversely, when an intracranial aneurysm does rupture it has a much more malignant clinical course. The annual incidence of aneurysmal SAH in the United States is estimated to be approximately 30,000. Approximately 20% to 25% of these life-threatening events occur in the elderly.[48] Once it has ruptured, an intracranial aneurysm has a high probability of rebleeding if it is not secured, often with catastrophic results. The risk of rehemorrhage is estimated to be from 3% to 13.6% in the first 24 hours followed by 1% to 2% per day for the first month, for an overall rate of rebleeding in the first month of 30% to 40%.[49,50] The risk of an early rebleed is just as high in the elderly as it is in younger patients.[48] Rehemorrhage is associated with a 70% to 80% fatality rate.[50] Even those patients whose ruptured aneurysms are successfully secured have a high incidence

(>50%) of death and dependency because of a number of factors, including cerebral injury from the initial hemorrhage, complications of surgery, delayed cerebral ischemia from vasospasm, increased intracranial pressure, hydrocephalus, and systemic complications.

SAH initiates a complex series of cerebral and systemic alterations, including reduced cerebral blood flow, decreased tissue oxygenation, impaired cerebral autoregulation, increased intracranial pressure, and decreased systemic blood volume. These effects are especially stressful on the aged brain that has limited reserve. Hydrocephalus occurs in 20% of cases caused by obstruction of the cerebrospinal fluid drainage pathways or arachnoid granulations. Vasospasm caused by degradation products from blood in the subarachnoid space causes delayed clinically significant cerebral ischemia in 25% of patients, of which 30% die and 50% of the survivors have permanent neurologic deficits. Massive sympathetic discharge can cause cardiac arrhythmias, myocardial ischemia, and pulmonary edema. Life-threatening gastrointestinal hemorrhage may result from gastric erosions or stress ulcers.[51]

The non–contrast enhanced head CT is the primary diagnostic imaging modality for SAH. High-attenuation blood is visualized in the subarachnoid space in more than 95% of cases when performed within 24 hours of the event; however, the CT scan becomes progressively less sensitive after the first day.[52,53] In the appropriate clinical setting (classically, abrupt onset of the worst headache of life) a normal-appearing non–contrast enhanced head CT does not entirely exclude the diagnosis of SAH, and a lumbar puncture is necessary to examine the cerebrospinal fluid for red blood cells and xanthochromia.[52] The head CT is also essential to identify associated early complications, such as cerebral hemorrhage and hydrocephalus. The pattern of hemorrhage on the CT often helps localize the site of the ruptured aneurysm.

MR imaging can also be used to detect acute SAH with sensitivity comparable with CT. Subacute SAH is detected with greater sensitivity on MR imaging than CT. Gradient-echo T2* and fluid-attenuated inversion recovery acquisitions are the most sensitive pulse sequences.[54,55] Nonetheless, MR imaging can also miss aneurysmal SAH that is identified by a positive lumbar puncture.[56]

Classically, conventional digital subtraction angiography has been considered the gold standard to diagnose intracranial aneurysms. Recent studies have shown that multidetector CT angiography can detect ruptured intracranial aneurysms with diagnostic accuracy equivalent to conventional digital subtraction angiography.[57] This may be useful to triage some elderly patients to surgical clipping without exposure to the risks of catheter-based digital subtraction angiography, and also to limit the extent of catheter manipulation during endovascular coiling. MR angiography is less applicable for older individuals with aneurysmal SAH because these critically ill patients are less accessible during the examination. MR angiography also is more time-consuming and more sensitive to motion artifacts.

The management of the elderly patient with aneurysmal SAH has evolved over the last several decades. The current therapeutic options include conservative treatment, surgical clipping, and endovascular coiling. With conservative management, the early mortality of a ruptured intracranial aneurysm in the elderly patient was unacceptably high, approximately 50%.[58] Five-year survival rates were less than 20%, primarily because of aneurysm rebleeding.[50]

In early surgical series elderly patients also had a very high mortality (approximately 50%) following aneurysm clipping, resulting in a reluctance to treat those patients.[29,59] More recent surgical series have reported improved outcomes in selected elderly patients as old as 75 to 80 years.[29] Rather than a direct result of advanced chronologic age, worse surgical outcomes are determined by a poor clinical grade (Hunt-Hess grades 4 and 5); the presence of significant atherosclerosis; aneurysm location in the posterior circulation; and medical comorbidities (especially ischemic cardiac disease). Carefully selected 60- to 70-year-old patients have had operative mortalities less than 10% for clipping of ruptured aneurysms.[29] Early surgery may be associated with better outcomes in older individuals, as is the case in younger patients.[60] Aggressive treatment may benefit elderly poor-grade patients in addition to good-grade patients.[48] Age alone should not be used to discriminate against aggressively treating elderly patients with aneurysmal SAH.[29,48,50]

In the last two decades, the endovascular treatment of intracranial aneurysms with detachable coils has been introduced and has undergone continuous refinements. This technique uses a very small, flexible microcatheter that is introduced directly into the aneurysm by an endovascular route with careful fluoroscopic guidance. The aneurysm is then carefully packed with platinum microcoils that are attached to a deployment mandril that permits repositioning or removal of the coil when necessary. The coil delivery system incorporates a detachment system (electrolytic, hydraulic, or mechanical) that releases the coil once it has been optimally positioned. Coils are placed until the aneurysm lumen completely thromboses or no additional coils can be deposited.

Detachable coil embolization of intracranial aneurysms has a number of theoretic advantages compared with conventional surgical craniotomy and clipping, including less physiologic stress in critically ill and fragile patients; the absence of manipulation or surgical trauma to the brain parenchyma during access to the aneurysm; ready access to some anatomic locations difficult to reach surgically (eg, the basilar tip); and more rapid recovery times. Nonetheless, there are also disadvantages compared with surgical clipping, including a lower percentage of aneurysms that are completely excluded from the arterial circulation; higher incidences of partial recanalization (caused by coil compaction) requiring follow-up surveillance imaging and some repeat coiling procedures; and higher rates of technical failures and thromboembolic complications in extremely tortuous and atherosclerotic vascular systems that are more often encountered in elderly individuals.

The introduction of detachable coil embolization of intracranial aneurysms led to considerable controversy and debate in the neuroscience community. Although accumulated anecdotal case series were generally positive, there was a reluctance to accept endovascular treatment as a viable alternative to traditional craniotomy and clipping. The International Subarachnoid Aneurysm Trial (ISAT) was a prospective multicenter randomized trial comparing endovascular coiling with neurosurgical clipping of ruptured intracranial aneurysms that has significantly changed that attitude, and has established detachable coil embolization as an important method to treat aneurysmal SAH.[61]

ISAT prospectively randomized 2143 patients judged equally suitable for both methods of treatment to endovascular coiling or craniotomy and clipping. Patients who were allocated to endovascular coiling had an absolute reduction of death or dependency at 1 year of 7.4% (relative risk reduction of 23.9%) compared with surgical clipping ($P = .0001$).[61] On long-term follow-up this relative benefit of coiling versus clipping has persisted to at least 7 years, with further follow-up currently in progress. As a result, many neurovascular centers now consider endovascular treatment to be the primary method to treat ruptured aneurysms that have anatomy favorable for coiling.

An ISAT subgroup analysis for treatment effect versus age group did not demonstrate a consistent trend; however, the study enrolled only a very small number of patients older than age 70 years, limiting the power of that analysis. The investigators theorized that elderly patients were less likely to be randomized in ISAT because of the perception they would do less well with surgery. This concern is supported by the International Study of Unruptured Intracranial Aneurysms trial data that demonstrated significantly higher 1-year morbidity from surgical clipping than from coiling of unruptured intracranial aneurysms in patients over age 50 years.[47] Of note, there was no evidence in the ISAT trial that the relative benefits of coiling did not apply to elderly patients.[61]

A number of case series analyzing detachable coil embolization of intracranial aneurysms in the elderly have reported favorable results when compared with conservative management and surgical clipping.[62–66] Cai and colleagues[62] reported 89% (25 of 28) of elderly patients with low-grade ruptured aneurysms had excellent outcomes following endovascular treatment, whereas 77% (10 of 13) of the high-grade patients did poorly. Lubicz and colleagues[66] reported good to excellent outcomes in 59% (40 of 68) of elderly patients. Sedat and colleagues[63] reported 48% of elderly patients had good or excellent outcomes with coiling, 29% had a fair or poor outcome, and 23% died. The authors' institutional experience has mirrored these results. The authors offer elderly patients with aneurysmal SAH early aggressive endovascular management of both posterior (**Fig. 3**) and anterior circulation aneurysms (**Fig. 4**) when they have favorable anatomic features.

The rupture of an aneurysm in the cavernous segment of the internal carotid artery results in a direct carotid-cavernous fistula. The clinical presentation usually includes pulsatile exophthalmos, ophthalmoplegia, chemosis, decreased visual acuity, and retro-orbital pain as a result of arterialized venous drainage through the superior ophthalmic vein into the orbit. Visual loss may be permanent unless the carotid-cavernous fistula is closed immediately. Cortical venous drainage may result in life-threatening intracranial hemorrhage. MR imaging typically reveals a dilated superior ophthalmic vein within the orbit and prominent flow voids within the cavernous sinus. Detachable coil embolization of the aneurysm and carotid-cavernous fistula while preserving the internal carotid artery is the preferred treatment (**Fig. 5**). Occasionally, the parent artery must be sacrificed either following a balloon test occlusion or surgical bypass.[67]

Hypertensive hemorrhage

Hypertension is the most common cause of primary ICH. The risk of hypertensive ICH is related to the duration and the severity of the blood pressure elevation. Hypertension primarily affects the small perforating arteries arising directly from the large basal arteries, causing pathologic changes defined as "lipohyalinosis"; this includes atherosclerosis of the larger (100–500 µm) perforators at vessel bifurcations manifested by subintimal fibroblast proliferation and deposition of lipid-laden macrophages, and arteriolosclerosis of the smaller (<100 µm) perforators with replacement of smooth muscle cells in the media by collagen. These histopathologic changes result in fragile, narrowed, and noncompliant vessels prone to occlusion (lacunar infarct) and disruption (ICH). Microaneurysms (Charcot and Bouchard) were previously believed to be the cause of hypertensive ICH, but have rarely been identified in pathologic specimens.[28]

Noncontrast head CT is the primary diagnostic modality for ICH, defining the size and location of the parenchymal hematoma, and the presence of subfalcine, uncal, or transtentorial herniation and associated complications (**Fig. 6**). Associated intraventricular, SAH, or subdural hemorrhage is also characterized. Hypertensive ICH is most common (50%–67%) in the basal ganglia and thalami; the lobar deep white matter, brainstem, and cerebellum are also common locations. Angiography is unnecessary in elderly patients with a history of hypertension and ICH in a characteristic location.[28]

Treatment is largely supportive. The recent International Surgical Trial in Intracerebral Hemorrhage found no value for early surgical evacuation of supratentorial hematomas compared with medical management.[68] Nonetheless, evacuation of a large posterior fossa hematoma may be lifesaving. Early ventricular catheter placement for obstructive hydrocephalus may also be beneficial.[28]

Cerebral amyloid angiopathy

CAA is the second most common cause of primary ICH, responsible for up to 10% of cases. Hereditary and sporadic forms of CAA both occur. The hereditary forms are rare and usually are autosomal-dominant; they display a broader spectrum of clinical manifestations and typically are evident clinically as early as the third decade of life. The sporadic form of CAA is primarily a disease of the elderly. The prevalence of sporadic CAA increases with age; it is estimated to cause more than 20% of ICH in patients over age 70 years. Most histologic specimens from patients over 90 years old demonstrate CAA.[28,69] CAA is becoming an increasingly common cause of ICH as the population ages and as hypertension is better medically managed.

Distinct from systemic amyloidosis, CAA is caused by deposition of a β-amyloid protein within the media and adventitia of small- and

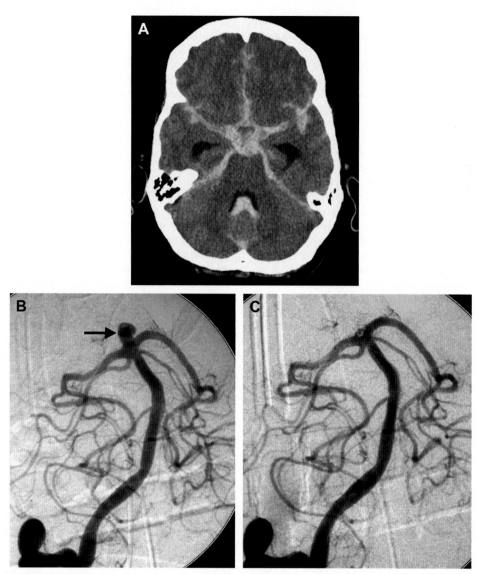

Fig. 3. Ruptured basilar tip aneurysm in a 71-year-old woman with Hunt-Hess grade 4 SAH. (*A*) The CT demonstrates diffuse SAH, blood in the 4th ventricle, and hydrocephalus. (*B*) Vertebrobasilar angiogram in a Waters projection reveals a 5-mm diameter basilar tip aneurysm (*arrow*). (*C*) Angiogram after detachable coil embolization of the aneurysm confirms complete occlusion of the aneurysm.

medium-size vessels in the cerebral cortex, the subcortical white matter, and the leptomeninges. The vessels in the deep white matter and deep gray nuclei are spared. The β-amyloid deposits stain with Congo red dye and exhibit yellow-green birefringence under polarized light. The β-amyloid deposition in the vascular wall causes fibrinoid necrosis, focal fragmentation of the vessel wall, and formation of microaneurysms. These histopathologic changes cause vascular fragility that can lead to repeated episodes of hemorrhage. Fibrinoid necrosis can also narrow or occlude the vessel lumen, causing ischemic changes.[70]

Despite its high prevalence in the elderly, CAA is often asymptomatic. When CAA becomes symptomatic, however, the clinical manifestations can include acute ICH, symptoms resembling an acute transient ischemic attack, and dementia. Acute ICH is the most common presentation. The specific symptoms and signs depend on the size and location of the bleed, and often include headache, nausea and vomiting, seizures, focal neurologic deficits, and a decreased level of consciousness.[28]

Neuroimaging features of CAA include acute parenchymal hemorrhage in a distinctive subcortical-cortical location, evidence of prior

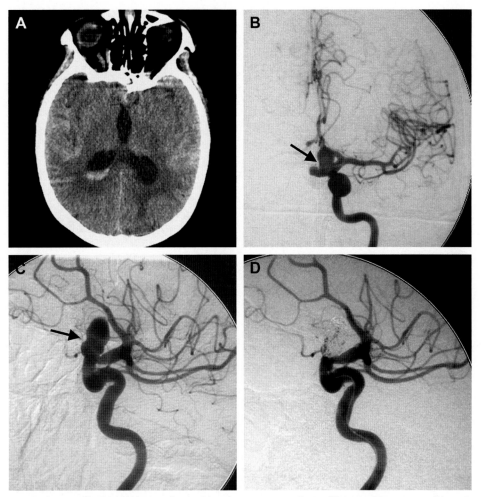

Fig. 4. Ruptured supraclinoid left internal carotid artery aneurysm in an 87-year-old woman with a decreased level of consciousness. (*A*) A CT demonstrates bilateral subarachnoid hemorrhage in both sylvian fissures (*arrows*), intraventricular hemorrhage in the right occipital horn (*arrowhead*), and hydrocephalus. AP (*B*) and oblique (*C*) left carotid cerebral angiogram reveals a large, bilobed supraclinoid carotid aneurysm (*arrows*). (*D*) Completion angiogram following detachable coil embolization documents successful obliteration of the aneurysm.

microhemorrhages on gradient-echo MR imaging, leukoencephalopathy, and atrophy. ICH associated with CAA occurs in a distinctive lobar distribution, involving the cerebral cortex and subcortical white matter. The deep white matter, deep gray matter, and brainstem are typically spared, in contradistinction to hypertensive ICH. CAA-related ICH can involve any lobe of the cerebral hemisphere, and rarely can involve the cerebellum. Both large and microhemorrhages demonstrate posterior (temporal and occipital) predominance.[71] These acute parenchymal hematomas tend to have irregular borders and may be associated with SAH, subdural hematoma, and less frequently intraventricular hemorrhage.[69]

A lobar hemorrhage in a normotensive elderly patient suggests CAA. The presence of chronic cortical-subcortical blood products from previous microhemorrhages strengthens the probable diagnosis of CAA (**Fig. 7**). These are demonstrated as focal areas of signal loss on T2*-weighted gradient-echo MR imaging that are caused by local magnetic field inhomogeneities from the paramagnetic effect of hemosiderin.[69] Susceptibility-weighted MR imaging (a velocity-compensated gradient-echo pulse sequence that combines magnitude and phase information) has been shown to be even more sensitive for chronic microhemorrhages.[72]

Unfortunately, similar to hypertensive hemorrhage the treatment for CAA-related ICH is largely supportive. There is no current therapy available to arrest or reverse the deposition of the β-amyloid protein. CAA patients have a higher risk of

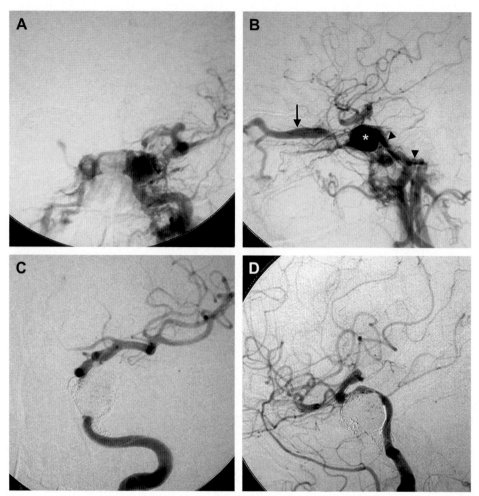

Fig. 5. Direct carotid-cavernous fistula (CCF) caused by rupture of a cavernous carotid aneurysm in an elderly woman presenting with an abrupt headache, proptosis, and acute loss of vision. AP (A) and lateral (B) left common carotid cerebral angiogram demonstrates a large cavernous carotid aneurysm (*) and a direct CCF draining into the left superior ophthalmic vein (arrow), the left inferior petrosal sinus (arrowheads), and across the intercavernous sinuses into the right cavernous sinus. AP (C) and lateral (D) completion angiogram after detachable coil embolization of the aneurysm demonstrates complete obliteration of the aneurysm and CCF, with preservation of the internal carotid artery.

hemorrhage during anticoagulation or thrombolytic therapy.[69]

Cerebral sinus thrombosis

Although cerebral venous and sinus thrombosis (CVST) is predominately a disease of the young and middle aged, there is also a significant incidence in the elderly population. In the International Study on Cerebral Vein and Dural Sinus Thrombosis, a prospective multicenter observational study of adults with symptomatic CVST, 51 (8.2%) of 624 patients were greater than or equal to 65 years of age. Presentations with depressed level of consciousness and mental status changes were more frequent in the elderly, whereas an isolated intracranial hypertension syndrome was less common than in younger patients. The prognosis of elderly patients was significantly worse, with complete recovery in only 49%; 22% were dependent and 27% were dead at the end of follow-up.[73]

Thrombosis of the cerebral veins or sinuses causes elevation of the local venous pressure, in turn impairing venous drainage. A number of variables affect the degree, including the location, extent, and rapidity of thrombosis modified by the availability of venous collateral routes. The elevated venous pressure is transmitted to the brain parenchyma causing interstitial edema and impaired tissue perfusion that can result in venous infarction, often associated with hemorrhagic transformation.[74]

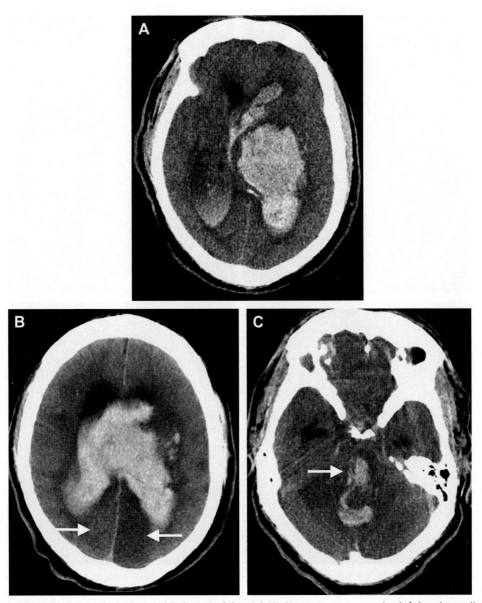

Fig. 6. Hypertensive hemorrhage in an elderly man. (A) Axial CT demonstrates a massive left basal ganglia hemorrhage with intraventricular extension. (B, C) A 16-hour follow-up CT reveals transtentorial herniation has caused bilateral posterior cerebral artery territory infarcts (*arrows* in B) by compression of the arteries against the free margin of the tentorium and Duret hemorrhages in the brainstem (*arrow* in C) caused by displacement and disruption of the perforating arteries. (*Courtesy of* Ronald Wolf, MD, PhD, Philadelphia, PA.)

Diagnostic imaging is essential to diagnose CVST. A number of signs have been described on CT, including high-density thrombus in cortical veins or dural sinuses (cord sign); parenchymal regions of low attenuation representing venous infarcts; and high density within these areas indicating hemorrhagic transformation. On contrast-enhanced CT, an enhancing sinus wall may surround hypodense thrombus within the sinus (empty delta sign). Unfortunately, these signs are often absent or equivocal.[75]

On MR imaging, abnormal signal intensity is typically seen within the dural sinuses associated with the absence of the usual flow voids. Most commonly, subacute thrombus in the extracellular methemoglobin state is seen as increased signal intensity on both T1- and T2-weighted images. Acute clot may be hypointense on all pulse sequences, however, and may be misinterpreted as a normal flow void. Of note, thrombus causes "blooming" at all ages of evolution on gradient-echo images because of its T2* effect. Similar to

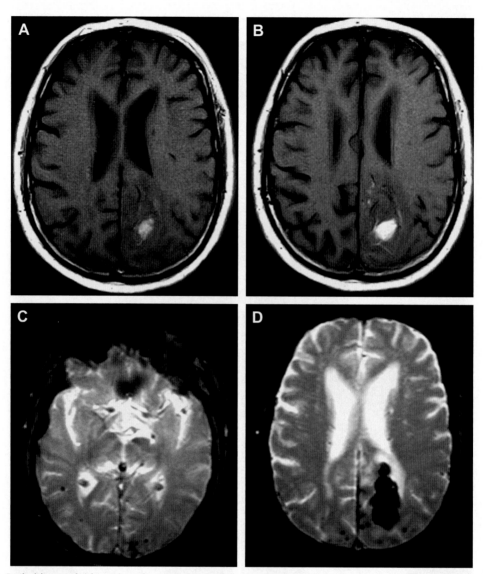

Fig. 7. Probable amyloid angiopathy in a normotensive 70-year-old man with a severe headache. Axial T1-weighted (*A, B*) and axial T2*-weighted (*C, D*) gradient-echo MR images demonstrate an early subacute hematoma in the left occipital lobe. In addition, scattered small cortical-subcortical hypointense foci (chronic microhemorrhages) are present on the gradient-echo images.

CT, contrast-enhanced MR imaging displays sinus wall enhancement around hypointense thrombus within the sinus. MR imaging identifies parenchymal abnormalities in 60% of cases; it is more sensitive than CT. Areas of increased T2 signal involving both the cortex and underlying white matter in a nonvascular pattern are seen in venous infarcts; hypointense areas within the infarcts on gradient-echo images represent hemorrhagic transformation. Time-of-flight, phase contrast, and contrast-enhanced MR venography and multidetector CT venography add to the accuracy of the imaging diagnosis; however, expert

knowledge of venous anatomy and variants, and imaging artifacts, is essential (**Fig. 8**).[75]

Although the treatment of CVST has been controversial, systemic anticoagulation is widely accepted as the standard therapy. Nonetheless, some high-risk groups still have poor outcomes, and the fate of an individual case is often uncertain. In the International Study on Cerebral Vein and Dural Sinus Thrombosis study, 13% of the patients fell into a clinically identifiable subgroup at increased risk of a poor outcome. Coma, cerebral hemorrhage, and malignancy were important prognostic factors for death or dependence. In

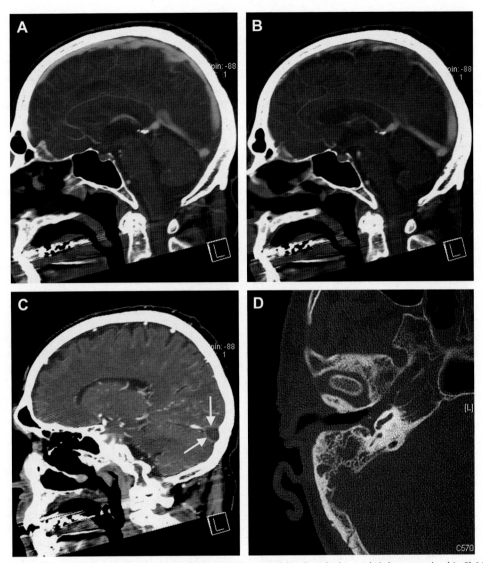

Fig. 8. Cerebral venous sinus thrombosis in a 74-year-old man with a headache and right ear pain. (*A, B*) Midline sagittal MPR images of a CT venogram demonstrate the superior and inferior sagittal sinuses, internal cerebral veins, vein of Galen, straight sinus, and torcular are all patent. (*C*) Sagittal MPR image to the right demonstrates thrombosis of an expanded, nonenhancing right transverse sinus (*arrows*). (*D*) Temporal bone CT demonstrates coalescent mastoiditis with opacification of the mastoid air cells and partial destruction of the bony septa.

addition, male gender, age greater than 37 years, decreased level of consciousness, deep venous thrombosis, and infection were variables associated with an increased risk of death or dependence.[76] Elderly patients who are at high risk for a poor outcome from CVST may benefit from endovascular recanalization procedures, such as intrasinus thrombolysis or rheolytic thrombectomy.[77]

SUMMARY

Neurovascular diseases are important causes of death and disability in the elderly, often presenting as life-threatening emergencies. Diagnostic imaging plays a central role in their initial clinical evaluation. Recent advances in the clinical neurosciences have improved the ability to treat many of these disorders; neurointerventional techniques are becoming increasingly valuable therapeutic options.

REFERENCES

1. Health, United States, 2007 with Chartbook on Trends in the Health of Americans. Hyattsville (MD): US Department of Health and Human Services; 2007.

2. Garcia JH, Brown GG. Vascular dementia: neuropathologic alterations and metabolic brain changes. J Neurol Sci 1992;109(2):121–31.

3. Choi JY, Morris JC, Hsu CY. Aging and cerebrovascular disease. Neurol Clin 1998;16(3):687–711.

4. Mooradian AD. Potential mechanisms of the age-related changes in the blood-brain barrier. Neurobiol Aging 1994;15(6):751–5.

5. Kasner SE, Chalela JA, Hickenbottom SL. Ischemic cerebrovascular disease. In: Sirven JI, Malamut BL, editors. Clinical neurology of the older adult. Philadelphia: Lippincott Williams & Wilkins; 2002. p. 214–27.

6. Wolf PA, Cobb JL, D'Agostino RB. Epidemiology of stroke. In: Barnett HJ, Stein BM, Mohr JP, editors. Stroke: pathophysiology, diagnosis, and management. New York: Churchill Livingstone; 1992. p. 3–27.

7. Williams GR, Jiang JG, Matchar DB, et al. Incidence and occurrence of total (first-ever and recurrent) stroke. Stroke 1999;30(12):2523–8.

8. Williams GR. Incidence and characteristics of total stroke in the United States. BMC Neurol 2001;1:2–7.

9. Hossmann KA. Viability thresholds and the penumbra of focal ischemia. Ann Neurol 1994;36(4):557–65.

10. Nakayama H, Jorgensen HS, Raaschou HO, et al. The influence of age on stroke outcome. The Copenhagen Stroke Study. Stroke 1994;25(4):808–13.

11. Hankey GJ, Jamrozik K, Broadhurst RJ, et al. Long-term risk of first recurrent stroke in the Perth Community Stroke Study. Stroke 1998;29(12):2491–500.

12. Adams HP Jr, del Zoppo G, Alberts MJ, et al. Guidelines for the early management of adults with ischemic stroke: a guideline from the American Heart Association/American Stroke Association Stroke Council, Clinical Cardiology Council, Cardiovascular Radiology and Intervention Council, and the Atherosclerotic Peripheral Vascular Disease and Quality of Care Outcomes in Research Interdisciplinary Working Groups: the American Academy of Neurology affirms the value of this guideline as an educational tool for neurologists. Stroke 2007;38(5):1655–711.

13. Schellinger PD, Thomalla G, Fiehler J, et al. MRI-based and CT-based thrombolytic therapy in acute stroke within and beyond established time windows: an analysis of 1210 patients. Stroke 2007;38(10):2640–5.

14. Albers GW, Thijs VN, Wechsler L, et al. Magnetic resonance imaging profiles predict clinical response to early reperfusion: the diffusion and perfusion imaging evaluation for understanding stroke evolution (DEFUSE) study. Ann Neurol 2006;60(5):508–17.

15. Tan JC, Dillon WP, Liu S, et al. Systematic comparison of perfusion-CT and CT-angiography in acute stroke patients. Ann Neurol 2007;61(6):533–43.

16. Mezzapesa DM, Petruzzellis M, Lucivero V, et al. Multimodal MR examination in acute ischemic stroke. Neuroradiology 2006;48(4):238–46.

17. Kidwell CS, Alger JR, Saver JL. Evolving paradigms in neuroimaging of the ischemic penumbra. Stroke 2004;35(11 Suppl 1):2662–5.

18. The National Institute of Neurological Disorders and Stroke rt-PA Stroke Study Group. Tissue plasminogen activator for acute ischemic stroke. N Engl J Med 1995;333(24):1581–7.

19. Hacke W, Donnan G, Fieschi C, et al. Association of outcome with early stroke treatment: pooled analysis of ATLANTIS, ECASS, and NINDS rt-PA stroke trials. Lancet 2004;363(9411):768–74.

20. Tanne D, Turgeman D, Adler Y. Management of acute ischaemic stroke in the elderly: tolerability of thrombolytics. Drugs 2001;61(10):1439–53.

21. Engelter ST, Bonati LH, Lyrer PA. Intravenous thrombolysis in stroke patients of > or = 80 versus <80 years of age: a systematic review across cohort studies. Age Ageing 2006;35(6):572–80.

22. Sylaja PN, Cote R, Buchan AM, et al. Thrombolysis in patients older than 80 years with acute ischaemic stroke: Canadian Alteplase for Stroke Effectiveness Study. J Neurol Neurosurg Psychiatry 2006;77(7):826–9.

23. Hills NK, Johnston SC. Why are eligible thrombolysis candidates left untreated? Am J Prev Med 2006;31(6 Suppl 2):S210–6.

24. Schumacher HC, Gupta R, Higashida RT, et al. Advances in revascularization for acute ischemic stroke treatment. Expert Rev Neurother 2005;5(2):189–201.

25. Furlan A, Higashida R, Wechsler L, et al. Intra-arterial prourokinase for acute ischemic stroke. The PROACT II study: a randomized controlled trial. Prolyse in acute cerebral thromboembolism. JAMA 1999;282(21):2003–11.

26. Kim D, Ford GA, Kidwell CS, et al. Intra-arterial thrombolysis for acute stroke in patients 80 and older: a comparison of results in patients younger than 80 years. AJNR Am J Neuroradiol 2007;28(1):159–63.

27. Lee WC, Joshi AV, Wang Q, et al. Morbidity and mortality among elderly Americans with different stroke subtypes. Adv Ther 2007;24(2):258–68.

28. Manno EM, Atkinson JL, Fulgham JR, et al. Emerging medical and surgical management strategies in the evaluation and treatment of intracerebral hemorrhage. Mayo Clin Proc 2005;80(3):420–33.

29. Elliott JP, Le Roux PD. Subarachnoid hemorrhage and cerebral aneurysms in the elderly. Neurosurg Clin N Am 1998;9(3):587–94.

30. Sacco RL, Wolf PA, Bharucha NE, et al. Subarachnoid and intracerebral hemorrhage: natural history, prognosis, and precursive factors in the Framingham Study. Neurology 1984;34(7):847–54.

31. van Gijn J, Kerr RS, Rinkel GJ. Subarachnoid hae-morrhage. Lancet 2007;369(9558):306–18.
32. Kim J, Smith A, Hemphill JC III, et al. Contrast extravasation on CT predicts mortality in primary intracerebral hemorrhage. AJNR Am J Neuroradiol 2008;29(3):520–5.
33. Furlan AJ, Whisnant JP, Elveback LR. The decreas-ing incidence of primary intracerebral hemorrhage: a population study. Ann Neurol 1979;5(4):367–73.
34. Gross CR, Kase CS, Mohr JP, et al. Stroke in south Alabama: incidence and diagnostic features. A pop-ulation based study. Stroke 1984;15(2):249–55.
35. Perret G, Nishioka H. Report on the cooperative study of intracranial aneurysms and subarachnoid hemorrhage. Section VI. Arteriovenous malforma-tions. An analysis of 545 cases of cranio-cerebral arteriovenous malformations and fistulae reported to the cooperative study. J Neurosurg 1966;25(4):467–90.
36. Weigele JB, Al-Okaili RN, Hurst RW. Endovascular management of brain arteriovenous malformations. In: Hurst RW, Rosenwasser RH, editors. Interventional neuroradiology. New York: Informa Healthcare USA; 2008. p. 275–303.
37. Ondra SL, Troupp H, George ED, et al. The natural history of symptomatic arteriovenous malformations of the brain: a 24-year follow-up assessment. J Neu-rosurg 1990;73(3):387–91.
38. Heros RC, Tu YK. Is surgical therapy needed for un-ruptured arteriovenous malformations? Neurology 1987;37(2):279–86.
39. Luessenhop AJ, Rosa L. Cerebral arteriovenous malformations: indications for and results of surgery, and the role of intravascular techniques. J Neuro-surg 1984;60(1):14–22.
40. Heros RC, Morcos J, Korosue K. Arteriovenous mal-formations of the brain: surgical management. Clin Neurosurg 1993;40:139–73.
41. Brown RD Jr, Wiebers DO, Torner JC, et al. Fre-quency of intracranial hemorrhage as a presenting symptom and subtype analysis: a population-based study of intracranial vascular malformations in Olmsted County, Minnesota. J Neurosurg 1996;85(1):29–32.
42. Crawford PM, West CR, Chadwick DW, et al. Arterio-venous malformations of the brain: natural history in unoperated patients. J Neurol Neurosurg Psychiatry 1986;49(1):1–10.
43. Harbaugh KS, Harbaugh RE. Arteriovenous malfor-mations in elderly patients. Neurosurgery 1994;35(4):579–84.
44. Hashimoto H, Iida J, Kawaguchi S, et al. Clinical fea-tures and management of brain arteriovenous mal-formations in elderly patients. Acta Neurochir (Wien) 2004;146(10):1091–8.
45. The n-BCA Trial Investigators. N-butyl cyanoacrylate embolization of cerebral arteriovenous malformations:
46. Rinkel GJ, Djibuti M, Algra A, et al. Prevalence and risk of rupture of intracranial aneurysms: a system-atic review. Stroke 1998;29(1):251–6.
47. Wiebers DO, Whisnant JP, Huston J III, et al. Unrup-tured intracranial aneurysms: natural history, clinical outcome, and risks of surgical and endovascular treatment. Lancet 2003;362(9378):103–10.
48. Laidlaw JD, Siu KH. Aggressive surgical treatment of elderly patients following subarachnoid haemor-rhage: management outcome results. J Clin Neuro-sci 2002;9(4):404–10.
49. Ohkuma H, Tsurutani H, Suzuki S. Incidence and significance of early aneurysmal rebleeding before neurosurgical or neurological management. Stroke 2001;32(5):1176–80.
50. Sarkar PK, D'Souza C, Ballantyne S. Treatment of aneurysmal subarachnoid haemorrhage in elderly patients. J Clin Pharm Ther 2001;26(4):247–56.
51. McKhann GM II, Le Roux PD. Perioperative and in-tensive care unit care of patients with aneurysmal subarachnoid hemorrhage. Neurosurg Clin N Am 1998;9(3):595–613.
52. van der Wee N, Rinkel GJ, Hasan D, et al. Detection of subarachnoid haemorrhage on early CT: is lumbar puncture still needed after a negative scan? J Neurol Neurosurg Psychiatry 1995;58(3):357–9.
53. Boesiger BM, Shiber JR. Subarachnoid hemorrhage diagnosis by computed tomography and lumbar puncture: are fifth generation CT scanners better at identifying subarachnoid hemorrhage? J Emerg Med 2005;29(1):23–7.
54. Mitchell P, Wilkinson ID, Hoggard N, et al. Detection of subarachnoid haemorrhage with magnetic reso-nance imaging. J Neurol Neurosurg Psychiatry 2001;70(2):205–11.
55. da Rocha AJ, da Silva CJ, Gama HP, et al. Compar-ison of magnetic resonance imaging sequences with computed tomography to detect low-grade subarachnoid hemorrhage: role of fluid-attenuated inversion recovery sequence. J Comput Assist To-mogr 2006;30(2):295–303.
56. Mohamed M, Heasly DC, Yagmurlu B, et al. Fluid-at-tenuated inversion recovery MR imaging and sub-arachnoid hemorrhage: not a panacea. AJNR Am J Neuroradiol 2004;25(4):545–50.
57. Papke K, Kuhl CK, Fruth M, et al. Intracranial aneu-rysms: role of multidetector CT angiography in diag-nosis and endovascular therapy planning. Radiology 2007;244(2):532–40.
58. Locksley HB, Sahs AL, Knowler L. Report on the co-operative study of intracranial aneurysms and sub-arachnoid hemorrhage. Section II. General survey of cases in the central registry and characteristics of the sample population. J Neurosurg 1966;24(5):922–32.

59. Sedat J, Dib M, Rasendrarijao D, et al. Ruptured intracranial aneurysms in the elderly: epidemiology, diagnosis, and management. Neurocrit Care 2005; 2(2):119–23.

60. Moriyama E, Matsumoto Y, Meguro T, et al. Progress in the management of patients with aneurysmal subarachnoid hemorrhage: a single hospital review for 20 years. Part II: Aged patients. Surg Neurol 1995; 44(6):528–33.

61. Molyneux AJ, Kerr RS, Yu LM, et al. International subarachnoid aneurysm trial (ISAT) of neurosurgical clipping versus endovascular coiling in 2143 patients with ruptured intracranial aneurysms: a randomised comparison of effects on survival, dependency, seizures, rebleeding, subgroups, and aneurysm occlusion. Lancet 2005;366(9488): 809–17.

62. Cai Y, Spelle L, Wang H, et al. Endovascular treatment of intracranial aneurysms in the elderly: single-center experience in 63 consecutive patients. Neurosurgery 2005;57(6):1096–102.

63. Sedat J, Dib M, Lonjon M, et al. Endovascular treatment of ruptured intracranial aneurysms in patients aged 65 years and older: follow-up of 52 patients after 1 year. Stroke 2002;33(11):2620–5.

64. Luo CB, Teng MM, Chang FC, et al. Endovascular embolization of ruptured cerebral aneurysms in patients older than 70 years. J Clin Neurosci 2007; 14(2):127–32.

65. Braun V, Rath S, Antoniadis G, et al. Treatment and outcome of aneurysmal subarachnoid haemorrhage in the elderly patient. Neuroradiology 2005;47(3): 215–21.

66. Lubicz B, Leclerc X, Gauvrit JY, et al. Endovascular treatment of ruptured intracranial aneurysms in elderly people. AJNR Am J Neuroradiol 2004; 25(4):592–5.

67. van Rooij WJ, Sluzewski M, Beute GN. Ruptured cavernous sinus aneurysms causing carotid cavernous fistula: incidence, clinical presentation, treatment, and outcome. AJNR Am J Neuroradiol 2006;27(1):185–9.

68. Mendelow AD, Gregson BA, Fernandes HM, et al. Early surgery versus initial conservative treatment in patients with spontaneous supratentorial intracerebral haematomas in the International Surgical Trial in Intracerebral Haemorrhage (STICH): a randomised trial. Lancet 2005;365(9457):387–97.

69. Chao CP, Kotsenas AL, Broderick DF. Cerebral amyloid angiopathy: CT and MR imaging findings. Radiographics 2006;26(5):1517–31.

70. Vonsattel JP, Myers RH, Hedley-Whyte ET, et al. Cerebral amyloid angiopathy without and with cerebral hemorrhages: a comparative histological study. Ann Neurol 1991;30(5):637–49.

71. Rosand J, Muzikansky A, Kumar A, et al. Spatial clustering of hemorrhages in probable cerebral amyloid angiopathy. Ann Neurol 2005;58(3):459–62.

72. Haacke EM, DelProposto ZS, Chaturvedi S, et al. Imaging cerebral amyloid angiopathy with susceptibility-weighted imaging. AJNR Am J Neuroradiol 2007; 28(2):316–7.

73. Ferro JM, Canhao P, Bousser MG, et al. Cerebral vein and dural sinus thrombosis in elderly patients. Stroke 2005;36(9):1927–32.

74. Mullins ME, Grant PE, Wang B, et al. Parenchymal abnormalities associated with cerebral venous sinus thrombosis: assessment with diffusion-weighted MR imaging. AJNR Am J Neuroradiol 2004;25(10): 1666–75.

75. Leach JL, Fortuna RB, Jones BV, et al. Imaging of cerebral venous thrombosis: current techniques, spectrum of findings, and diagnostic pitfalls. Radiographics 2006;26(Suppl 1):S19–41.

76. Canhao P, Ferro JM, Lindgren AG, et al. Causes and predictors of death in cerebral venous thrombosis. Stroke 2005;36(8):1720–5.

77. Zhang A, Collinson RL, Hurst RW, et al. Rheolytic thrombectomy for cerebral sinus thrombosis. Neurocrit Care, in press.

Index

Note: Page numbers of article titles are in **boldface** type.

Radiol Clin N Am 46 (2008) 837–843
doi:10.1016/S0033-8389(08)00136-X
0033-8389/08/$ – see front matter © 2008 Elsevier Inc. All rights reserved.

radiologic.theclinics.com

and bladder neoplasms, 778–779
and computed tomographic urography, 776
and excretory urography, 775–776
and prostate carcinoma, 779–781
and renal cell carcinoma, 773–776
Neurodegeneration with brain iron accumulation, 806
Neurodegenerative diseases, **799–817**
Neuropathic arthropathy, 716–717
Neurovascular emergencies in the elderly, **819–836**
Non-atherosclerotic arterial disorders, 677–678
Non-Hodgkin lymphoma, 723
Non-neoplastic genitourinary pathologies, 781–783

O

Olivopontocerebellar degeneration, 808–809
Oncohaematologic disorders affecting the skeleton in the elderly, **785–798**
Oropharyngeal incontinence
  and swallowing disorders, 757–758
Osteoarthritis, 704, 708–710, 713, 716–718
Osteomyelitis, 728–730
  and bone scintigraphy, 730
Osteomyelofibrosis and sclerosis, 795–796
  and magnetic resonance imaging, 796
  and multislice computed tomography, 795
  and radiography, 795
Osteoporosis, 703–704, 707, 715, 717–718, 722, 731, 735–749
  and appendicular skeleton, 740
  and axial skeleton, 738, 740
  and bone mineral density, 741–743, 746–747
  and broadband ultrasound attenuation, 745
  complications of, 737
  and conventional radiography, 737–738
  and cortical thinning, 738
  diagnostic imaging of, 737–747
  differential diagnosis, 747–749
  and dual x-ray absorptiometry, 740–742
  epidemiology of, 735–736
  etiology and risk factors of, 736
  and hypercortisolism, 747–748
  and hyperparathyroidism, 747
  and increased radiolucency, 737–738
  and infection, 749
  and magnetic resonance imaging, 746–747
  and malignant disease, 748–749
  and morphometric x-ray absorptiometry, 744–745
  and morphometry, 744–745
  physiopathology of, 736–737
  and post-traumatic deformity after compression fractures, 749
  and quantitative computed tomography, 742–744
  and quantitative ultrasound, 745–746

P

Paget's disease, 717–718
  and bone scintigraphy, 718
Palsy
  progressive supranuclear, 809
Parkinson disease
  idiopathic, 806–807
Parkinsonism
  secondary, 807
Pelvic floor pathologies, 759–763
  and cine colpo-cystodefecography, 760–761
  and dynamic magnetic resonance imaging, 761–762
  imaging techniques for, 760–762
  and pathological findings, 762–763
  and ultrasound, 760
Pelvic fractures, 706–707
Penetrating aortic ulcer, intramural hematoma, and dissection, 676–677
Perfusion weighted imaging
  and Alzheimer's disease, 803
Peripheral arterial disease, 664–668
  and ankle-brachial index, 664–665
  and computed tomographic angiography, 665–667
  and contrast-enhanced magnetic resonance angiography, 667
  and digital subtraction angiography, 665–666, 668
  and duplex ultrasound, 665
  and magnetic resonance angiography, 665, 667–668
  and multi-detector computed tomography, 665
  and time of flight imaging, 667–668
  and time resolved intravascular contrast kinetics imaging, 668
PET. See *Positron emission tomography.*
Pharyngeal retention
  and swallowing disorders, 758
Physiopathologic models, 692–699
Physiopathology of the aging heart, **653–662**
Pick's disease, 803–804
Pleural effusion, 686, 689, 694–695, 697
  and cardiac lung, 695
Positron emission tomography
  and Alzheimer's disease, 802–803
  and giant cell arteritis, 678
Positron emission tomography computed tomography
  and myeloma, 789
Progressive supranuclear palsy, 809
Prostate carcinoma
  and neoplastic genitourinary pathologies, 779–781
Pulmonary heart, 697
  versus cardiac lung, 697–699
PWI. See *Perfusion weighted imaging.*

Moving?

Make sure your subscription moves with you!

To notify us of your new address, find your **Clinics Account Number** (located on your mailing label above your name), and contact customer service at:

E-mail: elspcs@elsevier.com

800-654-2452 (subscribers in the U.S. & Canada)
1-407-563-6020 (subscribers outside of the U.S. & Canada)

Fax number: 407-363-9661

Elsevier Periodicals Customer Service
6277 Sea Harbor Drive
Orlando, FL 32887-4800

*To ensure uninterrupted delivery of your subscription, please notify us at least 4 weeks in advance of move.